# Advance Care Planning in End of Life Care

SECOND EDITION

Edited by

Keri Thomas

Ben Lobo

Karen Detering

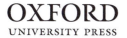
OXFORD
UNIVERSITY PRESS

Great Clarendon Street, Oxford, OX2 6DP,
United Kingdom

Oxford University Press is a department of the University of Oxford.
It furthers the University's objective of excellence in research, scholarship,
and education by publishing worldwide. Oxford is a registered trade mark of
Oxford University Press in the UK and in certain other countries

© Oxford University Press 2018

The moral rights of the authors have been asserted

First edition published 2011
Second edition published 2018

Impression: 1

Published in the United States of America by Oxford University Press
198 Madison Avenue, New York, NY 10016, United States of America

British Library Cataloguing in Publication Data

Data available

Library of Congress Control Number: 2017948692

ISBN 978–0–19–880213–6

Printed and bound by
CPI Group (UK) Ltd, Croydon, CR0 4YY

Oxford University Press makes no representation, express or implied, that the
drug dosages in this book are correct. Readers must therefore always check
the product information and clinical procedures with the most up-to-date
published product information and data sheets provided by the manufacturers
and the most recent codes of conduct and safety regulations. The authors and
the publishers do not accept responsibility or legal liability for any errors in the
text or for the misuse or misapplication of material in this work. Except where
otherwise stated, drug dosages and recommendations are for the non-pregnant
adult who is not breast-feeding

Links to third party websites are provided by Oxford in good faith and
for information only. Oxford disclaims any responsibility for the materials
contained in any third party website referenced in this work.

# Advance Care Planning in End of Life Care

# Foreword

Death will affect us all; it is the one certainty in life. Yet the subject of death remains something of a taboo, we rarely discuss what our preferences would be at end of life, what we would want, where we would want to be cared for, not even with loved ones. Therefore when a professional identifies that the person they are caring for is nearing the end of life, approaching these conversations can be hindered by worries of causing unnecessary distress and anxiety to them and their family members.

There is evidence in the literature that advance care planning improves end of life care, that satisfaction for both the person and their family improves and there is a reduction in stress in surviving relatives. By enabling discussion, people and their families have the opportunity to plan, to express their preferences, and have their care tailored accordingly.

*Advance Care Planning in End of Life Care* addresses a wide range of issues that are essential in the delivery of excellent care for people in the end stages of their life; from the importance of thinking about spirituality to looking after people who lack capacity, and end of life care for children and their parents. It suggests solutions and approaches to these complex scenarios and draws on experience not just from the UK, but also internationally. It considers the perspective of a broad range of healthcare professionals as well as service managers, commissioners and charities and looks at how the recommendations could be implemented in a variety of settings, from hospital to nursing home and hospice to own home.

The 'Ambitions for Palliative and End of Life Care: A national framework for local action: 2015–20' sets out six ambitions for improving end of life care. The concepts in this book focus on the first ambition in particular: each person is seen as an individual, and supports the others; fair access to care, maximising comfort and wellbeing, care is coordinated, staff are prepared to care, and communities are prepared to help. Both the ambitions framework and this book focus on the need for care for the person as an individual, not a disease.

We have the ability to change the way we talk about dying and death and prepare, plan, care, and support those who are dying and the people who support them. We have a duty to strengthen and improve our ability to provide care whatever the circumstances of whoever is dying.

Professor Sir Bruce Keogh
National Medical Director, NHS England

# Preface to Second Edition

'It seems we have failed to recognise that people have priorities . . . they want us to serve, besides just living longer. It seems obvious. . . . Well, the second important lesson I learnt was that the most reliable way to learn what peoples' priorities are—and there are highly technical studies on this—the most reliable way to learn is to ask . . . and we don't ask!'

*Atul Gwande, The Reith Lectures 2014, Lecture 3: The Problem of Hubris, BBC Radio*

Since the publication of the first edition of this book in 2010, advance care planning (ACP) has grown in and importance around the world, as an integral part of best practice for all, and particularly in care for people approaching the last stage of life. ACP has also grown in terms of acceptance, widespread usage and evidence of effectiveness and there is a developing understanding of how this complex intervention may achieve some of the desired outcomes. Many countries have integrated ACP (or equivalent terms representing the same process) into national policies, with many government-sponsored programmes to promote public and professional awareness and uptake, illustrated in the UK and international chapters included here. Now the arguments are less about whether ACP is acceptable, important and relevant and more about how to mainstream and implement ACP as part of quality care for all. It is heartening to see this worldwide movement gather pace.

One notable development since the first edition has been the growth of the International Society for Advance Care Planning and End of Life Care (ACPEL) in 2010, with now biannual international conferences held in different parts of the world, bringing together clinicians, researchers, policy, legal professionals, and others with the shared focus of increasing the uptake, use and evidence base of ACP across the world, and to better understand the most effective ways to achieve this. Two of the editors (Prof Keri Thomas and Dr Karen Dettereing) were founder members of ACPEL, and assisted in hosting several of these conferences, involving about 400–600 people from over 40 countries. Several of the chapters in this second edition have been written by other current or previous ACPEL Society members or conference participants, and represent some of the learning from these stimulating international conferences (see for example www.acpel2017.org). Although the book's primary focus is the UK, this strong international perspective, presenting current updates and insights from across the world, significantly increases the relevance and breadth of this book. Despite differences in contexts, legal frameworks, health and social care systems, and national cultures, one thing that we all have in common is the wish to listen more closely to peoples' wishes and priorities, and tailor care to better meet their needs particularly in their final stage of life.

The purpose of this fully updated second edition is to help readers explore a wide range of issues and practicalities in ACP for all people, providing a clear framework of shared understanding, whilst still acknowledging these differing contexts, terms, and approaches. The key message is that ACP is important, it works, is recommended and is possible in all settings and with people with all conditions and, despite variations in approach and implementation, is being recognised now as a vital part of care. With the challenges of the ageing population, and as possible medical interventions escalate, we increasingly meet the real dilemma summarised as *'just because we can, doesn't mean we should'*. This leads to the process of asking people in more detail about their priorities or 'trade-offs' as Atul Gwande puts it, through such ACP discussions, to determine the kind of care and the kind of life they really seek. There are of course views that counter these affirmations, with recommendations to tread carefully in this sensitive and complex area and we acknowledge the different opinions and variety of responses. But increasingly there is acceptance of the value of ACP, moves to adopt it appropriately in all settings, and to mobilise the public to have such conversations much earlier, before being introduced by doctors and nurses or medical events demand their necessity.

The book takes a comprehensive journey through ACP, framing the purpose, process, and outcomes and including contributions from experts from around the world. This book will be of great use for both the generalist and specialist professional in the provision of health and social care for people near the end of life, and those involved in policy, strategic planning, commissioning, or researching this area.

Each author takes a particular stance and focuses on a unique area, though there are likely to be some recurring themes, so that the consistency of the message may be affirmed in a variety of ways, and each chapter can be read independently or within the context of the whole. For ease of reference, the first section of each chapter describes the contents, key points and summarised key message along with a suitable quotation. This ensures easier scanning of the main messages, plus an invitation for a more detailed exploration as required, plus references and an Appendix of useful weblinks and resources. Although comprehensive, this is not exhaustive: for example we do not focus on such areas as euthanasia and physician assisted suicide, as we wish to site ACP discussions within the broadly positive context of the provision of active supportive quality care by all providers, to enable people to live well until they die.

The introduction and 'call to arms' (Chapter 1) provides an overview with a practical summary, and describes the evolving nature of ACP as a concept mirrored in other chapters balancing the personal (transformational) and more medical (transactional) aspects. There is now robust evidence of the benefits of ACP, despite it being a complex intervention (Chapter 2), it is well used in practice (Chapter 3), and it makes economic sense at every level in the development of person-centred care (Chapter 4). ACP gives us a vehicle as individuals to express this personally at the most important of junctures, as we age (Chapter 5), as we consider some deeper existential/spiritual challenges (Chapter 6), and as we face the final stage of our lives ourselves or with our families (Chapter 7). ACP is successfully happening in all settings, as described by frontline clinicians (Chapters 12–15), and for all conditions and ages, including for children (Chapter 16), learning disability (Ch 17) and the growing numbers with dementia (Chapter 18). National policy developments in the UK support ACP being adopted as part of mainstream practice on the ground (Chapters 8 and11), and it is also part of a world-wide movement successfully implemented within many countries across the world from Australia to Singapore (Chapters 19–24). Emerging developments mean we are using ACP better in line with discussions of capacity (Chapter 11), with resuscitation discussions (Chapter 10), with refusals of treatment (Chapter 9), and earlier in life with long-term conditions (Chapters 25 and 26), with better awareness of the required communication skills (Chapter 24). And its suggested that seeking person-centred care through ACP may be part of the public health solution at both the national population level as well as the individual level, by reducing overuse of unwanted interventions, facilitating the appropriate allocation of resources, and contributing to addressing some of the current ethical and economic challenges in healthcare (Chapter 28).

As co-editors, authors, and as clinicians we have particular experience within our fields of general practice, palliative care, geriatrics, respiratory medicine, education, and research in ACP and in caring for the people nearing the end of life. We divided the book according to our areas of expertise and experience, as lead editors and/or contributors for each chapter. Prof Keri Thomas was lead editor for Forward, Preface and chapters 1, 6, 7, 8, 12, 13, 14, 15, 25, and 28. Ben Lobo was lead editor for Chapters 3, 5, 9, 10, 11, 16, 17, and 18. Dr Karen Detering was lead editor for Chapters 2, 4, 19, 20, 21, 22, 23, 24, 25, and 26.

We would like to sincerely thank all the excellent chapter authors and contributors to the book who have worked wonderfully well with us in bringing this second edition to fruition – the book is so much stronger for the fact of its numerous contributors. Also thanks for our invaluable support from April Peake at OUP (without whom undoubtedly, we could not have completed the work), secretarial support from Jo Carwardine, Sue Richards, and all at The GSF Centre. Finally, we would like to thank our understanding and supportive families, to whom this book is dedicated:

Keri—my husband, the 'ever-fixed Mark' (Shakespeare Sonnet 116) and my wonderful five children Megan (and son-in-law Kurt, and my joyous life-affirming grandson Monty), Ben, Bethany, Sophie, and Imogen.

Ben—my wife Cheryl and Harriet my beautiful and brave daughter.

Karen—my husband Dave and my two amazing children Jia Jie and Bei Bei who continue to teach me so much.

We hope this updated second edition of the book makes a significant contribution to this national and international priority and that by promoting this systematic approach to ACP, more will be enabled to implement ACP in their area, thereby enabling more people to live well as they approach the end of life, and to die well in the place and manner of their choosing.

# Contents

# Contributors

**Chris Absolon**
GP Palliative Care Lead and GP Patient Safety Lead, Somerset Clinical Commissioning Group (CCG), UK

**Doris Barwich**
Executive Director, BC Center for Palliative Care, New Westminster, Canada

**Tony Bonser**
Trustee, National Council for Palliative Care, London, UK

**Simon Chapman**
Formerly Director of Policy and External Affairs, National Council for Palliative Care, London, UK

**Irwin C A Wai Hoong Chung**
Associate Consultant Family Physician and Director, Primary Care Academy, National Healthcare Group Polyclinics, Singapore

**Josephine Clayton**
Associate Professor of Palliative Care, Northern Clinical School, University of Sydney, Australia

**Karen Harrison Dening**
Head of Research and Publications, Dementia UK, London, Honorary Research Fellow, University of Liverpool, and Honorary Assistant Professor, School of Health Sciences, University of Nottingham, UK

**Karen Detering**
Medical Director, ACP Research and Evaluation, Advance Care Planning Australia, Austin Health, Heidelberg, Australia

**Josie Dixon**
Assistant Professorial Research Fellow, Department of Social Policy, London School of Economics and Political Science, UK

**Premila Fade**
Consultant in Geriatric Medicine, London North West NHS Trust, UK

**Scott Fraser**
Project Manager, ACP Research and Evaluation, Advance Care Planning Australia, Austin Health, Heidelberg, Australia

**Kornelia Götze**
General Practitioner, ACP Research Group, Institute of General Practice, Medical Faculty, Heinrich-Heine-University of Düsseldorf, Germany

**Muir Gray**
Consultant in Public Health, Oxford University Hospitals NHS Trust, and Organisational Lead, Better Value Healthcare (BVHC), Oxford, UK

**Karen Groves**
Consultant in Palliative Medicine, Southport and Ormskirk Hospitals NHS Trust, Southport, UK

**Louise Hanvey**
Director (Retired), Advance Care Planning in Canada, Canadian Hospice Palliative Care Association, Ottawa, Canada

**Claire Henry**
Director of Improvement and Transformation, Hospice UK, England

**Cari Borenko Hoffmann**
Project Implementation Coordinator for Advance Care Planning in Fraser Health, Surrey, Canada

**Ben Lobo**
Consultant Physician and Geriatrician, Sherwood Forest Hospitals NHS Foundation Trust and former National Clinical Lead for Advance Decisions to Refuse Treatment, Mid Trent Cancer Network, Nottingham, UK

**Leigh Manson**
ACP Programme Director, The National
Advance Care Planning Cooperative &
Auckland District Health Board, New Zealand

**Georg Marckmann**
Professor of Medical Ethics and Director,
Institute of Ethics, History and Theory of
Medicine, Ludwig Maximilians University of
Munich, Germany

**Clare Marlow**
Consultant in Palliative Medicine,
The Royal Wolverhampton NHS Trust,
Wolverhampton, UK

**Jonathan Martin**
Consultant in Palliative Medicine, Central
and North West London NHS Foundation
Trust, and National Hospital for Neurology
and Neurosurgery, University College London
Hospitals NHS Foundation Trust, UK

**Nigel Mathers**
Professor of Primary Medical Care and Head
of Academic Unit of Primary Medical Care,
University of Sheffield, UK

**Rammya Mathew**
National Medical Director's Clinical Fellow,
Royal College of Physicians, London, UK

**Shona Muir**
ACP Training Programme Manager, The
National Advance Care Planning Cooperative
and Auckland District Health Board,
New Zealand

**Anjali Mullick**
Medical Director and Consultant in Palliative
Medicine, St Peter's Hospice, Bristol, UK

**Scott Murray**
St Columba's Hospice Chair of Primary
Palliative Care, Primary Palliative Care
Research Group, The Usher Institute of
Population Health Sciences and Informatics,
University of Edinburgh, UK

**Pete Nightingale**
GP Advisor in End of Life Care, Macmillan
UK, London, UK

**Simon Noble**
Clinical Reader and Honorary Consultant in
Palliative Medicine, Royal Gwent Hospital,
Newport, UK

**David Pitcher**
Executive Committee Member and Past
President, The Resuscitation Council (UK),
London, UK

**Phillip Rodgers**
Associate Director of Clinical Programs,
Palliative Care Program, University of
Michigan, Ann Arbor, MI, USA

**Sarah Russell**
Head of Research, Hospice UK, London
Visiting Fellow, University of Southampton

**Jürgen in der Schmitten**
Professor of General Practice, Head, ACP
Research Group, Institute for General Practice,
Medical Faculty, Heinrich-Heine-University of
Düsseldorf, Germany

**Maria J. Silveira**
Associate Director of Research, Palliative Care
Program, University of Michigan, Ann Arbor,
MI, USA

**Jessica Simon**
Head, Division of Palliative Medicine,
Department of Oncology, University of
Calgary, Canada

**Craig Sinclair**
Research Fellow, Rural Clinical School of
WA, University of Western Australia, Albany,
Australia

**Maggie Stobbart-Rowlands**
RGN, RMN, IQA Trainer/Assessor

**Elizabeth Sutton**
Programme Manager, Austin Health,
Heidelberg, Australia

**Mark Thomas**
Development Director and Spiritual
Care Lead, The National Gold Standards
Framework Centre in End of Life Care, UK

**Keri Thomas OBE**
National Clinical Lead, The National Gold
Standards Framework Centre in End of Life
Care and Honorary Professor in End of
Life Care, University of Birmingham, UK,
and former Department of Health National
Clinical Lead for Palliative Care

**Angela Thompson**
Palliative Care Lead Paediatrician for
Coventry and Warwickshire, South
Warwickshire NHS Foundation Trust, UK

**Mandy Thorn**
Managing Director, Marches Care Ltd,
Shrewsbury, UK

**Martin J. Vernon**
Consultant Geriatrician, Central
Manchester University Hospitals NHS
Foundation Trust, UK

**Max Watson**
Director, Project ECHO Hospice UK,
Visiting Professor, University of Ulster
Honorary Consultant Palliative Medicine,
Princess Alice  Hospice

**John You**
Associate Professor, Department of Medicine,
McMaster University, Hamilton, Canada

# Abbreviations

| | | | | |
|---|---|---|---|---|
| ACMP | anticipatory clinical management plans | | EFPPEC | Educating Future Physicians in eLFH e-learning for healthcare |
| ACP | Advance Care Planning | | EOL | end of life |
| ACPEL | International Society for Advance Care Planning | | EoLC | end of life care |
| | | | EPA | Enduring Powers of Attorney |
| ACT | Association for Children's Palliative Care | | EPaCCS | Electronic Palliative Care Co-ordination Systems |
| AD | Advance Directive | | GP | General Practitioner (family physician) |
| ADRT | advance decision to refuse treatment | | | |
| AFMC | Association of Faculties of Medicine of Canada | | GSF | gold standards framework |
| | | | GSFCH | The Gold Standards Framework in Care Homes |
| ALS | Amyotrophic Lateral Sclerosis | | | |
| AS | advance statements | | HCA | healthcare assistants |
| BAPM | British Association of Perinatal Medicine | | ICD | implanted cardioverter-defibrillator |
| | | | IDT | interdisciplinary team |
| BC | British Columbia | | IMCA | Independent Mental Capacity Advocate |
| CAD | court appointed deputy | | | |
| CANH | clinically assisted nutrition and hydration | | L2 | Level 2 |
| | | | LPA | Lasting Power of Attorney |
| CARENET | Canadian Researchers at End of Life Network | | LPOA | Legal Power of Attorney |
| | | | LST | life-sustaining treatment |
| CHPCA | Canadian Hospice Palliative Care Association | | MCA | Mental Capacity Act |
| | | | MND | motor neurone disease |
| CKD | Chronic kidney disease | | MNDA | motor neurone disease association |
| CNS | community nurse specialist | | MOH | Ministry of Health |
| COPD | Chronic obstructive pulmonary disease | | NCEPOD | National Confidential Enquiry into Patient Outcome and Death |
| COPD | chronic obstructive pulmonary disease | | NCPC | The National Council for Palliative Care |
| CPCT | community palliative care teams | | | |
| CPR | cardiopulmonary resuscitation | | NEHR | National Electronic Health Record |
| CQC | The Care Quality Commission | | NGOs | non-governmental organisations |
| CYP | children and young people | | NHMRC | National Health and Medical Research Council |
| DES | Direct Enhanced Service | | | |
| DHBs | District Health Boards | | NHS | National Health Service |
| DoHEoLC | Department of Health End of Life Care | | NICE | National Institute of Health and Care Excellence |
| DoLS | Deprivation of Liberty and Safeguards | | NICU | neonatal intensive care unit |
| | | | NZ | New Zealand |
| DSM | Diagnostic and Statistical Manual of Mental Disorders | | OoH | out of hours |
| | | | OPG | Office of the Public Guardian |
| eFI | Palliative and End of Life Care electronic frailty index | | OT | Occupational therapist |

| | | | | |
|---|---|---|---|---|
| PCC4U | National Palliative Care Curriculum for Undergraduates | | RCT | randomised control trial |
| PCC4U | National Palliative Care Curriculum for Undergraduates | | ReSPECT | Recommended Summary Plan for Emergency Care and Treatment |
| PEG | percutaneous endoscopic gastrostomy | | RPC | respecting patient choices |
| PIG | Prognostic Indicator Guidance | | SLA | service level agreements |
| POLST | Physicians' Orders for Life Sustaining Treatment | | SPC | specialist palliative care |
| | | | SUPPORT | Study to Understand Prognoses and Preferences for Outcomes and Risks of Treatment |
| PPC | preferred priorities of care | | | |
| PSDA | patient self determination act | | TEP | treatment escalation plan |
| QALYs | Quality adjusted life years | | TfSL | Together for Short Lives |
| QI | quality improvement | | UK | United Kingdom |

Section 1

# Introduction to advance care planning

Chapter 1

# Overview and introduction to advance care planning

Keri Thomas

'Make sure that when your time comes to die, that dying is all you have left to do'
*Anon*

---

**This chapter includes**

- An introduction to advance care planning (ACP)
- Introduction to this book as an overview of ACP
- What is ACP—current and evolving models?
- Who can initiate ACP discussions and how? Our experience, tips, triggers, and examples in practice
- How has ACP evolved—medical and personal aspects, goals of care?
- The two conversations and five steps in public awareness of ACP
- Thoughts on the deeper significance of ACP conversations, hope, and resilience

---

**Key Points**

- ACP discussions are important as a key means of improving end of life care and of enabling better provision of care in line with peoples' wishes
- ACP is possible and is becoming accepted as part of standard practice in many settings in the UK, and in many countries, illustrated in the different chapters of this book
- ACP is part of recommended best practice for all involved in caring for people in their last stages of life. Many involved in health and social care could initiate such discussions, ideally following further training, to ensure care is proactive and person centred
- ACP is a process of supporting decision making by informing, empowering, and enabling people and can change the course of care leading to greater alignment with wishes
- There is a robust evidence base, extensive international usage, and widespread support for its use in policy and with the public, yet it can be complex, there are differing emphases, terminology, and evolving concepts within it which can cause confusion
- ACP in the UK, in line with the Mental Capacity Act, includes advance statements of wishes and preferences, advance decisions to refuse treatments including resuscitation, and the nominated spokesperson or Lasting Power of Attorney
- The process can be valuable in itself for all people in supporting preparation and delivery of more person-centred care, but also relates to the possible future development of

incapacity, so is particularly helpful with people who lack capacity, such as those with dementia.

◆ There are evolving ACP definitions, with a move from purely the medical aspects (treatments, transactional) towards a focus also on more personal aspects (personal, non-medical, transformational) of ACP discussions and a discussion of goals of care and less 'medicalised' outcomes framework related to our ageing population.

◆ Most health and social care professionals can undertake initial discussions of advance statements of preferences, not just those with specialist training or dedicated facilitators, though many find some teaching in ACP and communication skills helpful. ACP is a key feature of the Gold Standards Framework (GSF) training, cited here as an example and in our experience ACP discussions can become mainstreamed by generalist teams in a variety of different settings.

◆ ACP can be a process of conversations over time, with many of the discussions occurring with families and carers before or between discussions with healthcare providers. Public awareness campaigns are therefore key to the promotion and uptake of ACP, and their effectiveness nationally.

◆ In one example of a public-facing initiative (GSF 5 Steps to ACP), the first steps include personal discussions within families and friends to clarify wishes, (suggested steps one to three) which could be later be built upon and discussed further with those involved in their professional care (suggested steps four and five). Healthcare involvement therefore can builds upon earlier foundational discussions, but there needs to be greater public awareness and promotion of the importance of these discussions in most countries before this becomes fully effective.

◆ There can be a deeper significance of these discussions, in drawing closer to the person's sense of meaning, core values, and spirituality, enhancing preparedness and hope with transformational and therapeutic elements intrinsic within the process.

---

**Key Message**

Advance care planning is important—such discussions open up a space in which the changes that affect the wider context of a person's life can be discussed. ACP is a key part of quality care, has wide adoption in practice, a strong evidence base of effectiveness and economic value, growing acceptance by the public and recommended in policy as pivotal to the delivery of quality care. It has evolved from just a medical transactional model to a more personal transformational one that in itself can be therapeutic, and help people both live well and die well in concordance with their values, goals, and wishes. There are implications also for population-based approaches to meet the current national challenges of twenty-first-century healthcare provision.

---

## An introduction to advance care planning

Advance Care Planning (ACP) is as much about life as it is about death. It is about enabling people to live out the final stage of life as fully as possible, to make the most of each remaining moment, and when the time comes, to be able to die with dignity in the place and the manner of their choosing. Therefore it has the potential to be many things—in addition to a discussion of preferences and 'trade-offs' when faced with different options, it also has the potential to be a life affirming process over time, helping people to live well before they die, which in turn can help the bereaved to know that their loved one's wishes were known, honoured and respected.

ACP discussions open up a space in which the various possibilities and scenarios can be discussed within the wider context of a person's life. They help people hold both possibilities together—to 'hope for the best but prepare for the worst', as part of the kind of 'parallel planning' that is needed when faced with any life-limiting condition.

ACP has the potential to improve care by enabling patients to discuss and record their future health and care wishes and also to appoint someone as an advocate or surrogate, thus increasing the likelihood of these wishes being known and respected at the end of life. This subject is important both for those with the ability to make decisions now, to plan ahead, and to live life as fully as possible until they die. It is also important to anticipate a time when they may not be able to make such decisions in future, and to plan for this eventuality. This aspect is stressed as a priority more by some than by others, and refers to the legislation related to mental capacity and development of advocacy or best-interest decisions, particularly in the context of dementia.

In addition, it is considered by many that at best, the process of having this discussion is as important as the outcome. ACP discussions provide the possibility of clarifying future directions and choices so that the issues can be raised, examined, and fully discussed; fears both trivial and huge can be clarified and addressed, and a more realistic and pragmatic approach can be taken to living out the final stage of life in the way that is important to that individual person.

This book is essentially about having a conversation. It is a particularly important conversation between someone who faces a changing reality as they approach the end of their life and someone who cares for them—their family, or close loved ones—and their care provider. It is usually part of an ongoing dialogue over time within a trusted relationship, or it might be an opportunistic one-off conversation, but either way it can be one of the most important conversations that is undertaken, with both 'life changing' and 'death changing' consequences.

As such, at its simplest, it is a matter of facing a changing reality and exploring the views, choices, preferences, understanding, and expectations of the person approaching the end of their life, with their family and carers, with the aim of informing and directing the care provided and the quality of life lived. Though essentially simple, within this lie multifaceted complexities that have an enormous impact on all involved in end of life care. This book is an exploration of this conversation and of some of the facets that underlie it.

## This book as an overview of advance care planning

This book includes aspects, evidence, experiences, and views on advance care planning (ACP) as a mosaic across many settings, subjects, and perspectives, with a particular focus on the UK, but including a strong international contribution and perspective as part of a world-wide movement. There are of course some justified concerns about approaching these discussions and recommendations to tread carefully in this sensitive area. But increasingly there is an acceptance of the value of ACP and a move to adopt it appropriately in all settings as an integral part of care. There is also an evolving movement towards affirming the importance of clarifying personal values, goals, and preferences before describing these in the medical context of completed documents, important as this is, and different groups place different emphases on these, as described later in this chapter and within this book.

There is now a robust evidence-base of the benefits of ACP, despite it being an evolving concept with challenging complexity (Chapter 2), it makes practical and economic sense at every level (see Chapters 3 and 4). With the challenges of the ageing population, and as we become increasingly focussed on self-determination, control, and personalised care, ACP gives us a vehicle as individuals to express this personally at the most important of junctures, as we age (Chapter 5), as we consider some deeper existential/spiritual challenges (Chapter 6) and as we face the final stage of our lives for ourselves or for our own families (Chapter 7). ACP is happening in all settings (Chapters 12–15) and for all conditions and ages (Chapters 16, 17) including for the growing numbers with dementia (Chapter 18). National policy developments in the UK support it now becoming adopted as part of mainstream practice on the ground (Chapters 8–11), and it is also part of a world-wide movement successfully used within many countries across the world (Chapters 19–24). Emerging developments mean we are using ACP better in line with discussions of capacity (Chapter 11), with resuscitation discussions (Chapter 10), refusals of treatment (Chapter 9), and earlier in life with long-term conditions (Chapters 25 and 26), with better awareness of the required communication skills (Chapter 24). And ACP can be part of the solution at both the individual, and the national population, and economic level (Chapter 4), by reducing overuse of unwanted interventions, facilitating the appropriate allocation of resources, and a low-cost means of addressing the current ethical and economic challenges in healthcare (Chapter 27).

In addition to the stated benefits, seeing this as a process, part of an evolving conversation, enables us to see that there is more to this than meets the eye—that it is in itself therapeutic and the process is itself part of the reward. Whilst taking heed of the warnings of avoiding a tick-box policy-driven formulaic response, how can listening, really listening, to people ever be wrong, and why might we find it so difficult? This conversation should never for forced, but those with responsibility for the care for our patients should be able to offer these discussions more openly and with the sensitivity to respond as needed. Many people express relief following these discussions, pleased that there is greater clarity on the way forward, that their feelings have been heard, their choices aired and noted. There is greater satisfaction with care following ACP discussions, with reduced anxiety from bereaved carers (1).

## What is advance care planning—the current and evolving models?

There has been some evolution and possible confusion of definition over the years. Within the UK, ACP was defined within the NHS End of Life care Programme and Strategy in 2008 (2,3) (see Chapter 8), and by the Royal College of Physicians Guidance (4) as **a process of discussion between a patient and professional carer, which may include family and friends,** leading to broadly three different outputs and main outcomes in line with the UK Mental Capacity Act (5) (see Figure 1.1). Firstly this includes an '**advance statement**', which describes the patient's positive preferences and aims for future care; and secondly an '**advance decision to refuse treatment**' or ADRT (see Chapter 8), which provides informed consent for refusal of specific treatment if the patient is

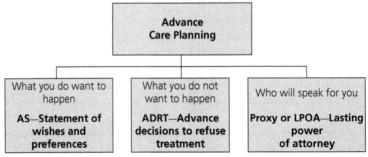

**Figure 1.1** Advance Care Planning discussions in the UK in relation to the Mental Capacity Act
Available from www.goldstandardsframework.org.uk/advance-care-planning
Reproduced courtesy of The National Gold Standards Framework Centre

---

## Box 1.1 The GSF Thinking Ahead ACP example

### GSF Thinking Ahead Advance Statement

Thinking Ahead . . .

- At this time in your life, what is important to you?
- What elements of care are important to you and what WOULD you like to happen in future?
- What would you NOT want to happen? Is there anything that you worry about or fear happening?
- Who would speak for you if you could no longer speak for yourself—your nominated proxy spokesperson or Lasting Power of Attorney?

In addition it asks:

- If your condition deteriorates where would you like to be cared for (at least two options)?
- Do you have an legal advance decision to refuse treatment (ADRT)?
- Do you have any special requests, preferences, or other comments?
- Are there any comments or additions from other people you are close to? (please name)
- NB See also any separate DNACPR/AND/Respect or ADRT documents

Reproduced courtesy of The National Gold Standards Framework Centre

---

not competent to make such a decision in the future. In addition to both of these, a further output is the **'nomination of a proxy spokesperson or advocate'** for the person, including, in England, the legal status of the Lasting Power of Attorney. As with other countries (see Chapters 19–24), the focus of ACP is shifting increasingly towards everyone having the opportunity to discuss the first i.e. what they do want to happen, (advance statements), with an appropriate minority wishing or needing to discuss the second—what they do not want to happen, or a refusal of treatment.

Further details of current policy recommendations in the UK on ACP are given in Chapters 8 and 11, illustrating growing national and government support for clarification of peoples' wishes through these discussions, enabling greater choice for people nearing the end of life.

NHS England and the current Right Care Programme affirms the importance of shared decision making, an area with great overlap and commonality with ACP, (see Box 1.1) (6).

There are many examples of advance statements used in the UK, (see Appendix). One example is the GSF 'Thinking Ahead' ACP document, which includes the four simple questions that have been a good starter to discussions for many thousands of people using it in GP practices, hospitals, care homes, and domiciliary care for over a decade (see Box 1.1).

ACP discussions can be a place for contemplating future outcomes and eventualities within a safe environment in order to maximise life in the present. This is a 'liminal' space, a pause in the journey at which different routes and options can be explored and confirmed. This should be at the pace of the individual person and responded to appropriately, to be able to ensure that care is delivered in alignment with the person's requests and wishes. The conversation can be visualised rather like a waltz, with each person moving harmoniously in step with each other, responding to the movement and direction of the other, never treading on each other's toes or overwhelming them with more than they can cope with at the time. In this sense, the ACP discussion can only be good.

Though this might appear at first sight possibly a simple and easy process, it would not take long to realise that despite sounding straightforward, it requires skill and sensitivity due to the deep significance of the subject. We are talking about something as big as death, as terrifying as loss of all we hold dear, the most threatening subject known to the human race. The death of a loved one can be the most painful and devastating event that we ever face, so it is unsurprising that we naturally would avoid the discussion—whether as patients, carers, families, or as professionals. Like other animals, our survival instincts are strong, and contemplating death is counter-intuitive, and for some, denial is a legitimate coping mechanism.

There will always be complexities; sensitivities about how to approach and handle the subject; how to say the right words; how to respond to heartfelt longings or deep-seated fears; how to maintain hope despite the declining reality; how to handle back-lash or denial; how to respond appropriately to optimistic expectations—how to waltz effectively with our patients. The so called 'death denying' instincts of us all are intrinsic in our makeup, part of our survival DNA and we are right to tread carefully in this area and not demean their significance. Their family may regret this 'collusion of silence' but we must at all times respect the views of the person concerned, and never force the conversation. However many are relieved and empowered to gain some control within this new reality once such open discussions are initiated.

## Who can initiate advance care planning discussions and how? Our experience and examples in practice

There is a growing belief that we, as health and social care providers, have a responsibility to open up this dialogue in a sensitive and open way, because the benefits of doing so greatly outweigh the disadvantages and personal cost. And in addition, there is a move to greater public awareness of the need to consider this discussion at an earlier stage before decisions about medical care become prominent (see Box 1.2).

ACP is a key part of the **Gold Standards Framework (GSF)** quality improvement programmes used extensively in the UK across different settings and across boundaries of care (7). In our experience working with many hundreds of care homes, primary care teams, and in hospitals, the early introduction of this discussion to patients and families eases the path and normalises the process—helping people in 'thinking ahead', so that they can provide best care in line with their hopes and expectations (8,9). GSF focuses on enabling 'generalists' or the usual frontline healthcare provider, and **helps** improve the early identification of patients, triggering increased uptake of ACP. The **GSF Summary Statement of ACP**, used across all settings is that 'Every appropriate person should be offered the chance to have ACP discussions' (mainly Advance Statements) by their chosen/usual healthcare provider which then becomes an action plan against which quality of care is assessed' (10).

Therefore, in our experience, over the last two decades, working in primary care, hospitals, care homes, hospices, domiciliary care services, and prisons, ACP can be integrated as a normal part of care, can be initiated by the usual care provider—the GP, ward nurse, hospital doctor, care home staff member, and, in some cases, the trained lay volunteers enabling earlier consideration and clarification of patients' values, goals, and preferences, that determine and inform care across the whole system (11). See Box 1.2, Box 1.3, and Chapter 7 for examples in practice. Our reflection is that ACP is possible to do by all, important to the mainstream, and should become a standard part of care in all settings that later determine the outcomes-based assessment of progress across a wider population (12). Other countries may take different views, recommending independent facilitators who do not have continuing relationships with these people, (see international chapters) but largely in our UK experience, enabling the front-line care provider to have this conversation as part of the longer term relationship has worked well.

People's priorities for a good death have been described in many different ways: key elements include being with people they love, a sense of being prepared, of not being a burden on others,

## Box 1.2  Overview of advance care planning

### Why do it? What are the benefits of advance care planning?

◆ Enables greater autonomy, choice, and control—respects the person's human rights, enabling a sense of retaining control, self-determination, and empowerment

◆ Improves the quality of end of life care provided for individuals and populations

◆ Care is more person-centred: there is greater concordance with wishes if they have been discussed, for example, enabling more to die where they choose

◆ Potential for reducing unwanted or futile invasive interventions, treatments, or hospital admissions, guiding those involved in care to provide appropriate levels of treatment

◆ Economically cost-effective in reducing unwanted interventions and admissions

◆ Enhanced proactive decision making reduces later burden on family and relieves anxiety

◆ Enables better planning of care, including provision by care providers

◆ Greater satisfaction, reduced anxiety and depression in bereaved relatives

◆ The process can itself be therapeutic and enable resolution of relationships

◆ Enables deeper discussions and consideration of spiritual or existential issues, reflection on meaning and priorities, and encourage resilience and realistic hope

### Why not do it? Barriers and difficulties

◆ Fear of causing distress, having difficult discussions, reducing sense of hope, facing anxiety

◆ Difficulty in initiating the discussion, finding the right words, requiring sensitivity

◆ Making time and space for the discussion, and 'emotional energy'

◆ Unpredictable response—differences within families causing conflict

◆ Over optimistic expectations of prognosis, or care provision by family

◆ Concern about repeating difficult discussions too often—sometimes left to junior staff

◆ Difficulties of being asked about exact prognostication

◆ Lack of information about ACP discussions e.g. on hospital discharge, need for electronic documentation

◆ Peoples' preferences and priorities may change as they approach death

◆ 'Death anxiety' or personal loss of staff

◆ There may be cultural barriers restricting open communication

and of retaining some control including in place of care (13,14). The usual understanding of the benefits of ACP are respect for autonomy, preparation for possible future incapacity, and completion of formal directives. But in addition, people see the potential benefits of ACP to include preparation for end of life care and death, relieving anxiety, dealing with unfinished business, avoiding prolongation of dying, strengthening of personal relationships, relieving burdens placed on family, and the communication of future wishes (15). Some find the timing of the discussion a crucial factor in its success, and for some this can be particularly relevant, indicating that ACP for younger cancer patients or with children facing life-limiting illnesses might be a rather different issue than for the elderly in care homes or those with long-term non-cancerous conditions.

# Box 1.3 Overview of advance care planning—tips for a successful advance care planning discussion

- ACP is a process, not usually a single event, a 'relationship' discussion on several occasions (over days, weeks, months) and usually not on a single visit
- The discussion can be introduced with open exploration of the issues, further discussions planned or recording of decisions and a summary close with invitation for later review
- Essentially this includes using open questioning and clarification of what is important to them, their experience so far, what they want to happen or not to happen and who will speak for them plus any other concerns, preferences or issues
- The person needs to be ready for the discussion—it cannot be forced but only offered—they can refuse, defer, avoid, or wish to discuss other issues
- It takes time and effort and should not be done as a checklist, but in comfortable, unhurried surroundings
- An ACP leaflet to give family and friends before the discussion and an ACP document to guide the discussion are both helpful, and communication skills teaching may be useful
- Clear information should be given; clarify, check, and reflect with the patient—a 'waltz'
- The discussion is characterised by truthfulness, respect, time, compassion, and empathy
- Look out for cues that they wish to end the discussion, summarise and check understanding with the patient, and plan for a review
- The discussion could result in a completed document if the patient so wishes or this could be given for later completion
- Not all people will be able to document their wishes, but may well be able to nominate their preferred decision maker and discuss their long-term values

## How—policy and tools

- National public awareness campaigns e.g. 'Dying Matters' Let's Talk campaign
- Staff may need special training support in identifying the right patients (as in GSF Programmes), communication skills etc
- They mad need leaflets or guidance materials to give to families before the discussion
- Region-wide ACP documents to be used and agreement as to when they should be used
- Information transfer—health and social care providers including out of hours, emergency services, and ambulance, especially related to preferred place of care and DNAR status e.g. Electronic Palliative care Coordinating Systems (EPaCCS)
- Make both advance statements and ADRTs accessible as needed

## When—triggers

Specific examples

- At an earlier stage e.g. retirement or following a life-changing event such as move to a care home, death of spouse
- Following a new diagnosis of life-limiting condition
- Consideration and reflection after repeated hospital admissions

- Proactively included on GP's palliative care register, or Locality Register/EpaCCs considered to be in their final year/s of life, GSF or 'gold' patients
- Expressed need of patient or family
- Making or changing a will, preparing a LPOA or other legal preparation

## Who

- Patient and family—supporting patients and their families to discuss this early e.g. using an introductory leaflet e.g. Planning Your Future Care (18) or GSF five steps video (25)
- The usual healthcare provider who has a long standing relationship e.g. GP, care home staff, community nurse, or other care provider
- Secondary care—specialist consultant hospital ward staff who knows the patient well
- Palliative care specialist or hospice team
- Sometimes trained non-clinical facilitator or volunteer

**Where**—For recommendations in different settings see relevant chapters

- For all settings—following consultation, agree a policy, plan triggers for inclusion and means of communication across the area, involve family, carers, and all health/social care providers
- Back policy up with systematic education
- Audit the proportion of people offered ACPs and concordance with their wishes e.g. proportion dying in their preferred place of care and other end of life care metrics
- Note and communicate resuscitation status where appropriate

## How has advance care planning evolved? Emerging models

As detailed in other chapters in the history of ACP, historically the use of advance directives dominated, particularly in the US. However, some who have been using ADs for many years in the US were from about the year 2000 becoming sceptical about the benefit of focussing on the refusal decision exclusively. '. . . Unexpected problems often arise to defeat ADs. ACP should emphasise not the completion of directives but the emotional preparation of patients and families for future crises' (16).

There was a growing feeling that the discussion could potentially be over-medicalised and an agreement that things were shifting towards the discussion being focussed more on personal aspects of care, being better prepared, and the conversation being initiated earlier between the patient and family.

## Box 1.4 Consensus definition of advance care planning

'Advance care planning is a process that supports adults at any age or stage of health in understanding and sharing their personal values, life goals, and preferences regarding future medical care. The goal of advance care planning is to help ensure that people receive medical care that is consistent with their values, goals and preferences during serious and chronic illness.'

(Sudore et al. 2017)

Reprinted from *Journal of Pain and Symptom Management*, Sudore RL, 'Defining Advance Care Planning for Adults: A Consensus Definition From a Multidisciplinary Delphi Panel', Copyright © 2017 American Academy of Hospice and Palliative Medicine, with permission from Elsevier, www.sciencedirect.com/science/article/pii/S0885392416312325

| **Medical**<br>**What's the matter with you ?**<br>**'Transactional model'** | **Personal**<br>**What matters to you ?**<br>**'Transactional model'** |
|---|---|
| Secondary responsive discussions<br>Medical issues, patient choices<br>leading to treatment planning | Foundational values discussions<br>Personal issues, relational, leading to<br>reconfiguring life and care planning |
| *Pathology/Disease Agenda—biomedical perspective*<br><br>• Pathology, differential diagnosis, further investigations and monitoring<br>• Options for treatment<br>• Documents completed e.g. Refusals of treatment ADRT, emergency plans, DNAR cellings of care, treatment escalation plans<br><br>• Tasks to do | *Wellbeing/Illness Agenda—person's perspective*<br><br>• Ideas, concerns, expectations,<br>• Feelings, thoughts, fears<br>• Goals of care, priorities<br>• Holistic-physical social emotional spiritual<br>• Effects and impact on the person and family<br>• Subjective experience and perception<br>• Deeper spiritual/ existential issues<br><br>• Triggers for further discussion |

**Figure 1.2** The evolving balancing of both the medical 'transactional' and personal 'transformational' models of advance care planning. Available from: http://www. goldstandardsframework.org.uk/advance-care-planning

Reproduced courtesy of The National Gold Standards Framework Centre

This culminated in a 2017 consensus definition of ACP, developed by a large, multi-disciplinary Delphi panel of international ACP experts (17) (see Chapter 2 for more details), which helps us to embrace this wider more inclusive definition (see Box 1.4).

This 2017 definition however demonstrates the growing movement towards the less medicalised model, moving away from the clinician–patient transactional medically based conversation about treatment and care options towards the foundational person–family/carer conversation about alignment with goals, values, and wishes, supporting people to reflect and prepare, where possible, and to live and die as they would choose (see Figure 1.2).

## Goals of care and changing priorities with ageing

As people live longer with multi-morbidities, there are changes in our medical approach as a whole, not just in the proposal of ACP. Tinetti (18), points out that as we move from the clinically focussed 'disease-orientated' model of care to the era of an integrated, individually tailored model, we need to refocus our care on the patient's goals of care, in line with a less medicalised view of the kind of care they require. In the medical disease-focussed model, survival is the main goal, but with the tailored individually tailored model, survival is not the only goal. Indeed a study of goals of care and priorities affirmed that 'living as long as possible was not the most important value for many people', and that priorities other than merely prolonging life should be considered when considering end of life treatment options (19), (see Figure 1.3).

This discussion can dovetail with a specific enquiry about the goals of care or treatment. Different countries use this term in varying ways, but one way is to balance the discussion of quality and quantity of life issues, seeking the person's underlying aims and ensuring these are met within such planning. This is reflected in the UK's updated emergency and resuscitation discussions and

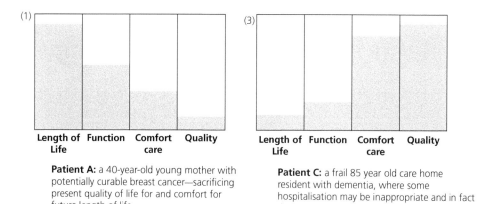

Patient A: a 40-year-old young mother with potentially curable breast cancer—sacrificing present quality of life for and comfort for future length of life

Patient C: a frail 85 year old care home resident with dementia, where some hospitalisation may be inappropriate and in fact detrimental to health

**Figure 1.3** Examples of different scenarios for discussing goals of care

From The National Gold Standards Framework  Centre ACP Guidance

development of 'Respect' (20). Considerations could include length of life, functioning, comfort care, and quality of life, as in the examples in Figure 1.3.

## The two conversations—the personal and the medical

The balance and shifting focus of the two conversations is now more apparent. With the early growth of ACP predominantly focussing on the medical clarification of preferred treatment options, there is now, as discussed, further affirmation of the other deeper conversation, between the foundational person/family values-based conversation, that can both pre-empt this, as well as follow this. Through public awareness campaigns, many countries including the UK are encouraging people to have these discussions at an earlier stage, before they need to consider them in the light of impending decline. There has been much progress and many lessons to learn from countries such as New Zealand, Singapore, Canada, and Australia (see Chapters 18–23) with government-funded campaigns to raise public awareness of ACP.

One such model (see Figure 1.4) as produced as part of the work of The GSF Centre, illustrates this and encourages public awareness of the need for this discussion, through Five Steps in two stages:

1. Firstly the personal foundational discussion, encouraging people to have this conversation early, record and review it (steps one, two, and three).

2. Then secondly for the discussion on steps four and five, directed more to health and social care providers, to be shared with their relevant care provider and others involved in their care.

Much policy and teaching focusses on the healthcare provider initiating the discussion (from steps four and five), and may not take into account any formalised discussions that might have previously occurred (steps one to three).

If more people could initiate such foundational discussions before they become seriously unwell, this would help the communication of these discussions once the person has deteriorated or following a major incident. This is one of the aims of public awareness campaigns and there are encouraging signs of increasing uptake and completion of ACP and even of them being held on digital records on admission to hospital (21). See also the GSF Five Steps animated video on the ACP section of the GSF website—www.goldstandardsframework.org. uk/advance-care-planning

**Advance Care Planning (ACP)**

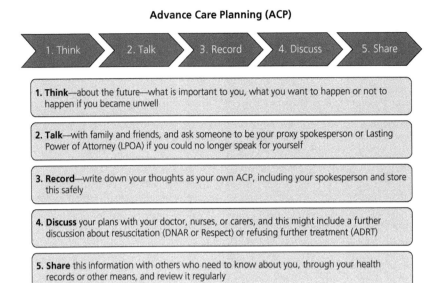

1. Think  2. Talk  3. Record  4. Discuss  5. Share

**1. Think**—about the future—what is important to you, what you want to happen or not to happen if you became unwell

**2. Talk**—with family and friends, and ask someone to be your proxy spokesperson or Lasting Power of Attorney (LPOA) if you could no longer speak for yourself

**3. Record**—write down your thoughts as your own ACP, including your spokesperson and store this safely

**4. Discuss** your plans with your doctor, nurses, or carers, and this might include a further discussion about resuscitation (DNAR or Respect) or refusing further treatment (ADRT)

**5. Share** this information with others who need to know about you, through your health records or other means, and review it regularly

**Figure 1.4** Five simple steps to Advance care Planning—a public awareness campaign (vii). Available from http://www.goldstandardsframework.org.uk/advance-care-planning (25)

Reproduced courtesy of The National Gold Standards Framework Centre

## Thoughts on the deeper significance of ACP discussions

Despite the shock of a life threatening diagnosis or event, some people express thankfulness for the jolt such an experience might give to reawaken their sense of values and priorities and enable them to live life to the full. They have a new perspective with more appreciation of the now, less anxiety about the trivial, and a reawakened sense of what matters in life. In facing death, there is much we can learn about life.

Death focuses the mind on what is important in life—the end of life (time) points to the end of life (meaning). If we were able to face the reality of death, overcoming our fundamental death-denying delusion, could we live in the context of our dying and would our lives be better for this?

Therefore at a deep level, such conversations are not about death but about life, not about how we want to die but how we want to live, and can in themselves reset the compass to ensure we live now in accordance with our values, goals, and aspirations.

This is the experience of many working in palliative care—that patients become our teachers and deeper lessons are there if we choose to see them. Likewise, we can discover this during these important ACP discussions, we can help people live fuller lives, of better quality, more in tune with their wishes and preferences in the time remaining to them, and help to bring their lives to a fitting and respectful conclusion.

The conversation can also trigger something very important within families, and help create the opportunity to say those things that otherwise may be left unspoken. People approaching death can find it easier than their families to discuss meaningful things, and yet such affirmations of a sense of pride, of approval, of shared memories, of forgiveness, of love, can be with them in the memory for years to come. Ira Byock in his book, *The Four things that Matter Most*, suggests these four great affirmations are: I'm sorry, I forgive you, thank you, I love you (22). This brings about a sort of ending that may befit the life led. Initiation of such a discussion for the many is increasingly seen as being more valuable than specific refusal of treatment for the few (see Chapter 6).

## Hopes and expectations

Realistic information, sensitively provided, helps patients and their families to maintain a feeling of normality and allows them to adapt and develop new coping strategies. Such discussions engender hope rather than diminish it.' Davison and Simpson describe the importance of these discussions in normalising life and enhancing hope, even when, to the outsider, it seems that all hope is lost (23). Planning for death with our patients may be an uncomfortable concept but is likely to engender longer-term resilience, realistic hope in many rather than dispel it (24).

## Conclusion

In conclusion, ACP is considered of benefit to people in the final stage of life as a key means of improving care in any setting at any age and with any condition. The goal of ACP is to help ensure that people receive medical care that is consistent with their values, goals, and preferences during serious and chronic illness.

An evolving model of ACP now incorporates both aspects—the medical-focused transactional aspects ensuring clarification of wishes related to treatment options, with the more person–focussed transformational aspects, encompassing deeper values-based reflections enabling people to be better prepared for decision making in the future and more likely to receive care concordant with their values, goals, and preferences.

ACP therefore has a benefit far greater than is at first apparent, in supporting deeper reflection and communication, greater quality of life, and enabling the person and their family or carers to live life more fully in the way they wish to live. ACP, skilfully undertaken, integrated into standard practice, respectfully delivering care aligned with the person's wishes, can be a life-enhancing experience, and play a major role in enabling best end of life care for all.

This book includes many examples of good practice in ACP in different settings and scenarios from around the world, and paints a picture of a time when ACP might become the norm, and might routinely inform all areas of care. This might therefore act as an encouragement, a resource and a 'call to arms' for all striving to implement ACP within their area of care, and enable more to be able to live well and die well in the place and the manner of their choosing.

So, whilst acknowledging some reservations, but encouraged by the common experience of others across the world, this is a plea to colleagues in health and social care, to the public, to policy makers, to those in power—let us be courageous and open up this conversation, listening to and acting upon the responses, so that our care can be in concordance and aligned with peoples' wishes and end of life care is the best we can possibly provide.

## References

1. **Detering KM, Hancock AD, Reade MC, and Silvester W** (2010). 'The impact of advance care planning on end of life care in elderly patients: randomised controlled trial'. *BMJ* **340**: c1345.
2. **Department of Health, London** (July 2008). *Department of Health End of Life Care Strategy.* Available from: www.dh.gov.uk/en/Healthcare/IntegratedCare/Endoflifecare/DH_299
3. *Advance Care Planning: A guide for health and social care staff* (Aug 2008). NHS End of Life Care, UK.
4. **Royal College of Physicians** (Feb. 2009). *Advance Care Planning—Concise Guidance to Good practice, no. 12.* Available from: www.bookshop.rcplondon.ac.uk
5. **Office of the Public Guardian** (September 2014). *Mental Capacity Act: making decisions.* Available from: https://www.gov.uk/government/collections/mental-capacity-act-making-decisions
6. **NHS England** (2017). *Shared Decision Making* [Internet]. Available from: https://www.england.nhs.uk/ourwork/pe/sdm/

7. **Gold Standards Framework** *Advance Care Planning* [Internet]. Available from: http://www.goldstandardsframework.org.uk/advance-care-planning

8. **Gold Standards Framework**, *Evidence* [Internet]. Available from: http://www.goldstandardsframework.org.uk/evidence

9. **Gold Standards Framework** (Sept. 2016). *GSF Update on Evaluations and Evidence No. 2*, [Internet]. Available from: https://tinyurl.com/hlvh4bz

10. **Gold Standards Framework** [Internet]. Available from: http://www.goldstandardsframework.org.uk/home

11. **Gold Standards Framework**, *Cross Boundary Care Training* [Internet]. Available from: http://www.goldstandardsframework.org.uk/cross-boundary-care-training

12. **Thomas K** (2003). *Caring for the dying at home. Companions on a journey*. Oxford: Radcliffe Medical Press.

13. **Smith R** (2000). 'A good death "age concern debate of the age"' *BMJ*, **320**: 129–30.

14. **Gomes B** and **Higginson IJ** (2006). 'Factors influencing death at home in terminally ill patients with cancer: systematic review'. *BMJ* **332**: 515–21.

15. **Steinhauser KE, Clipp EC, McNeilly M, Christakis NA, McIntyre LM, and Tulsky JA** (2000). 'In search of a good death: observations of patients, families, and providers'. *Annals of Internal Medicine* **132**(10): 825–32.

16. **Perkins HS** (2007). 'Controlling death: the false promise of advance directives experience of dying'. *Annals of Internal Medicine* **147**: 51–7. www.annals.org

17. **Sudore RL, Lum HD, You JJ, Hanson LC, Meier DE, Pantilat SZ**, et al. (Jan 2017). 'Defining advance care planning for adults: a consensus definition from a multidisciplinary delphi panel'. *J Pain Symptom Manage* **53**(5): 821–32.

18. **Tinetti M and Fried T**, (2004). 'The end of the disease era'. doi: j.amjmed. 2003.09.031.

19. **Milnes S** et al. (2014). 'Patient values informing medical treatments'. *BMJ Support Pall care* doi: 10.1136/bmjspcare-2016-001177

20. **Pitcher** et al. (2017). 'Emergency care and resuscitation plans'. *BMJ* **356**: j876.

21. **NHS England** (2016). *Coordinate my care: a complete guide* [Internet]. Available from: http://coordinatemycare.co.uk/cmc/wp-content/uploads/2014/06/cmc-complete-guide-2016.pdf

22. **Byock I** (2003) *The Four things that matter most*, London: Atria Books, Simon & Schuster.

23. **Davison SN** and **Simpson C** (2006). 'Hope and advance care planning in patients with end stage renal disease: qualitative interview study'. *BMJ* **333**: 886.

24. **Murray SA, Sheikh A, and Thomas K** (2006). 'Advance care planning in primary care uncomfortable, but likely to engender hope rather than dispel it'. Editorial *BMJ* **333**: 868–914.

25. **GSF 5 Steps to ACP** animation. The National GSF Centre—http://www.goldstandardsframework.org.uk/new-5-steps-advance-care-planning-film or https://www.youtube.com/watch?v=i2k6U6inIjQ

Chapter 2

# What are the benefits of advance care planning and how do we know?

Sarah Russell and Karen Detering

'Just to have time to listen and to see me as a person and not just a name on a piece of paper where they tick things off and scribble things down'
*Research participant* (1)

---

**This chapter includes**

- A brief outline of the development of advance care planning (ACP) and a selective summary of the current evidence base of its benefits and challenges
- The variety of policy, clinical, and legal definitions is discussed
- The interface between decision making and documentation, conversations and discussions, to help patients and their families prepare for death, review their immediate goals and hopes for the future, and strengthen their relationships is considered
- ACP as a complex intervention and outcome measurements

---

**Key Points**

- ACP has an established history in the literature, but with multiple terms, definitions, practice, policy, and legal frameworks
- ACP is not solely concerned with decisions and documentations—it also encompasses discussions about living with and preparing for dying, hopes, fears, and relationships
- ACP is a complex intervention involving multiple concurrent factors
- Outcome measurements should be multifactorial

---

**Key Message**

The convincing evidence base for advance care planning is now well established, and despite international variations in definitions and forms of implementation there is robust evidence of its benefits. The concept has evolved over the years towards a broader relational communication, including both clinical and individual considerations, preparing people who are approaching the end of their life. This is reflected in advance care planning research as a complex intervention, whilst affirming advance care planning as a key intervention within person-centred end of life care.

## Introduction

Advance care planning (ACP) as a process, intervention, and outcome is a key part of international palliative care and policy. From the 1960s it has challenged us as patients, carers, clinicians, commissioners, policy makers, researchers, and educators to define, deliver, and evaluate it in a consistent and effective way. What are the benefits of ACP and how do we know?

## A whistle-stop tour of the history of advance care planning

ACP has been present in the literature for some time. In 1967, Luis Kutner, a human rights lawyer representing the Euthanasia Society of America described a document called 'a living will'. Made in advance it described the extent to which an individual might want treatment to be used when they were no longer able to make a healthcare decision themselves (2).

In 1989–91 the *Study to Understand Prognoses and Preferences for Outcomes and Risks of Treatment* (SUPPORT) in the United States of America aimed to improve decision making in order to address the growing concern over the loss of control that patients had near the end of life and to reduce the frequency of a mechanical, painful, and prolonged process of dying (3). The study prompted further discussion about ACP. This was pertinent as one of the outcomes of the SUPPORT study was to highlight that improving clinicians' communication skills on their own did not improve care (4).

The rationale for the SUPPORT study was illustrated by a number of seminal cases such as Karen Ann Quinlan, Nancy Cruzan, Terri Schiavo, and Tony Bland (1). These highlighted the need for clarity of legislative, clinical, and decision-making frameworks in the event of future incapacity (1). Central to this was consideration of the decision-making process for the circumstances of when an individual was unable to express or consent themselves for interventions, the right to refuse treatments in advance for one self, as well as decisions to withdraw or withhold treatments based upon precedent autonomy of previously expressed wishes or preferences.

Attorneys (an individual legally empowered to act on another's behalf i.e. surrogate decision maker) have been within the international legal frameworks for some time. In Virginia, US, 'Durable Power of Attorneys' for property have been in force since 1954 (5). In England and Wales, general powers of attorney represented by 'Enduring Power of Attorney' were replaced by the more specific property and affairs or health and welfare 'Lasting Power of Attorney' in 2005 (6). Surrogate decision makers enabled further detail and authority; for example, 'best interest' decisions at the end of life when the individual was unable to communicate their wishes or choices about care or interventions.

ACP also developed within several international end of life clinical strategies (see Chapters 18–23). However, national strategies and legal frameworks varied widely in terms of definitions, clinical focus, legal requirements, and choice aspects (5). For example, a comparison of palliative care across seven European countries reported significant differences in the presence of legislation and regulations for ACP (7).

## Benefits of advance care planning

Studies reporting ACP benefits stemmed from a variety of international clinical audit, service evaluation, and research literature (8). This reflected the diverse and often competing needs of patients, health professionals, legislature and health systems (9). Evidence is predominately based upon patient, family, clinician or organisational interventions, and experiences in anticipation of an individual's future loss of capacity and the need to plan for that eventuality. Much literature is from institutional settings such as hospitals, care homes, and intensive care units (4). There is a regular focus on where people want to die (preferred place of death), the anticipation of the loss of capacity (and appointment of surrogate decision makers) and the completion of documents identifying what treatments individuals do not want in the future (for example, advance decision variations).

Studies report that ACP increases the achievement of the preferred place of death (often assumed to be at home) with less invasive or costly treatments (10,11). Much research is concerned with advance decisions (12). Benefits include the enhancement of autonomy and decision making in anticipation of future loss of capacity, relieving family anxiety by removing the burden of decision making, reducing futile interventions, reduction of inappropriate hospital admissions (4,10), as well as economic cost savings (13,14).

ACP may decrease the use of cardio-pulmonary resuscitation, increase hospice and palliative care services, reduce family distress (4) as well as increase the concordance between preferences for and delivered care (11). Also reported is an increase in patient and surrogate shared decision making (4). Studies comment that ACP improves the quality of end of life care, patient and family satisfaction, reducing stress, anxiety, and depression in surviving relatives (10). The process in itself can be therapeutic (15).

## Some challenges

ACP is repeatedly presented as a measure of successful end of life conversations, activity, and interventions. However, there are many contextual factors (Box 2.1). These illustrate the value in recognising its complexity and the need for different outcome measurements.

The success of ACP remains unclear in terms of what are the patients, families, clinicians or systems barriers, blocks, processes, or goals of ACP (8). Studies report a low uptake of ACP (16). Furthermore, the contextual factors of ACP are poorly understood (17) and there are a number of challenges to its effectiveness (18,19). A focus on advance directives has not necessarily reduced

---

### Box 2.1 Other examples of factors influencing advance care planning

Different terms, definitions, legal frameworks and documents (5,12)

Public or patient (e.g. engagement or understanding), systems (e.g. multiple initiatives), resources (e.g. time for conversations or communication systems), healthcare provider factors (e.g. staff discomfort and education) (23)

Measuring economic benefits (14)

Access to palliative care for hidden or hard to reach populations (24)

Diagnosis inequity (13)

Physical functioning, symptom control and perception of suffering (25)

Social networks and friendships (26)

Concerns over being a burden (27)

Accuracy of decisions by surrogate decision makers (28)

Ethnicity, race and cultural aspects (9,13)

Demographic factors such as age, gender, marital and socio economic status (9,12)

Written and health literacy (29,30)

Uncertainty about timing of ACP conversations (31)

hospital admissions or improved care (20) with further comments that improving patient–physician communication on its own is not sufficient with a need to improve systems both within and across organisations (9).

Commentators report that clinicians and patients are uncertain of terms, definitions, and documents (12,17). Questions have been raised about the value of documents (5). Some research advocates a focus on on-going discussions rather than encouraging binding advance decisions (21). Recent systematic reviews remind us that conceptualising ACP as a complex intervention may be more effective than written documents alone (4). Moreover, the assumptions that documentation will lead to higher physicians' confidence or engagement in communicating with patients/families cannot be objectively demonstrated (22). (See Box 2.1).

The reasons why ACP activity is successful (or not) remain unclear and there continues to be calls to recognise ACP as a complex intervention with a need for a broader evidence base to understand all its elements (32). Evaluation needs to consider not only whether an intervention worked, but how it worked.

## Defining advance care planning

Despite the recognition of the importance of ACP, there is significant variation in its definitions in the clinical, legal, research, and policy literature. This has philosophical and practical relevance. Terminology and definitions matter as clarity at an academic and policy level and shared or agreed understandings of care structures, interventions, and goals help organise and evaluate policy, experience, clinical, and research practice (33).

The historical development of ACP is of interest here. Gysels et al.'s (34) review of end of life care definitions make a point relevant for ACP. They argue that definitions evolve over time reflecting changes in meaning as research and practice develops (34). Moreover, end of life definitions and concepts represent historical, geographical, institutional, professional, personal, and cultural developments (34). It is not unreasonable to suggest that ACP has also experienced evolution of its meaning and understanding from a narrower clinician based focus on advance decisions and surrogate decision making to wider social, emotional, and spiritual considerations about facing death.

In 2016, in order to address the issue of ACP definition variety, Sudore et al. (35) convened a large, multidisciplinary Delphi panel of international ACP experts to create a consensus on a definition to be used by clinicians, researchers and policy makers. The panel achieved a final consensus one-sentence definition and accompanying goals statement: 'Advance care planning is a process that supports adults at any age or stage of health in understanding and sharing their personal values, life goals, and preferences regarding future medical care. The goal of advance care planning is to help ensure that people receive medical care that is consistent with their values, goals and preferences during serious and chronic illness.' This definition can provide critical guidance in clinical interventions, research studies, and policy initiatives; however, to ensure generalisability to a larger international audience and lay public, this definition may still require some modifications (35).

## Advance care planning is more than decisions and documentation

The focus of much ACP clinical and research activity has been on advance decision and surrogate decision-maker variations (4,9). However, this activity on its own does not improve end of life care (20). Studies remind us to explore better the stability of choices (36) as well as not make assumptions of the validity of precedent autonomy (37). Michael and colleagues point out the 'grey zone' of decision making due to fluctuating cognitive capacities with arguments for an ACP model with conversations occurring at key points across a person's lifespan (38).

Indeed, there are persistent arguments that ACP should move towards a social, health, behavioral, and contextual process, with conversations about preparing for death, reviewing immediate goals, hopes for the future, and strengthening relationships (3,5,9). This is seen in other literature with reminders that not only should doctors treat the disease but that they should also care about the patient's attitude to the disease (41). Whilst we will all die eventually there are comments that dying has *blurred into a more disease-estimated view of dying* (42). This can be seen in a clinical and policy focus as end of life care is broadened to include last year of life and prediction of patients who may be in the last year of life being one of the triggers for ACP and palliative care.

There is support for the view that ACP should be more than just documents, decisions, and place of death. Sinclair et al. (43) reminds us not to focus solely on prognostic risk in ACP conversations. Sabatini (5) argues the importance of a move away from a legal transactional model of ACP (for example: decisions and documents) toward a relational communications model. Fins et al. (39) question the adherence to narrow notions of self-determination arguing that judgements are contextually informed. Rietjens et al. (32) comment that ACP should be seen as a complex intervention because it includes reflection and communication as well as the completion of documents. Sudore and colleagues report on the relevance of a health behavioural lens on ACP conversations and decisions (44). Borgstrom (40) observe that ACP tools have become tasks to do as opposed to triggers for conversations with those tasks overshadowing relational aspects such as care as an on-going process and relationships forged through connections to others. Furthermore, there are observations that the complexity of individuals and sociocultural factors and the legal health system is underestimated in ACP (9). There is debate if place of death is the most important aspect of end of life care (45) implying the importance of the quality of *living with* as well as *actively dying* (rather than just place of death). Furthermore, there are observations that the focus on the place of death has detracted from how death is experienced (19). Broom and Kirby (46) point out the necessity to view the dying process situated within the cultural and family environment, arguing that 'the focus on individual preferences and management of disease in palliative care contexts must be augmented with sophisticated and nuanced understandings of the family context' (46).

These comments illustrate the breadth of the debate about ACP itself. Is it solely concerned with planning for dying (for those with an identifiable short prognosis); within a medical gaze (47) paradigm of choice and control through anticipation of biomedical death, future incapacity, foreseeing of future decisions, and subsequent documentation with the appointment of surrogate decision makers (1)? Or is it something wider, broader, less planned, and related to how people contemplate and live within their social worlds with the knowledge of their future deaths with choice and control not only concerned with the where and when of death but also rooted in how people choose to live with and talk about their dying (1)? ACP conversations can (and perhaps should) happen earlier or at any time in chronic and life-limiting illness representing a personalised rather than diagnosis/prognosis approach toACP.

## Advance care planning as a complex intervention and outcome measurements

There are calls to recognise ACP as a complex intervention with a broader evidence base to understand all its elements (32). The theories of complex adaptive systems and complex interventions are helpful here. They point out that complex interventions are made up of many components that act both on their own and in conjunction with each other (48). In other words, complex interventions are not linear, nor confined to only understanding processes because there are interacting components including those delivering (e.g. clinicians) or receiving (e.g. patients and families) an interaction and evaluation outcomes (48). This has resonance for ACP especially if it is situated within the paradigm of a person-centred approach (with all its physical, social, emotional, and spiritual interlinking components) such as 'what matters to you, rather than what's the matter with you' as described by Maureen Bisognano in 2012 (49).

ACP presents challenges when evaluating implementation processes and outcomes. There are issues considering the generalisability of findings because of the variety of interconnected components (e.g. type of intervention, by whom, when and where). Some of the discussions illustrated by the MORECare statements identify such challenges such as (a) moving from feasibility and piloting to implementation without robust evaluation; (b) failing to develop the feasibility of the evaluation methods alongside the feasibility of treatment/intervention; and (c) lack of a theoretical framework underpinning treatment/intervention (50). What this means in real terms is that in the evaluation of complex interventions such as ACP it is important to determine whether an intervention is effective, what the theoretical underpinning is, and how and why it actually works. Evaluation of ACP interventions may include discussion regarding structure, and measurement of process, and outcomes. This maybe for both receiver of the intervention as well as those that are delivering it. Structure, or the context of care, includes anything external to the actual intervention that may act as a barrier or facilitator to its implementation or effects. Thus, an ACP model of implementation may be effective in a particular setting, sector, or location, but may be less effective elsewhere due to contextual factors.

A specific intervention may have limited effects either because of weaknesses in its design or because it is not properly implemented. Similarly, positive outcomes may occur even when an intervention was not delivered fully as intended. Thus, evaluation of ACP interventions ideally need process measures to capture fidelity (whether the intervention was delivered as intended), dose (the quantity of the intervention implemented) and reach of the intervention (whether the intended audience comes receives the intervention).

In evaluation of ACP interventions, clinicians', researchers, educators and commissioners need to decide what outcomes are most important and which are secondary. Biondo and colleagues systematic review of the evaluation of ACP interventions highlighted that the most common outcome measures relate to document completion, followed by healthcare resource use (51). Patient/family/healthcare provider reported outcomes are less commonly measured and concordance measures (e.g. dying in place of choice) were reported by only 26% of studies (51). Other outcome measurement approaches include Detering and colleagues (10) who report outcomes such as known end of life wishes, patient satisfaction, and impact on family. Sampson et al. (52) utilised carer reported outcomes e.g. Kessler Distress Scale, Decision Satisfaction Inventory, Client Satisfaction Questionnaire, Euroqol-5D and The Satisfaction with End of Life Care in Dementia Scale. Houben (11) reported upon the occurrence of ACP discussions. The reduction of hospital admissions, bed days or hospital deaths (particularly from the nursing or care home setting) is also often reported as an ACP outcome measure (53).

What this tells us is not only the variety of outcome measures used to demonstrate the benefits of ACP, but also the necessity to think systematically through the lens of a complex intervention. Viewing ACP outcome measurements in this way is illustrated by a recent report from Oregon. Tolle and Teno (54) point out that the intervention 'Physicians Orders for Life Sustaining Treatment Programme' may have benefited from a complex intervention approach that included state-wide education, coordination, research, and a registry (54). Moreover, they argue that to transform care; complexity, multifaceted interventions, and a public health strategy needs to be embraced with interventions aimed at individuals, local healthcare systems, state government levels and local champions, and state collation (54). The Oregon example illustrates system wide outcomes and a multiple components approach aimed at individuals, organisations, and region.

## Summary

ACP has an established place in the clinical literature. It encompasses discussion, decisions, and documentation about clinical care as well as wider broader considerations about how an individual (and their family) contemplate their future death. There is robust evidence of its benefits. A planned, systematic, and consistent manner to measuring its outcomes from a variety of perspectives, lends itself to a complex intervention approach.

## References

1. **Russell S.** (2016). *Advance care planning and living with dying: the views of hospice patients*, [Internet]. University of Hertfordshire. Available from: http://hdl.handle.net/2299/17474

2. **Kutner L** (1969). 'Due process of euthansia: the living will, a proposal'. *Indiana Law J* **44**(4): 539–54.

3. **Hamel MB, Davis RB, Teno JM, Knaus WA, Lynn J, Harrell FJ,** et al. (Nov 1999). 'Older age, aggressiveness of care, and survival for seriously ill, hospitalized adults. SUPPORT Investigators. Study to understand prognoses and preferences for outcomes and risks of treatments'. *Ann Intern Med* **131**(10): 721–8.

4. **Brinkman-Stoppelenburg A, Rietjens JA, and van der Heide A** (2014). 'The effects of advance care planning on end-of-life care: A systematic review'. *Palliat Med* **28**(8): 1000–25.

5. **Sabatino CP** (Jun 2010). 'The evolution of health care advance planning law and policy'. *Milbank Q* **88**(2): 211–39.

6. **Lyne M.** *The Mental Capacity Act 2005* (2010). 33–6. Available from: http://eprints.bournemouth.ac.uk/16782/1/licence.txt

7. **Van Beek K, Woitha K, Ahmed N, Menten J, Jaspers B, Engels Y,** et al. (2013). 'Comparison of legislation, regulations and national health strategies for palliative care in seven European countries (results from the Europall Research Group): a descriptive study'. *BMC Health Serv Res* **13**: 275.

8. **Russell S** (2014). 'Advance care planning: Whose agenda is it anyway?' *Palliat Med* **28**(8): 997–9.

9. **Lovell A and Yates P** (Sep 2014). 'Advance Care Planning in palliative care: a systematic literature review of the contextual factors influencing its uptake 2008–2012'. *Palliat Med* **28**(8): 1026–35.

10. **Detering KM, Hancock a. D, Reade MC, and Silvester W** (Mar 2010). 'The impact of advance care planning on end of life care in elderly patients: randomised controlled trial'. *BMJ* **340** (1): c1345–c1345.

11. **Houben CHM, Spruit M, Wouters EFM, and Janssen DJ** (2014). 'A randomised controlled trial on the efficacy of advance care planning on the quality of end-of-life care and communication in patients with COPD: the research protocol'. *BMJ Open* **4**(1): e004465–e004465.

12. **Institute of Medicine of the National Academies** (2014). *Dying in America: Improving Quality and Honouring Individual preferences Near End of Life*. PSSRU Discussion Paper 2894, London School of Economics.

13. **Dixon J, King D, Matosevic T, Clark M, and Knapp M** (Apr 2015). 'Equity in the Provision of Palliative Care in the UK : Review of Evidence'. Personal Social Services Research Unit London School of Economics and Political Science.

14. **Klingler C, In der Schmitten J, and Marckmann G** (Aug 2015) 'Does facilitated Advance Care Planning reduce the costs of care near the end of life? Systematic review and ethical considerations'. *Palliat Med* **30**(5): 423–33.

15. **Thomas K** (2011). 'Overview and introduction to Advance Care Planning'. In: Thomas K, (ed.) *Advance Care Planning in End of Life Care*. Oxford: Oxford University Press. Pp. 4–15.

16. **Gillick MR** (Jun 2010). 'The challenge of applying advance directives in hospital practice'. *Hosp Pract (1995)*. **38**(3): 45–51.

17. **Rhee JJ, Zwar NA, and Kemp LA** (Apr 2013). 'Advance care planning and interpersonal relationships: a two-way street'. *Fam Pract* **30**(2): 219–26.

18. **Mullick A., Martin J, and Sallnow L** (Oct 2013). 'An introduction to advance care planning in practice'. *BMJ* **347** (3): f6064–f6064.

19. **Pollock K and Wilson E** (Jul 2015). 'Care and communication between health professionals and patients affected by severe or chronic illness in community care settings: a qualitative study of care at the end of life'. *Health Services and Delivery Research* **3**(31): Southampton (UK).

20. **Prendergast TJ** (Feb 2001). 'Advance care planning: pitfalls, progress, promise'. *Crit Care Med* **29**(2 Suppl): N34–9.

21. **MacPherson A, Walshe C, O'Donnell V, and Vyas A** (Mar 2013). 'The views of patients with severe chronic obstructive pulmonary disease on advance care planning: a qualitative study'. *Palliat Med* **27**(3): 265–72.

22. **Lewis E, Cardona-Morrell M, Ong KY, Trankle SA, and Hillman K** (Oct 2016). 'Evidence still insufficient that advance care documentation leads to engagement of healthcare professionals in end-of-life discussions: A systematic review'. *Palliat Med* **30**(9): 807–24.

23. **Hagen NA, Howlett J, Sharma NC, Biondo P, Holroyd-Leduc J, Fassbender K, et al.** (Aug 2015). 'Advance care planning: identifying system-specific barriers and facilitators'. *Curr Oncol* **22**(4): e237–45.

24. **Song J, Ratner ER, Wall MM, Bartels DM, Ulvestad N, and Petroskas D, et al.** (Jul 2010). 'Effect of an End-of-Life Planning Intervention on the completion of advance directives in homeless persons: a randomized trial'. *Ann Intern Med* **153**(2): 76–84.

25. **Ruijs CDM, Kerkhof AJFM, van der Wal G, and Onwuteaka-Philipsen BD** (2013). 'Symptoms, unbearability and the nature of suffering in terminal cancer patients dying at home: a prospective primary care study'. *BMC Fam Pract* **14**(1): 201.

26. **Leonard R, Horsfall D, and Noonan K** (2015). 'Identifying changes in the support networks of end-of-life carers using social network analysis'. *BMJ Support Palliat Care* **5**(2): 153–9.

27. **Akazawa T, Akechi T, Morita T, Miyashita M, Sato K, Tsuneto S, et al.** (Aug 2010). 'Self-perceived burden in terminally ill cancer patients: a categorization of care strategies based on bereaved family members' perspectives'. *J Pain Symptom Manage* **40**(2): 224–34.

28. **Meeker MA** (2004). 'Family Surrogate Decision Making at the End of Life: Seeing them Through with Care and Respect'. *Qual Health Res* **14**(2): 204–25.

29. **Waite KR, Federman AD, McCarthy DM, Sudore R, Curtis LM, Baker DW, et al.** (Mar 2013). 'Literacy and race as risk factors for low rates of advance directives in older adults'. *J Am Geriatr Soc* **61**(3): 403–6.

30. **Sudore RL, Landefeld CS, Barnes DE, Lindquist K, Williams BA, Brody R, et al.** (Dec 2007). 'An advance directive redesigned to meet the literacy level of most adults: a randomized trial'. *Patient Educ Couns* **69**(1–3): 165–95.

31. **Holley JL** (Jun 2012). 'Advance care planning in CKD/ESRD: an evolving process'. *Clin J Am Soc Nephrol* **7**(6): 1033–8.

32. **Rietjens J, Korfage I, and van der Heide A** (2016). 'Advance care planning: Not a panacea'. Vol. **30**, *Palliat Med* London: Sage Publications. Pp. 421–2.

33. **Gott M, Seymour J, Ingleton C, Gardiner C, and Bellamy G** (Apr 2012). '"That's part of everybody's job": the perspectives of health care staff in England and New Zealand on the meaning and remit of palliative care'. *Palliat Med* **26**(3): 232–41.

34. **Gysels M, Evans N, Menaca A, Higginson IJ, Harding R, and Pool R** (2013). 'Diversity in defining end of life care: an obstacle or the way forward?' *PLoS One* **8**(7): e68002.

35. **Sudore RL, Lum HD, You JJ, Hanson LC, Meier DE, Pantilat SZ, et al.** (Jan 2017). 'Defining advance care planning for adults: a consensus definition from a multidisciplinary delphi panel'. *J Pain Symptom Manage* **53**(5): 821–32.

36. **Wittink MN, Morales KH, Meoni LA, Ford DE, Wang N-Y, and Klag MJ, et al.** (Oct 2008). 'Stability of preferences for end-of-life treatment after 3 years of follow-up: the Johns Hopkins Precursors Study'. *Arch Intern Med* **168**(19): 2125–30.

37. **Seymour J and Horne G** (2011). 'Advance Care Planning for the end of life:an overview'. In: Thomas K and Lobo B, eds *Advance Care Planning in End of Life Care*. Oxford: Oxford University Press. Pp. 16–27.

38. **Michael N, O'Callaghan C, and Sayers E** (Jan 2017). 'Managing "shades of grey": a focus group study exploring community-dwellers' views on advance care planning in older people'. *BMC Palliat Care* **16**(1): 2.

39. **Fins JJ, Maltby BS, Friedmann E, Greene MG, Norris K, Adelman R**, et al. (Jan 2005). 'Contracts, covenants and advance care planning: an empirical study of the moral obligations of patient and proxy'. *J Pain Symptom Manage* **29**(1): 55–68.

40. **Borgstrom E** (Nov 2015). 'Being mortal: illness, medicine, and what matters in the end, by Atul Gawande'. *Anthropol Med* **22**(3): 333–5.

41. **Frankl V** (1967). *Psychotherapy and Existentialism*. New York: Washington Square Press.

42. **Kellehear A** (2009). 'On dying and human suffering'. *Palliat Med* **23**(5): 388–97.

43. **Sinclair C, Gates K, Evans S, and Auret KA** (Apr 2016). 'Factors influencing australian general practitioners' clinical decisions regarding advance care planning: a factorial survey'. *J Pain Symptom Manage* **51**(4): 718–27.e2.

44. **Sudore RL, Stewart AL, Knight SJ, McMahan RD, Feuz M, Miao Y**, et al. (2013). 'Development and validation of a questionnaire to detect behavior change in multiple advance care planning behaviors'. *PLoS One* **8**(9): e72465.

45. **NIHR Dissemination Centre** (2015). *Better Endings: Right Care, Right Place, Right Time* [Internet]. Available from: http://www.dc.nihr.ac.uk/highlights-and-reviews/end-of-life-care

46. **Broom A and Kirby E** (2013). 'The end of life and the family: hospice patients' views on dying as relational'. *Sociol Health Illn* **35**(4): 499–513.

47. **Foucault M** (1973). *The Birth of the Clinic: An Archaeology of Medical Perception*. New York: Pantheon Books.

48. **Craig P, Dieppe P, Macintyre S, Michie S, Nazareth I, Petticrew M**, et al. (2008). 'Developing and evaluating complex interventions : new guidance'. *BMJ* **337**: a1655.

49. **Bisognano M**. 'An Ounce of Prevention'. In: *IHI International Summit 2012 Keynote Presentation at IHI 13th Annual International Summit on Improving Patient Care in the Office Practice & the Community*, 19 March 2012. Available from: http://www.ihi.org/resources/Pages/AudioandVideo/BisognanoSummit2012Keynote.aspx

50. **Higginson IJ, Evans CJ, Grande G, Preston N, Morgan M, McCrone P**, et al. (2013). 'Evaluating complex interventions in end of life care: the MORECare statement on good practice generated by a synthesis of transparent expert consultations and systematic reviews'. *BMC Med* **11**: 111 doi: 10.1186/1741-7015-11-111.

51. **Biondo PD, Lee LD, Davison SN, and Simon JE** (2016). 'How healthcare systems evaluate their advance care planning initiatives: Results from a systematic review'. *Palliat Med* **30**(8): 720–9.

52. **Sampson EL, Jones L, Thuné-Boyle IC V, Kukkastenvehmas R, King M, Leurent B**, et al. (2011). 'Palliative assessment and advance care planning in severe dementia: an exploratory randomized controlled trial of a complex intervention'. *Palliat Med* **25**(3): 197–209.

53. **Martin RS, Hayes B, Gregorevic K, and Lim WK** (Apr 2016). 'The effects of advance care planning interventions on nursing home residents: a systematic review'. *J Am Med Dir Assoc* **17**(4): 284–93.

54. **Tolle SW, Teno JM** (Mar 2017). 'Lessons from Oregon in embracing complexity in end-of-life care'. *N Engl J Med* **376**(11): 1078–82.

# Chapter 3

# An introduction to advance care planning: practice at the frontline

Anjali Mullick and Jonathan Martin

'. . . our most cruel failure in how we treat the sick and the aged is the failure to recognise that they have priorities beyond merely being safe and living longer; that the chance to shape one's story is essential to sustaining meaning in life; that we have the opportunity to refashion our institutions, our culture, and our conversations in ways that transform the possibilities for the last chapters of everyone's lives'.
*Atul Guwande* (1)

---

**This chapter includes**

- A useful definition of advance care planning (ACP) that can be applied to clinical practice
- An overview of the benefits, challenges, and limitations of ACP
- Practical information on when and how to carry out ACP discussions including specific communication tips
- A summary of the potential outcomes of an ACP discussion and a general guide on writing ACP statements
- An illustration of how ACP decisions might be applied in clinical practice through a variety of case studies

---

**Key Points**

- ACP is a process that aims to help patients establish decisions about future care that take effect when they lose capacity. This can include formal decisions
- Benefits include: increasing patient autonomy, preparing families for the future, and a sense of professional satisfaction
- Setting realistic expectations of ACP with patients is important, as it is not possible to anticipate and plan for every eventuality
- An adequate knowledge of the Mental Capacity Act and good communication skills will be necessary to successful discussions
- Possible outcomes of ACP discussions include, but are not limited to, writing an Advance Statement, an Advance Decision to Refuse Treatment (ADRT) or appointing a Lasting Power of Attorney (LPA)

> **Key Message**
>
> The key to success with ACP is to focus on the process, in an open exploration of patient's concerns and preferences, as it may result in a different outcome to the one envisaged by the professional. The process of ACP discussions can enhance the relationship between professional and patient through a deeper understanding of the patient's wishes, beliefs and values. Patient and family centred outcomes are more likely to be achieved using this approach.

## Deciphering the definition

For the busy clinician, making sense of advance care planning (ACP) and its various definitions can be challenging. These definitions often have a bureaucratic tone distant from the daily reality of clinical care and the experience of ACP in practice. We favour a definition of ACP as a process of formal decision making that aims to help patients establish decisions about future care that take effect when they lose capacity (2) or, in other words, making decisions in advance. In clinical practice, patients may have a range of views about their future care and treatments. Examples of future interventions might include cardiopulmonary resuscitation (CPR) and use of medication such as antibiotics or analgesics. ACP discussions will also often highlight wider issues, which may be of equal or greater importance to a patient, such as place of care, and who they would want involved in their care. Understandably some professionals feel nervous about engaging with a process defined as 'formal', that requires knowledge of the Mental Capacity Act (MCA) (3), a working concept of mental capacity, and an idea of what clinical and other scenarios may face the patient with their particular constellation of diagnoses and circumstances. The aim of this chapter is to shed light on what the ACP process actually entails in clinical practice and to give tips to help bring theory into practice. We will demonstrate some of the key concepts of ACP through three case vignettes. Some of the areas, such as the MCA and advance decisions to refuse treatment (ADRT) will be covered in more detail.

## Benefits in practice

ACP has been the subject of an active and extensive international research agenda. Early evidence did not show the anticipated advantages of undertaking ACP but more recent evidence has demonstrated wide-ranging benefits for individual patients, their loved ones, healthcare workers, and the healthcare economy. The benefits for which there is some evidence fall into a number of distinct categories which may be useful to have in mind during ACP discussions.

### Preparing for the patient's future

Whilst some patients do not want to think about the future, in our experience many value the opportunity to prepare for decisions that may face them in times ahead (4). Honest and open conversations about the likely future impact of an illness can be empowering for patients, and discussions may cover many issues, including their quality of life and life expectancy; patients frequently gain an increased sense of control, not least in avoiding interventions that he or she would not want. Withholding the opportunity for such discussions, perhaps on the basis of not wanting to remove hope or through fear of difficult conversations, could be viewed as sidestepping our professional responsibilities; we will later suggest ways of offering ACP discussions in a sensitive manner that allows the patient to emerge unscathed, should they choose not to engage in the process.

## Preparing the family

Overall the weight of evidence is in favour of family benefit, both in preparing for their loved one's death and in reaching decisions at a time when the patient has lost capacity (5). A common example concerns the admission of someone with dementia to a care home: ACP can reduce guilt about such decisions, and may lead to a better bereavement with lower levels of psychological morbidity for those left behind (6). Overall the families of those who undertake ACP show greater satisfaction with care, presumably because they can see that the care was aligned to the wishes of their loved one.

## Benefits for the health service

At a practical level our experience is that making best interests decisions is far easier for those who have an advance care plan. This is true even if the plan did not pertain to the situation now being faced by the patient; the simple fact of its presence often means that families are more prepared to engage in best interests conversations and may have some understanding of the processes involved. Importantly, the evidence for ACP also shows a reduction in needless resource use, such as unwanted hospital admissions (7).

# Preparing for pitfalls

There are a number of practical and philosophical concerns around ACP, of which we will focus mainly on the former.

## Patient concerns

Before beginning ACP, patients must have the necessary mental capacity to consider the topics under discussion. In addition, given that ACP may be an emotionally taxing process, patients must have a willingness to contemplate and plan for their own deterioration and demise (8). Against this patients may believe that ACP is unnecessary, for instance, that they will receive the right care by default or that a loved one will know their wishes without prior discussion, something that turns out to be true less frequently than most believe (9).

## Professional concerns

There is evidence to suggest that some healthcare professionals outside palliative care do not feel equipped to offer or undertake ACP work with their patients; partly this relates to differing views about who should do the work. For example, hospital professionals may believe that GPs are well placed to facilitate ACP given their long-standing and holistic relationships with patients, whilst GPs might have concerns about the level of knowledge and information they have about a patient's illness, especially if care has been largely delivered in a specialist setting. Both groups are rightly apprehensive about time pressures. In practice we favour a shared approach, although we acknowledge the difficulties inherent to achieving this.

Concerns may also relate both to the degree of experience with ACP and the communication skills needed to start a sensitive conversation that may 'bring death into full view' (10). These are all entirely legitimate anxieties, which we hope to alleviate in part in 'Communication tips'.

In our experience, ACP is a process and rarely completed in one sitting; certainly our view is that a 'tick box' approach cannot achieve a high enough quality of discussion, and therefore outcome. In addition, once ACP has been completed, information sharing can also be challenging, so we offer our suggestions for this later on in the chapter.

Finally, we need to avoid giving the impression that we can accurately predict the future. Nor is it possible to capture every nuanced wish the patient may have for their future care: in our view the quality and accuracy of a best interests decision, even one based on ACP, is unlikely to match a capacitous decision made in the here and now.

Despite these limitations our experience of ACP is that it not only enhances the future autonomy of patients, but also improves decision-making in the present, reflecting the strengthened relationship between patient and professional that is achieved through a deeper understanding of the person's beliefs and values.

## ACP discussions in practice

ACP is usually undertaken with patients who have a progressive illness and an anticipated deterioration that may result in a future loss of mental capacity. If you encounter patients who may benefit do not assume that other professionals have already had ACP conversations; instead you should check. The process is voluntary, so do not press them if it is clear from initial exploration that the patient is not willing to engage with discussions at that moment; conversations can be revisited in the future, if appropriate.

Box 3.1 suggests some triggers for ACP discussions.

### Communication tips

We find that the process of ACP often works best when discussion initially focusses on a patient's goals, values, and beliefs, rather than on particular treatments, interventions, or outcomes. Box 3.2 gives some example triggers for these discussions.

Mahon suggests two questions that you may find useful as a basis for initiating an ACP discussion:

1. If you cannot, or choose not to, participate in healthcare decisions, with whom should we speak?

2. If you cannot, or choose not to, participate in decision making, what should we consider when making decisions about your care? (11)

We include some further tips that we have used in our clinical practice in Box 3.2.

---

## Box 3.1 Triggers for initiating or reviewing advance care planning discussions

### Triggers for initiating or reviewing advance care planning discussions

- Patient initiates the conversation
- Diagnosis of a progressive condition which is likely to result in a loss of capacity, such as dementia or motor neurone disease
- A change or deterioration in condition
- Change in the person's personal circumstances, such as moving into a care home or loss of a family member
- Routine clinical review of the patient, such as clinic appointments or home visits
- When a previously agreed review interval elapses

Adapted from Mullick A, Martin J, & Sallnow L, 'An introduction to advance care planning in practice', *The British Medical Journal*, 347, Copyright © 2013 *BMJ Publishing Group*, doi: 10.1136/bmj.f6064, with permission from BMJ Publishing Group Ltd

## Box 3.2 Communication tips

### Starting the conversation

Use general open questions and be guided by the patient's cues and responses to know whether to explore further.

Examples:

- How have you been coping with your illness recently?
- Do you like to think about or plan for the future?
- When you think of the future, what do you hope for? (12)
- When you think about the future, what worries you the most? (12)
- Have you given any thought to what kinds of treatment you would want (or not want) if you become unable to speak for yourself? (13)
- What do you consider you quality of life to be like now? (13)

### During the conversation

Use language that patients can understand and any other communication aids you might need.

Give patients enough information to make informed choices without overloading them.

Clarify any ambiguous statements that patients make—for example:

- Patient: 'I don't want heroics.'
- Professional: 'What do you mean by heroics?'

### Ending the conversation

Summarise what has been discussed to check mutual understanding, or ask the patient to do so.

Screen for any other problems—for example: 'Is there anything else you would like to discuss?'

Arrange another time to continue, complete or review the discussion if necessary—for example if the patient would like help completing an ADRT.

Document the contents of the discussion in the patient record.

Share the contents (with the patient's permission) with anyone else who needs to know.

## Potential outcomes of advance care planning discussions

1. Patient does not wish to engage in ACP at that moment

   Make it clear that the patient is welcome to reopen an ACP discussion at any time, and reoffer in the future if appropriate

2. Patient makes an Advance Statement (variously known as a 'Statement of Wishes' or a 'Statement of Wishes and Preferences')

The NHS End of Life Care Programme states that this is a 'summary term embracing a range of written and/or recorded oral expressions, by which people can, if they wish, write down or tell people about their wishes or preferences in relation to future treatment and care, or explain their feelings, beliefs and values that govern how they make decisions. They may cover medical and non-medical matters' (14). This type of statement is not legally binding but, as per the Mental Capacity Act, must be considered when making best interests decision about that person.

For example:

'The quality of my life is really important to me—I don't want to be kept alive just for the sake of it.'

'I've been in and out of hospital too many times. If I become ill again I want to stay and home and die in peace.'

'So far the antibiotics help me feel better each time I get ill, so I'd like to receive them until they stop working.'

'I'd like people to talk to my daughter if I'm not able to make decisions myself–she understands where I am coming from.'

In practice, these conversations are often recorded in the patient's medical records, but may need to be shared more widely depending on local information-sharing systems.

The first case study relates to an Advance Statement.

3. Patient writes an ADRT

This form of written or oral statement is specific to treatment refusals: it enables a person to affirm ahead of time that there are particular treatments that they do not wish to have. It does not cover place of care. Many treatment refusals are contingent on circumstances ('I don't want to be tube fed if my dementia is so severe that I am unable to recognise my family'), so it is advisable that these circumstances are specified. Some refusals will apply whatever the circumstances, such as a Jehovah's Witness' refusal of blood products, and often CPR refusal; in these cases specific circumstances are irrelevant. Note that there is a checklist of validity and applicability factors to consider, including extra requirements for refusals of potentially life-sustaining treatments, when deciding whether to act on an ADRT. A valid and applicable ADRT carries legal weight and must be followed; therefore best interests do not apply.

The second case study involves application of an ADRT.

4. Patient draws up a Lasting Power of Attorney (LPA)

A patient appoints an attorney to whom they give decision making powers should they lose mental capacity to make decisions. There are two types of LPA: 'property and financial affairs' and 'health and welfare'.

The third case study covers LPAs in more detail.

Many patients will not have a clear outcome in mind when they embark upon ACP discussions and will often not be aware of the possibilities, although some may have an awareness of the options if they have done their own research. In our experience, the most common outcome of an ACP discussion is an Advance Statement.

There may be other outcomes that arise from an ACP discussion that were not anticipated. For example, a patient may decide to make a will, or talk to a loved one about something that, previously, they did not have the confidence to do. In our experience, focussing on a formal outcome alone is not necessarily the key to success in ACP discussions. In particular, open exploration of a person's concerns and preferences may lead you in a different direction to the one that either you or the patient had envisaged, even if the patient instigated an ACP conversation with a particular outcome in mind.

## A general guide to writing advance care planning statements

There is no one right way in which to write an Advance Statement or ADRT, nor any legal requirement that clinicians, lawyers or others are involved in the process. Our view, however, is that patients should be encouraged to seek the advice of clinicians to help shape the document so that what the patient is trying to achieve is more likely to be immediately clear to other clinicians. In this way an Advance Statement or ADRT will be of use both in circumstances where an unpressured, thoughtful application of the best interests framework is possible, and those in which urgent decisions are necessary in a medical emergency.

Our experience in relation to ADRTs in particular is that the intention of the patient is not always clear. For example, a statement such as 'I do not want antibiotics' provides little insight into the quality and scope of the decision-making process, and whether the patient has made an informed decision. We advise writing ADRTs using simple language and in such a way that gives insight into the intention of the patient behind his or her wishes for care and for refusing particular treatments. For example, someone might not wish to be given antibiotics for a life-threatening chest infection where the intention of the treating team is to prolong life, whereas the same person might accept antibiotics where the intention is symptom control or comfort care, even if life is prolonged as a result. This illustrates the point that ACP may appear to offer the patient more certainty and security than is possible to deliver in practice.

In the example already given, it is a clinician that would guide the decision-making process by determining whether the chest infection was life threatening, often in a context of a high degree of uncertainty, and would assess other benefits such as symptom control. In addition, it is not possible to foretell every eventuality, which is something that should be made explicit to the patient. For this reason, a statement outlining the person's overall goal of care (such as 'I value quality of life over length of life') would be a very useful addition to an ADRT. Indeed, when patients seek our help with ADRTs, we recommend that they include within the ADRT documentation an Advance Statement of this nature. This might include a record of their diagnosis, their quality of life now, a nominated person for the decision maker to prioritise in discussions about best interests and information about preferred place of death.

Generally, it is our experience that it is difficult to encapsulate all a person's nuanced wishes for future care into an Advance Statement or ADRT. It is important, therefore, to be very clear with patients about the various limitations of ACP at the time of discussion.

### Information sharing

Once the ACP process has been completed the information within it needs to be shared, which can be challenging; only LPA instruments have a central repository (at the Office of the Public Guardian). We ask our patients to consider who should receive a copy e.g. carers, relatives, and loved ones and relevant healthcare professionals, and to list this on the documentation with appropriate contact details. We also advise them to keep a copy at home and perhaps even on their person. Some areas may have a specific means of ACP information sharing, such as an Electronic Palliative Care Coordination System, or data sharing through electronic patient records, so check local practice. It is important to ensure information is updated if changes are made.

# Applying the outcomes of advance care planning—case studies

## Case study
### Mary's advance statement

Mary is an 88-year-old lady with advanced metastatic breast cancer. She is known to have bone metastases. You are her GP providing medical input in partnership with the local community palliative care team. She is in a nursing home, has an estimated prognosis of several months and is largely nursed in bed. Mary has said on several occasions that she does not wish to go to hospital in the future and would like to die in the nursing home. She has previously shown a good understanding of her illness. She has no close family.

One day, after turning in bed, Mary develops excruciating leg pain and you have a strong clinical suspicion of a pathological hip fracture. At this stage, she has become confused, is unable to make sense of the situation and does not have relevant mental capacity. She is distressed and crying out in pain.

### How would you proceed?

Mary's verbally expressed preference to die in the nursing home has previously been recorded in her medical notes by both you and the palliative care team. This is an example of an advance statement.

In this case, you do not have time to instruct an Independent Mental Capacity Advocate, but you do liaise with the palliative care team to determine the best course of action. Whilst both of you want to respect Mary's wish to remain in the nursing home if possible, neither of you believe that Mary had anticipated the sort of clinical event that has now occurred. Whilst both parties realise that surgical intervention will not offer an improvement in function, it might offer good pain control.

In the first few hours after the suspected fracture, in light of her previously expressed preferences, it is decided to try and manage Mary's pain control within the nursing home setting with strong painkillers. However, it becomes apparent that her pain does not respond to medication and she is extremely distressed both at rest and on slight movement. You decide to send her to hospital for surgical assessment, making it clear to hospital colleagues that the intended goal of intervention is pain relief. Mary receives surgery and is sent back to the nursing home a few days after the operation. Her pain is well controlled following the operation and she dies peacefully six weeks later in the nursing home.

## Case study
### Interpreting Jean's advance decision to refuse treatment

Jean, a 71-year-old lady with advanced dementia, is admitted to hospital from a nursing home with a chest infection. The admitting doctor notes that her medical record contains an ADRT, written four years previously. It outlines that Jean was aware of her dementia diagnosis and that she feared increasing dependency. It states that, should she ever be dependent on nursing home care and develop a chest infection, she would not want antibiotics to treat the infection where the intention of the treating team is to prolong her life. It is signed by her, a witness and it is dated.

Jean's daughter arrives at the hospital. She says that she is aware of Jean's ADRT, but as her next of kin she insists that the team give antibiotics.

### How should you, as the treating doctor, approach this issue?

Assuming antibiotics are an appropriate treatment to offer, an assessment of Jean's mental capacity to make decisions around antibiotic use needs to be made. The Mental Capacity Act tells us to assume that a person has capacity to make a decision unless it can be demonstrated otherwise, and to do everything reasonably possible to help him or her make a capacitous decision. Capacity assessments should be carefully recorded.

In this case Jean does not have the mental capacity to make this decision, so you must decide whether the ADRT is both valid and applicable. Consider whether the clinical situation now facing Jean is that which she envisaged when making the ADRT. Relevant questions to consider when a prolonged period of time has elapsed since the document was written or reviewed are:

1. *Does the ADRT exist?* Have you seen the written document and does it comply with the requirements of the Act (especially if this relates to life sustaining treatment)?
2. *Is it valid?* e.g. Has Jean done anything since that is clearly inconsistent with the decision set out in the ADRT?
3. *Is it applicable?* e.g. Are there any new circumstances that might have altered Jean's decision had she anticipated them?

Time permitting these need to be explored carefully with those who know her. If the ADRT is either not valid or not applicable, you would be faced with taking a best interests approach. If, however, the ADRT is found to be valid and applicable, then Jean's stated decision must be followed. The idea of 'next of kin' has no legal relevance to the Mental Capacity Act but it will be critical to sensitively explore the daughter's understanding of her mother's wishes and also her own views. It will be helpful to keep her informed of the procedures you are following and to explain the legal framework you must adhere to. It is sometimes necessary to seek a second opinion or even an urgent judgement from the Court of Protection. To avoid issues such as these we advise patients to talk to their families about ADRTs they have made.

## Case study
## Ahmed's Lasting Power of Attorney

Ahmed, a 75-year-old gentleman with mild dementia is under your care on the ward having had a stroke. His daughter shows you an LPA for issues pertaining to health and welfare, and tells you that Ahmed should not be for CPR. This is not in keeping with the current medical decision that CPR would be attempted in the event of a cardiac arrest.

## What should you do next?

Ahmed's Health and Welfare LPA will only come into force if he does not have mental capacity to make a decision about CPR, so an assessment of his capacity in this regard is key. In contrast, a Property and Welfare LPA can come into force even if the patient has not lost capacity, at their choosing (unless the LPA states otherwise). Assuming that Ahmed does not demonstrate the relevant capacity, you should then examine his LPA document.

Before you can act in accordance with the contents of his Health and Welfare LPA you should:

- Check that the document has been registered with the Office of the Public Guardian (OPG)
  *If so, each blank box on the form will be marked with an OPG stamp which prevents additions being made after registration*
- Contact the Office of the Public Guardian, using the form 'OPG 100' accessed via the OPG website, to instigate a search of the OPG's records. The OPG search certificate will tell you other important information including:
  - Whether the document is registered
    *If Ahmed's LPA document has not been registered, or it has been revoked subsequently, it cannot be acted upon. However, it may still contain information useful for a best interests decision*
  - The name(s) of his attorney(s) (i.e. the people to whom Ahmed, the donor, has given decision-making powers)
  - The types of power (Health and Welfare and/or Property and Financial Affairs)
  - The type of appointment of the attorneys if more than one
    *In Ahmed's case his daughter is his only attorney, but if there had been two or more attorneys, and these were appointed 'jointly', then decisions must be agreed between them, whereas if appointed 'jointly and severally' then decisions may be made by a single attorney*

This information should be cross-referenced with his LPA documentation.

Ideally the original LPA document should be available for your inspection since a photocopy could have been altered. Each page of the original document will have 'VALIDATED—OPG' embossed along the bottom edge. Our preference is to see the original and take a copy for our records, initialling each page to show colleagues that it is an authentic copy.

Having established that you have the original, or an authentic copy, you need to verify the limits of decision-making authority that Ahmed has given to his daughter by reading the whole document. The main distinction is whether his daughter has the authority to give or refuse consent to life sustaining treatment or not. This is indicated by the signature box: Ahmed has signed Option A, which does give that authority; signing Option B does not.

It is also important to know what, if any, other advance decision documents Ahmed may have drawn up, since these may influence his daughter's decision making. In particular, note that an ADRT written and dated before an LPA is superseded by the LPA (assuming that the LPA covers the same decisions), whereas one written and dated after the LPA may put limitations on the decisions that attorneys can make.

Finally, you need to establish to your satisfaction that the person claiming to be an attorney is who they say they are. In practice, we ask for a form of photo identification such as a passport or driving licence, again taking a copy for the medical records.

Following a conversation with Ahmed's daughter you are convinced that her decision that he should not be for cardiopulmonary resuscitation is the correct best interests decision and is in keeping with what he would want. However, the existence of an LPA does not remove a doctor's duty of care. It is important that you and the attorney cooperate in establishing what is in the donor's best interests in any given situation since attorneys are under the same obligation to make best interests decisions as you are. The Court of Protection must ultimately adjudicate disagreements that cannot be resolved by the usual processes.

# References

1. Guwande, A (2015). *Being mortal.* London: Profile Books. P. 243.
2. Hayhoe B and Howe A (2011). 'Advance care planning under the Mental Capacity Act 2005 in primary care'. *Br J Gen Pract* **61**: e537–41.
3. Mental Capacity Act 2005 (c.9) London: HMSO.
4. Dunphy EJ, Conlon SC, O'Brien SA, Loughrey E, and O'Shea B (2016). 'End-of-life planning with frail patients attending general practice: an exploratory prospective cross-sectional study'. *Brit J Gen Pract* doi: 10.3399/bjgp16X686557
5. Poppe M, Burleigh S, and Banerjee S (2013). 'Qualitative evaluation of advanced care planning in early dementia (ACP-ED)'. *PLOS One* **8**: e60412.
6. Detering KM, Hancock AD, Reade, MC, and Silverster W (2010). 'The impact of advance care planning on end of life care in elderly patients: randomised controlled trial'. *BMJ* **340**: c1345.
7. Abel J, Pring A, Rich A, Mailk T, and Verne J (2013). 'The impact of advance care planning of place of death, a hospice retrospective cohort study'. *BMJ Support Palliat Care* **3**: 168–73.
8. Halpern, S (2012). 'Shaping end-of-life care: behavioral economics and advance directives'. *Semin Respir Crit Care Med* **33**: 393–400.
9. Seckler A, Meier D, Mulvihill M, and Crammer B (1991). 'Substituted judgement: How accurate are proxy predications'? *Ann Intern Med* **115**: 92–8.
10. Barnes K. Jones L, Tookman A, and King M (2007). 'Acceptability of an advance care planning interview schedule: a focus group study'. *Pall Med* **21**: 23–8.
11. Mahon MM (2011). 'An advance directive in two questions'. *J Pain Symptom Manage* **41**: 801–7.
12. Pantilat S and Steimle A (2004). 'Palliative care for patients with heart failure'. *JAMA* **291**: 2476–83.
13. Quill T (2000). 'Initiating end-of-life discussions with seriously ill patients—addressing the elephant in the room'. *JAMA* **284**: 2503–7.
14. Henry C and Seymour J (2008). *Advance Care Planning: A Guide for Health and Social care Staff.* Leicester: Department of Health.

## Chapter 4

# Person-centred care: how does advance care planning support this and what are the economic benefits?

Josie Dixon

'It is well established now that one can in fact improve the quality of healthcare that is delivered and reduce the costs at the same time.'
*Susan Dentzer, former Editor-in-Chief, Health Affairs* (1)

---

**This chapter includes**

◆ discussion about person-centred care, its benefits, its place in policy, and its relevance in end of life care

◆ consideration of the role that ACP plays in promoting person-centred care at end of life

◆ comments about the relevance of person-centred outcomes in the economic case for ACP

---

**Key Points**

◆ Person-centred care emphasises compassion and dignity, is well-coordinated and respects individual needs and preferences

◆ ACP helps to facilitate person-centred care by allowing people to have a say in decisions about their end of life care, as well as being associated with a range of person-centred outcomes

◆ Economic evaluations of ACP have tended to focus on hospital cost savings. However, such studies are too limited and more comprehensive economic evaluations are needed, taking into account not just financial costs and savings, but also wider person-centred benefits

---

**Key Message**

ACP is a key aspect of delivering person-centred care in advanced illness and at end of life. It allows people to consider and voice their preferences for future care, helps people to receive more of the care they want (and less of what they don't want), and is associated with higher levels of carer satisfaction with the end of life care received by their relative. It may also be associated with hospital-related cost savings. Both person-centred outcomes and financial costs and savings are equally important to the economic case.

# Introduction

Advance care planning (ACP) has, as its primary purpose, the aim of making a person's voice heard, even when that person can no longer speak for themselves directly. Terminology and legal frameworks vary from country to country, but people can:

- complete advance directives, advance health directives or advance decisions to refuse or limit medical treatment
- write down broader wishes about future care in advance directives, advance care plans or advance statements
- discuss healthcare and wider preferences with doctors and other professionals
- assign power of attorney to give someone they trust legal authority to make decisions on their behalf

Use of these different ACP tools and processes can facilitate person-centred care in advanced illness and at end of life and help ensure that care is delivered according to a person's individual needs and preferences.

The concern to ensure that care is tailored to people's individual needs and preferences may seem remote from consideration of the economic implications of ACP. However, these two different perspectives on ACP are much more closely related than may be commonly thought.

This chapter will explore person-centred care, its benefits, its place in policy and its relevance in end of life care. It will consider the particular role of ACP in promoting person-centred care at end of life and look at how effective it appears to be at doing this. Finally it will consider the economic implications of ACP, arguing that its role in promoting person-centred care is an integral part of the economic case.

# Person-centred care and its benefits

There is no single authoritative meaning of the term 'person-centred care'. It refers to a range of different approaches for ensuring that care is focused on the individual rather than on the needs of professionals or the health and care system. Person-centred care emphasises compassion and dignity, and is well coordinated. It is personalised and respects a person's individual needs and preferences, rather than being delivered in a 'one size fits all' way. While there is a professional obligation upon doctors and other service providers to take account of people's wishes, a person-centred approach makes this explicit. It rejects the idea that professionals should simply do what they think is best for someone and, instead, promotes a partnership model in which people are enabled to play an active role in determining their own care and support needs (Box 4.1).

Person-centred care is based upon a biopsychosocial model of health (2). It recognises the often significant impact of psychological, emotional and social factors on health and well-being outcomes, and recognises that people significantly affect their own health and well-being, through the daily decisions they make in their lives and in how they make use of healthcare and other types of support.

A wide range of terms are used to refer to person-centred care, including user-centred, family-centred, patient-centred, client-centred, individualised, or personalised care. These can refer to a general approach to providing care. There are also specific person-centred initiatives. In England, these include, collaborative care and support planning, the NHS 'house of care' model for people with long-term conditions (3), personal health budgets and self-management support for people with long-term conditions.

---

### Box 4.1 Four principles of person-centred care

The Health Foundation in England identify four principles of person-centred care:

- Care is delivered with dignity, compassion and respect
- Care is well coordinated
- Care is personalised and takes account not just of clinical needs, but also of wider social, emotional and practical needs
- Care is enabling, allowing people to participate, as far as possible, in shaping, and potentially even delivering (in the form of self-management), their own care

Source: data from The Health Foundation, 'Person-centred care made simple: what everyone should know about person-centred care', 2014, available from http://www.health.org.uk/publication/person-centred-care-made-simple

---

Conducting research into person-centred care is methodologically difficult and, so far, there are only a limited number of well-conducted outcome studies (4). However, evidence suggests that it can lead to care that is more appropriate to people's needs, improve people's experiences of care, improve health outcomes and help health and care professionals feel more confident in delivering care (5–8). It is likely that there are also economic benefits; improved self-management of long-term conditions can reduce emergency hospital admissions and, when well informed (including through the use of decision aids), people tend to be more risk adverse and opt for less surgery and fewer invasive procedures than their doctors (9).

## Person-centred care in policy and practice

The idea of person-centred care is not new (10,11), but its prominence in policy has grown in recent years, largely as a response to increasing levels of long-term chronic illness. There is a clear emphasis on the right for people to be actively involved in decisions about their care and treatment. The Government's mandate for NHS England (12) requires it to, 'ensure the NHS becomes dramatically better at involving patients and their carers, and empowering them to manage and make decisions about their own care and treatment' (p. 9). The NHS constitution (13) has person-centred care as one of its seven core principles, stating that, 'patients, with their families and carers where appropriate, will be involved in and consulted on all decisions about their care and treatment'. Person-centred care is also secured in legislation, in particular in the Health and Social Care Act, 2012, and the Care Act, 2014. The Mental Capacity Act, 2005, also underpins person-centred care by supporting people's rights to make their own decisions and to be helped to do so wherever needed and, if they cannot make their own decisions, for these to be taken in their best interests and in consultation with people important to them.

Person-centred care is similarly prominent in healthcare policy in other comparable countries. In the United States (US), for example, the Institute of Medicine, in 2001 (10), established person-centred care as central to ensuring quality improvements in patient care and made proposals for how it should be promoted (14). It is also prominent in the Affordable Care Act (2010) and in the evolution of accountable care organisations, in the US (15) and in Europe, in countries such Spain (16). Similarly, in Australia, person-centred care is promoted in a range of national and state initiatives, including the Australian Charter of Healthcare Rights (17), the National Safety and Quality Health Service Standards (18), and the Australian Safety and Quality Framework for Healthcare (19).

In practice, however, progress towards person-centred care has been slow. In 2015, the Health Foundation found that, in England, only five per cent of people with a long-term condition had a written care plan (a key indicator of person-centred care for people with long-term conditions) and almost 20% of inpatients felt that they were not always treated with dignity and respect (20). In a 2016 review of how people are involved in their care (21), the Care Quality Commission concluded that,

> 'the trends in national surveys of patients and people using services over the last five to 10 years high-light there has been little change in people's perceptions of how well they are involved in their health or social care, despite the national drive for person-centred care' (p. 3).
> Contains public sector information licensed under the Open Government
> Licence v3.0. © Care Quality Commission 2017, http://www.cqc.org.uk

## Person-centred care at end of life

Person-centred care is as relevant in advanced illness and at end of life as at any other time, and possibly more so. This includes that people should receive care that is well-coordinated, compassionate and personalised. It also includes patients and their carers having the opportunity to be involved in decision-making about their care and treatment. The NHS Constitution (12) states that, 'you have the right to be involved in planning and making decisions about your health and care with your care provider or providers, including your end of life care', adding that, 'Where appropriate, this right includes your family and carers'.

However, person-centred care at end of life is far from universal and there have been a range of reports that have highlighted poor communication and poor quality care (22–7). In comparable countries, similar problems have been identified. In 2014, for example, a report by the Institute of Medicine, *Dying in America: Improving quality and honoring individual preferences near the end of life* (28), found evidence of undertreatment of pain and other symptoms, unwanted medical treatments and poor coordination and continuity of care and concluded that there was 'a mismatch between the services patients and families need most and the services they can readily obtain.' (p. 25).

## The role of advance care planning in promoting person-centred care

What marks out ACP from other forms of person-centred care is that people's priorities and preferences are elicited ahead of time, in anticipation of later deterioration. ACP conversations include discussion of a person's health condition and their wider social circumstances, decisions that may need to be taken in future and exploration of a person's priorities for future care. In a person-centred care framework, such conversations are intended to be 'activating' and 'enabling' allowing people to develop more understanding of their condition and prognosis, as well as of possible future care options, and for them and their families to be supported to be involved in decision-making about their future care, to the degree that they want to be (29).

In England, ACP is emphasised in the *The end of life care strategy for England*, 2008 (23) and in a wide range of subsequent national guidance, professional guidance and policy documents. Similarly, the report, *Dying in America* (27), in discussing solutions to poor and inappropriate end of life care devotes around 70 of its 380 pages to person-centred and family orientated care and a further 100 pages to clinician-patient communication and ACP. More recently, Medicare in the US has also introduced new billing codes to allow healthcare professionals, for the first time to claim for discussions with patients about ACP.

As yet, however, we know that ACP is not routinely conducted in practice, particularly in England where progress towards establishing ACP in practice has been slower than in other countries such as the US, Australia, Canada, and New Zealand (30).

## The effectiveness of advance care planning in promoting person-centred care

Researchers have used various approaches for assessing the effectiveness of ACP in supporting person-centred care. One seemingly straight-forward way used in some studies has been to look at whether people's stated preferences are met in practice (known as 'concordance'). In the case of a legally binding decision to refuse treatment this is closer to audit than research. However applied more generally, this approach is more problematic than it appears. People's preferences may not be documented. Alternatively, they may not be specific enough, and the decision needed may involve too much uncertainty to determine whether a particular treatment was concordant or not. Furthermore, while often willing to have discussions about end of life care and/or to assign power of attorney, there are many people who do not wish to make written plans for fear that these might 'tie the hands' of those caring for them (31).

An alternative approach taken by many researchers has been to rely on evidence about the outcomes that *most* people prefer to achieve at end of life. We know, from the Health and Retirement Study (a US panel study of approximately 25,000 people aged 51 and upwards) that most people with advance directives use them to limit treatment in certain circumstances and to opt for care aimed at comfort rather than prolonging life (32). It makes sense, therefore to see if people who undertook ACP tended to experience less life-prolonging treatment at the end of life received more palliative or hospice care and/or spent less time in hospital or in intensive care units (ICU). Most people also want to die at home provided that they are well supported (33), so it may also make sense to consider place of death. Where it is possible to gather such data, carer, or patient satisfaction is likely to indicate that care met people's individual needs and preferences. Quality of life and quality of death measures may also be important in, more broadly indicating a person-centred approach.

Brinkman-Stopellenberg et al. (2014) undertook a systematic review of the evidence on the effectiveness of ACP (34). Although there were mixed results (reflecting the methodological difficulties of research in this area), they found that written advance directives (or other written plans) tended to be associated with out of hospital care and care aimed at increasing comfort, as well as a lower likelihood of ICU- or hospital-based death. ACP interventions appeared to be more effective that written documents alone. These were associated with out of hospital care, care aimed at increasing comfort, less ICU use, greater concordance between written plans and patient wishes, a lower likelihood of ICU- or hospital-based death, better quality of life and greater carer and patient satisfaction with care. Evidence about the precise mechanisms underlying these associations, however was more limited.

## A quick guide to economic evaluation

Before moving on to consider the economic implications of ACP, it will be helpful to identify different types of economic study.

A cost minimisation study looks only at monetary inputs and tries to identify the least costly intervention between two or more alternatives. This is only appropriate when we know that the alternatives being compared are equally effective. A cost-savings study also only takes account of monetary factors including inputs (e.g. staff salaries) and the financial savings that are thought to arise as a result of the intervention. These types of study take no account of non-monetary benefits and outcomes.

A cost benefit analysis considers all costs and all of the important benefits of an intervention. However, a monetary value is attached to all non-monetary benefits so the costs of the intervention and the benefits can be summed to give a net-benefit figure. Methods for attaching monetary values to non-monetary benefits attempt to determine what people would, in principle be willing to pay or trade off for these benefits. However, these methods are controversial and cost benefit analyses are not much undertaken in social policy, except in certain areas such as transport where there is sufficient 'real world' data to inform these approaches.

A cost-effectiveness study takes account of the costs of the intervention and the main outcome, which it measures using natural units (e.g. days in hospital). A cost consequence study is similar but uses more than one outcome. Because these different outcomes are all measured in their own natural units, the results may be difficult to interpret and different interventions can be hard to compare.

A cost-utility study is a form of cost-effectiveness study, but one which uses a utility measure (a measure of overall 'usefulness') for an outcome. This is a summary composite measure in which weights, usually taken from population surveys are attached to different states or outcomes. Quality adjusted life years (QALYs) is the most commonly used utility measure in health-economic analyses. This includes both quality and length of life and is expressed using a scale ranging from zero (dead) to one (perfect health). The advantage of QALYs is that they can be compared across different interventions, conditions, or patient groups. Some health systems have attached a 'social willingness to pay' threshold for QALYs. In England it is between £20,000 to £30,000 per QALY (35).

However, QALYs may be less relevant for certain conditions or at end of life (36). The National Institute of Health and Care Excellence (NICE) in England recommends use of QALYs (e.g. using the EQ-5D tool) or social care QALYs (using the ASCOT tool), alongside capability measures such as ICECAP (37). Capability measures reflect people's capability to achieve certain desired outcomes and are measured using a scale of 'no capability' to 'full capability' (38,39). The ICECAP-SCM for end of life care is currently in its later stages of development (40,41). It covers making decisions about one's life and care, love and affection, pain and suffering, emotional suffering, dignity, feeling supported, and being able to make preparations. A related measure, the ICM close person measure, which considers outcomes for carers at end of life is also currently in development (42). This covers good communication with services, privacy and space to be with ones loved one, emotional support, practical support, being able to prepare and cope, and being free from emotional distress related to the condition of the decedent (Box 4.2).

## Economic implications of advance care planning

What is hopefully clear from the previous section is that different types of economic study measure outcomes in different ways. More limited designs such as cost-minimisation and cost-savings are only appropriate in very limited circumstances where there is already good information about other aspects. The more comprehensive types of study are more complete. These attempt to include all important quality as well as financial impacts. Economic evaluation, therefore is not just about finding cost savings, even though the current literature on the economics of ACP might inadvertently give that impression.

A systematic review of the economic evidence for ACP by Dixon et al. (2015) found 18 relevant studies, ten of which measured the impacts of specific ACP interventions and eight of which measured the impacts of ACP more generally (e.g. having an advance directive) (43). There were no

## Box 4.2 Types of economic evaluation

### Cost-minimisation study

The simplest type of economic evaluation is a cost-minimisation study. This compares the costs of delivery for two (or more) interventions to identify the least-costly alternative.

### Cost-savings study

In a cost savings study, financial savings associated with an intervention (e.g. from reduced use of hospital care) are identified. These are combined with the costs of the intervention to give a net savings figure. Such studies are often seen as limited types of cost-benefit analysis. They take no account of non-monetary benefits.

### Cost-effectiveness study

A cost-effectiveness study identifies the costs of the intervention and measures outcomes in natural units, such as life years gained. Interventions can be compared in terms of their respective cost per unit of benefit gained.

### Cost-utility study

A cost utility study is a type of cost-effectiveness analysis. The costs associated with the intervention are identified and outcomes are measured with a measure of utility (or 'usefulness'). Different circumstances (e.g. health states) are given different 'utility weights', usually based on preference surveys of the general population. A commonly used utility measure for healthcare is the quality adjusted life year (or QALY) which takes account of both quality and length of life.

### Cost-consequence study

A cost-consequence study is a type of cost effectiveness analysis. It is used where it would be inappropriate to focus on just one outcome. It measures both the costs associated with the intervention and a range of different outcomes, measured in natural units.

### Cost-benefit analysis

In a cost-benefit analysis, measures both the costs associated with the intervention and all benefits, but converts all benefits into monetary terms. If benefits exceed the costs, then the intervention is worthwhile. Methods for attaching monetary costs to non-monetary benefits attempt to determine what people would, in principle, be willing to pay or trade-off for them.

---

cost-effectiveness studies amongst these. Instead, studies could be loosely characterised as cost-savings studies or given that other outcomes were commonly reported, cost-consequence studies. As economic evaluations, however, the studies had important limitations.

Only four of the intervention studies reported the cost of the ACP intervention (two more included partial information) and in the non-intervention studies, no account was taken of costs involved in undertaking ACP or of producing a written advance directive. With regard to outcomes, it was generally not clear whether researchers thought all important outcomes had been included. Data availability appeared to restrict the choice of outcomes but this was only occasionally explicitly discussed as a limitation. No study took a societal perspective. Rather, the studies tended to focus narrowly on healthcare, and particularly hospital-based cost savings. This meant, for example, that the costs of alternative care in the community in place of hospital care or the economic impacts on carers were not addressed. Despite these limitations, many of the studies were otherwise well conducted and provided information that is potentially useful, particularly concerning whether ACP is associated with hospital-based cost savings.

Around half of the studies including three randomised controlled trials found that ACP was associated with healthcare, usually hospital-based, cost savings. These savings appeared to be related to reduced hospitalisation, shorter hospital stays and fewer invasive treatments. There was stronger evidence of savings for some particular groups who are, arguably, most likely to receive unwanted medical treatment at end of life. These include people with dementia living in the community, people living in areas with high levels of end of life care spending and people living in nursing homes.

## Conclusion

ACP is a key aspect of delivering person-centred care in advanced illness and at end of life, since it provides an important opportunity for people to consider and express their wishes and preferences for future care. There is promising evidence that it can promote person-centred care more generally, with people receiving more of the care they want (and less of what they don't want) and with higher levels of carer satisfaction with the care received by their relative at the end of life. It also appears, in some cases to be associated with hospital-related cost savings.

All of these aspects are equally important to the economic case if not equally easy to measure. Economic evaluation is not about trying to save money and a focus solely on financial costs is likely to be distorting. The cost to the health system of an emergency hospital admission, for example, is not the same as that which people, or society at large, would be prepared to pay to avoid someone being admitted to hospital in their last week of life. It is quite possible, indeed, that an intervention could actually cost *more* and yet still be more cost effective. Rather than be seen as something to be resisted, those working in and researching ACP should focus on developing fuller economic evaluations that incorporate the full range of person-centred benefits that ACP promises.

## References

1. **Susan Dentzer** (19 October 2011). 'Opening Remarks', *Saving Money And Improving Patient Care In Medicare: Ideas For The Joint Select Committee, Symposium*, Washington D.C., Available from: http://www.healthaffairs.org/events/2011_10_19_saving_money_and_improving_patient_care_in_medicare/
2. **Engel GL** (1977). 'The need for a new medical model: A challenge for biomedicine'. *Science* **196**: 129–36.
3. **McShane M and Mitchell EW** (9 July, 2013). 'Put individuals at the centre of care'. *Health Service Journal* **123**(6539): 26–7.
4. **Dwamena F, Holmes-Rovner M, Gaulden CM, Jorgenson S, Sadigh G, Sikorskii A, Lewin S, Smith RC, Coffey J, and Olomu A** (2012). 'Interventions for providers to promote a patient-centred approach in clinical consultations'. *Cochrane Database Syst Rev* **12**: CD003267.
5. **McMillan SS, Kendall E, Sav A, King MA, Whitty JA, Kelly F, and Wheeler AJ** (2013). 'Patient-centered approaches to health care: A systematic review of randomized controlled trials'. *Med Care Res Rev* **70**(6): 567–96.
6. **Olsson LE, Jakobsson Ung E, Swedberg K, and Ekman I** (2013). 'Efficacy of person-centred care as an intervention in controlled trials: A systematic review'. *J Clin Nurs* **22**(3–4): 456–65.

7. van den Pol-Grevelink A, Jukema JS, and Smits CH (2012). 'Person-centred care and job satisfaction of caregivers in nursing homes: A systematic review of the impact of different forms of person-centred care on various dimensions of job satisfaction'. *Int J Geriatr Psychiatry* **27**(3): 219–29.

8. Mead N and Bower P (2002). 'Patient-centred consultations and outcomes in primary care: A review of the literature'. *Patient Educ Couns* **48**(1): 51–61.

9. Mulley A, Trimble C, and Elwyn G (2012). *Patients' preferences matter: Stop the silent misdiagnosis.* London: The King's Fund.

10. Wagner EH (1998). 'Chronic disease management: What will it take to improve care for chronic illness'? *Effective Clinical Practice* **1**(1): 2–4.

11. Institute of Medicine, Committee on Quality of Health Care in America (2001). *Crossing the Quality Chasm: A New Health System for the 21st century,* Washington: National Academy Press.

12. Department of Health (2012). *The Mandate: A mandate from the Government to the NHS Commissioning Board: April 2013 to March 2015.* London: Department of Health.

13. NHS England. *NHS constitition: The NHS belongs to us all.* Available at: https://www.gov.uk/government/publications/the-nhs-constitution-for-england/the-nhs-constitution-for-england (Accessed 21st October 2016.)

14. Care Quality Commission. *Guidance for providers. Health and Social Care Act 2008 (Regulated Activities) Regulations 2014: Regulation 9.* Available at: http://www.cqc.org.uk/content/regulation-9-person-centred-care (Accessed 15 October 2016.)

15. Rickert J (2012). *Patient-centered care: what it means and how to get there.* Available at: http://healthaffairs.org/blog/2012/01/24/patient-centered-care-what-it-means-and-how-to-get-there/ (Accessed 21 October 2016.)

16. Royal College of General Practitioners (2014). *An Inquiry into Patient Centred Care in the 21st Century.* London: Royal College of General Practitioners.

17. Australian Commission on Safety and Quality in Healthcare (2008). *Australian Charter of Health Care Rights.* Available at: http://www.safetyandquality.gov.au/national-priorities/charter-of-healthcare-rights (Accessed 21 October 2016.)

18. Australian Commission on Safety and Quality in Healthcare (2010). *Australian Safety and Quality Framework for Healthcare.* Available at: http://www.safetyandquality.gov.au/national-priorities/australian-safety-and-quality-framework-for-health-care (Accessed 21 October 2016.)

19. Australian Commission on Safety and Quality in Healthcare. (2012). *Patient-centred care: Improving quality and safety through partnerships with patients and consumers.* Available at: http://www.safetyandquality.gov.au/wp-content/uploads/2012/03/PCC_Paper_August.pdf (Accessed 21 October 2016.)

20. Wood S, Collins A, and Taylor A (2015). *Is the NHS becoming more person-centred?* London: The Health Foundation.

21. Care Quality Commission (2016). *Better care in my hands: A review of how people are involved in their care.* Newcastle upon Tyne: Care Quality Commission.

22. Care Quality Commission (2016). *A different ending: Addressing inequalities in end of life care. Overview report.* Newcastle upon Tyne: Care Quality Commission.

23. Health Care Commission (2008). *Spotlight on complaints. A report on second-stage complaints about the NHS in England.* London: Health Care Commission.

24. Department of Health (England) (2008). *The end of life care strategy for England: promoting high quality care for all adults at the end of life.* London: Department of Health.

25. Cooper H, Findlay G, Goodwin APL, et al. (2009). *Caring to the End? A review of the care of patients who died in hospital.* London: National Confidential Enquiry into Patient Outcome and Death.

26. Parliamentary and Health Service Ombudsman (2015). *Dying without dignity: Investigations by the Parliamentary and Health Service Ombudsman into complaints about end of life care.* London: Parliamentary and Health Service.

27. **Royal College of Physicians** (2016). The *end of life care audit—Dying in hospital: National report for England 2016*. London: Royal College of Physicians.

28. **Institute of Medicine, Committee on Approaching Death** (2014). *Dying in America: Improving quality and honoring individual preferences near the end of life*. Washington, DC: The National Academies Press. Available at: http://iom.edu/Reports/2014/Dying-In-America-Improving-Quality-and-Honoring-Individual-Preferences-Near-the-End-of-Life.aspx.

29. **Hibbard** and **Greene J** (2013). 'What the evidence shows about patient activation: better health outcomes and care experiences; Fewer data on costs'. *Health Aff (Millwood)* **32**(2): 207–14.

30. **Harrison-Dening K, Jones L, and Sampson L** (2011). 'Advance care planning for people with dementia: A review'. *Intl Psychogeriatr* **23**(10): 1535–51.

31. **Robinson L, Dickinson C, Bamford C, Clark A, Hughes J, and Exley C** (2013). 'A qualitative study: Professionals' experiences of advance care planning in dementia and palliative care, "a good idea in theory but ..."'. *Palliat Med* **27**(5): 401–8.

32. **Silveira MJ, Scott MPH, Kim YH,** and **Langa KM** (2010). 'Advance directives and outcomes of surrogate decision making before death'. *N Engl J Med* **362**: 1211–8.

33. **Gomes B Calanzani N, and Higginson IJ** (2011). *Local preferences and place of death in regions within England 2010*. London; Cicely Saunders International.

34. **Brinkman-Stoppelenburg A, Rietjens JA, and van der Heide A** (2014). 'The effects of advance care planning on end-of-life care: A systematic review'. *Palliat Med* **28**(8): 1000–25.

35. **Dillon A.** (2015). *Carrying NICE over the threshold*. Blog. National Institute for Health and Care Excellence. Available at: https://www.nice.org.uk/news/blog/carrying-nice-over-the-threshold (Accessed 21 Oct 2016.)

36. **Normand, C** (2009). 'Measuring outcomes in palliative care: limitations of QALYs and the road to PalYs'. *J Pain Symptom Manag* **38**(1): 27–31.

37. **The National Institute of Health and Care Excellence.** (2016). *The social care guidance manual: Process and methods* [PMG10]. Available at: https://www.nice.org.uk/process/pmg10/chapter/incorporating-economic-evaluation (Accessed 15 October 2016.)

38. **Mitchell PM, Roberts TE, Barton PM, and Coast J** (2015). 'Assessing sufficient capability: A new approach to economic evaluation'. *Soc Sci Med* **139**: 71–9.

39. **Mitchell PM, Roberts TE, Barton PM, and Coast J** (2016). 'Applications of the capability approach in the health field: A literature review'. *Soc Indic Res* First online : 1–27 [open access].

40. **Coast J, Bailey C, Orlando R, Armour K, Perry R, Jones L, and Kinghorn P** (2015). ' "The ICECAP-SCM tells you more about what I'm going through": Measuring quality of life amongst patients receiving supportive and palliative care'. *BMJ Support Palliat Care* **5**: 110–11.

41. **Coast J, Bailey C, Canaway A, and Kinghorn P** (2016). 'Measuring and valuing outcomes for care at the end of life: the capability approach'. In Round J (ed.) *Care at the end of life: An economic perspective*. Heidelberg: Springe. Pp. 89–101.

42. **Canaway A, Al-Janabi H, Kinghorn P, Bailey C, and Coast J** (3 Jun 2016). 'Development of a measure to capture the benefits of end of life care to those close to the dying for use in economic evaluation'. *Pall Med* pii: 0269216316650616. [Epub ahead of print.]

43. **Dixon J, Matosevic T, and Knapp M** (2015). The economic evidence for advance care planning: Systematic review of evidence. *Pall Med* **29**(10): 869–84.

Chapter 5

# Advance care planning for an ageing population

Martin J. Vernon

---

**This chapter includes**

- The impact of changing population age structure on worldwide healthcare policy
- Summary of UK government policy in response to multiple long-term conditions and disabilities in older people
- Discussion of frailty and frailty assessment, advance care planning (ACP) in care homes and among people with dementia

---

**Key Points**

- Population ageing is driven by decline in fertility and improved life expectancy
- Current government policy is focused on healthy ageing and extending disability-free life
- More people are surviving to later life with multiple long-term conditions
- Disability trajectories in people living with frailty can assist with ACP
- Older people living with frailty have increased risk of acute and unexpected health decline
- Routine frailty identification by severity can assist with ACP
- ACP should be prompted in anticipation of health decline and imminent lost mental capacity
- Recognising potential professional and organisational barriers to ACP could improve its uptake
- Guided serious illness conversations could assist with ACP in older people
- ACP in care homes and among people with dementia is likely to be beneficial

---

**Key Message**

A rapidly ageing world population creates new demands for health and social care policy and planning. ACP must be prompted in anticipation of health decline and lost mental capacity, and the changing shape of societies and families should be fully considered when initiating discussions with an older person.

---

## Worldwide ageing

The World Bank estimates that between 1960 and 2015 the population proportion of people aged 65 and over rose from five to eight per cent (1). In real terms this means that the number of people in the world aged 65 and over rose from 249 million to 690 million. In the European Union, in line with high-income countries in general this rose from ten to 19%.

In heavily indebted poor countries, although the overall proportion has previously remained stable at around three per cent, the most rapidly ageing populations are now in less developed areas of the world. Between 2010 and 2050, the number of people in less developed countries is projected to increase by over 250% compared to 71% in developed countries (2).

Simultaneous decline in fertility and improved life expectancy are thought to be the principle factors driving this impressive change in population age structure. Fewer children are now entering the population, particularly in less developed countries, while adults are living longer which means that older people represent an increasing proportion of the total population. In consequence the future care of older people, especially those nearing the end of their natural life in great numbers has rapidly assumed newfound prominence in worldwide healthcare policy.

While successful human ageing is something to celebrate, particularly for those achieving greater numbers of disability free life years, the greater numbers of people surviving to later life with multiple long-term health conditions and increased levels of social care and support need, will pose significant challenges for governments, economies and health and social care systems around the world. Global disease burden has shifted from communicable (infectious) to non-communicable diseases and from premature death to years lived with disability (3).

In 2010 the leading causes of disability adjusted life years (the number of years lost due to ill health, disability or early death) were ischaemic heart disease, lower respiratory infection and stroke. Rising levels of mental health and behavioural disorder, musculoskeletal disorder and diabetes are now expected to put health systems under even greater pressure (3). By 2050 the worldwide prevalence of Alzheimer's dementia is expected to quadruple from the estimated 26.6 million in 2006. There will be an estimated one in 85 people living with dementia (4) in the absence of clear therapeutic intervention or prevention strategies for dementia.

In shaping health and social care policy for future generations, it is crucial to understand and define the populations of older people who are living added life years in either good or poor health. Current projections suggest that health and social care systems should prepare themselves for meeting the needs of older people whose leading causes of disability will be depression, hearing loss, musculoskeletal disease, dementia, falls, chronic obstructive lung disease, and diabetes mellitus (5). This will have significant impacts on how we approach ACP in later life.

## UK ageing

To successfully approach advance care planning ACP for older people we must first understand the structure, diversity, circumstances and economic, health and social needs of the population of people entering their final years of life.

In the UK there are now 11.6 million people aged 65 or over (6). By 2040 nearly one in seven people will be aged over 75 (6). The proportion of the working age population aged between 50 and state pension age will increase from 26% in 2012 to 35% in 2050 (7). Challenges facing the ageing UK workforce include supporting older people to lead fuller and longer working lives, through maintained fitness and skills development through lifelong learning.

By 2037 there are projected to be 1.42 million more households headed by someone aged 85 or over (7). Poor housing has been estimated to cost the National Health Service £2.5 billion per year across all ages and so maintaining suitable housing, neighbourhoods and communities suitable for an ageing population has become an increasing priority. In addition families play a major role in maintaining support across generations: 73% of older people living with disability do so with support of a spouse or family member (7). The shape of families is also becoming more diverse with an increase in lone parent households in the last ten years to three million and 'verticalisation' of families with more generations alive simultaneously in the same family unit than ever before.

Within the older population there are currently two million people, the majority women, aged over 75 and living alone (8). There are estimated to be one million lesbian, gay and bisexual people aged over 55 (9) and 14 million grandparents (10). An estimated 80% of people aged over 65 give their religious affiliation as Christian and nine per cent 'no religion' (11).

Current estimates for female life expectancy at birth are 82.8 years and 79.1 years for men (12). Healthy life expectancy in the UK is 66 years for women and 64 years for men. At age 65, women in the UK can expect to live on average for another 12 years in good health and men another 10.7 years. Put another way, men and women aged 65 can expect 60% of their remaining life expectancy to be in good health. This means however that for women aged 65, on average just under ten of their last years of life, and for men 7.5 years will be spent living with a disability.

Together, the current and projected future profiles of the ageing UK population will increasingly put governments, policy makers and public services under pressure to meet their health and social care needs. In addition families and individuals will find themselves increasingly under pressure to enable society as a whole to continue to provide care and support to older relatives while remaining in paid employment and maintaining adequate housing across the generations. In particular these factors will become of increasing importance to people planning for and making decisions about their present and future care and support arrangements.

## Healthy ageing

Current UK government policy is focused on addressing the needs of a society whose structure is changing (13). This includes improving recruitment and retention of an ageing workforce by encouraging a positive attitude to working into later life and removal of the default retirement age, which means that in most cases employers cannot force people to retire just because they reach the arbitrary age of 65.

Among other things this will mean that people will be encouraged to stay healthier and fitter as they age to enable them to remain employed and contribute positively to the economy. This is important when considering the expected rising levels of need for care and support for increasing numbers of older people in the last few years of life. While some of this will need to be met by an ageing care workforce in paid employment, family members and those in their social networks will also meet some of it informally.

Increasingly older people are living in a digital age, which is having influence on the way social interaction occurs. Current government policy sets out how high quality digital services people prefer to use will be provided (14). Reliable digital connectivity to family and social networks will be of crucial importance to older people who are making, updating and sharing plans which detail preferences for how their care and support is provided as they move towards the last year of their life.

Loneliness, isolation and loss of physical connectivity to society are expected to present particular difficulty to older people in the future. The increased likelihood of dying as a result of social isolation, loneliness or living alone has been reported to be up to 30% (15). In recognition of this the UK Government commissioned an 'Age Well' programme to support councils to provide local services to meet the needs of older people helping them to remain active both now and in the future (16).

## Multi-morbidity and multiple long-term conditions

When considering how to approach ACP for older people it is of key importance to ensure that scarce resources for engaging in care planning discussions are appropriately targeted. This requires us to think about risk stratification of the older population to as a means of identifying those anticipated to be at most risk of entering the final years of life, and yet retain the capacity to make decisions and offer views about their preferences for future care. The systematic and proactive recognition of those who have accumulated multiple health deficits provides one such means of doing this at scale.

Multi-morbidity refers to the presence of two or more long-term health conditions. These can include physical and mental health conditions, on-going conditions such as learning disability, symptom complexes such as frailty or chronic pain, sensory impairments such as sight or hearing loss, or alcohol and substance misuse (17). The prevalence of multi-morbidity varies across world primary care populations from 13% to 95% and has a significant positive association with age and lower socioeconomic status. It is also positively associated with female gender and mental health disorder (18). The most frequent patterns of multi-morbidity include osteoarthritis together with cardiovascular and/or metabolic disorders such as diabetes.

Guidance issued in 2016 by the National Institute for Clinical Excellence (NICE) (17) set out an approach to optimising care for adults with multi-morbidity by reducing treatment burden associated with taking multiple medications and attending multiple health care appointments. Its aim is to improve quality of life by promoting shared decisions based on what is important to each person in terms of treatments, health priorities, lifestyle and goals. Triggers to beginning a conversation with a person to tailor the approach to their care include:

- Request from the person themself
- Finding it difficult to manage their managing treatment or day to day care
- Receiving care and support from multiple services and needing additional services
- Having both long-term mental health and physical conditions
- Having frailty or falls
- Frequently seeking unplanned or emergency care
- Prescribed multiple (ten to 14) regular medications

Identifying people with multi-morbidity can occur opportunistically during routine care or proactively using electronic health records. Best practice guidance supports the use of validated tools to identify adults with multi-morbidity who are at risk of adverse events such as unplanned hospital admission or admission to care homes.

## Frailty

Frailty is aligned to multi-morbidity in older people and has been described as an especially problematic component of population ageing (19). The concept of frailty concerns those people who are at greater risk of adverse health outcomes (such as unplanned hospital admission, care home admission or death) compared with people of the same age (20). The overall prevalence of frailty in the English population aged 60 or over is 14% (21) and it is more common in women than men (16% versus 12%). However its prevalence rises from 6.5% in those aged 60–69 to 65% in those aged 90 or over. Two thirds of these people report difficulties in performing activities of daily living.

Typically the presence of frailty predisposes a person to unexpected and significant deterioration in their health and function from which recovery is more likely to be prolonged and/or incomplete. This is likely to occur after a comparatively minor stress event such as an acute infection or injury. Older people with frailty who develop acute illness requiring hospital care are especially vulnerable to this unanticipated sequence of events. In addition the presence of frailty and high acute illness severity has been independently associated with high risk (20%) of inpatient mortality (22). Early identification of the co-existence of frailty and severe acute illness could therefore assist in personalised planning for care and its escalation, in the knowledge that the episode carries a high risk of adverse outcome.

Routine identification of people at risk by determining whether frailty, in varying degrees of severity, is present or absent can help with population risk stratification and for those at greatest risk can be used to prompt further assessment, diagnosis and where appropriateACP. Counting cumulative health deficits gives a way of identifying the presence (or absence) frailty in older populations.

In 2016 an electronic frailty index (eFI) which uses routinely available English primary care electronic health record data was validated as a means of easily identifying populations of people aged 65 or over who are at varying degrees of risk of adverse health outcomes (19). This tool makes it possible to identify mildly frail people, comprising 35% of the population aged 65 or over who, compared to their fit counterparts, are twice as likely over the coming year to require unplanned hospital admission, care home admission or die. For severely frail people comprising 3% of the population aged 65 or over, the risk of these adverse outcomes compared to their fit counterparts is increased by almost five times. These individuals have on average two co-morbidities and take eight medications.

Frailty assessment should be considered in people with multi-morbidity and in 2017, NHS England began to require the routine identification and diagnosis of frailty in primary care (23). It is recognised that optimally organising urgent care systems for older people with frailty can reduce hospital bed occupancy and relative risk of hospital mortality by nearly 20% without increasing the risk of readmission (24).

## Disability trajectories for older people in the last year of life

During the last year of life hospital admissions can have a significant but complex impact on the disability trajectories of older people. These provide both opportunity and challenge to the timing of ACP discussions. Six distinct trajectories have been identified in one prospective cohort study of people aged 70 or above (25):

1. No disability (17.2%)
2. Catastrophic disability (11.1%)
3. Accelerated disability (9.6%)
4. Progressively mild disability (11.1%)
5. Progressively severe disability (23%)
6. Persistently severe disability (28.1%)

Most people had one hospital admission in the last year of life and 45% had multiple admissions. It is known that the course of disability does not follow a predictable pattern for older people at the end of life. Understanding which trajectory an older person is on could therefore facilitate clinical decision making and ACP for some older people at the end of their life.

## Health and social policy context for older people

Decisions about the care and support people receive must take into account both their needs and preferences. People have a right to be involved in discussions and make decisions about the way they are cared for in collaboration with health and care professionals. This includes ensuring that information about their care and treatment is provided in a way that a person can understand

(26). Intrinsic to this process is the need for health and care professionals to understand key information about the person they are caring for which includes what is important and matters to them most, and what worries them most.

For older people living with multiple long-term conditions which include cognitive and sensory impairment, and who may be living along and/or in isolated circumstances meeting these requirements poses particular challenges. For people unable to understand or make decisions for themselves there are legal frameworks setting out the duties of health and care professionals to act at all times in the best interests of the person to whom they are providing care (27). Key to this is ensuring that a person is assisted and supported to make decisions.

People involved in providing care are equally discouraged from being overly restrictive or controlling. The purpose of this approach is to keep the person at the centre of decisions about their care and treatment. This requires balancing a person's right to make decisions for themselves with their right to be protected from harm. For people who lack the capacity to make specific decisions about their current and future care, due diligence must be taken to ensure involvement of those with valid Lasting Powers of Attorney, court appointed deputies and, where not befriended or represented, an Independent Mental Capacity Advocate.

## Approaches to advance care planning for older people

ACP is defined as a voluntary process of discussion between an individual (accompanied by family and friends if they wish) and their care providers to identify that person's concerns and wishes, values, or personal goals for care, their understanding about their illness and prognosis, and their preferences for future care and treatment that may be beneficial. Its purpose is to help an individual with the capacity to make decisions and to anticipate how their condition may affect them in future, and if they wish, record their choices about care, treatment, and future decisions (28). The principle difference between ACP and routine care planning is that ACP will usually occur in the context of anticipated deterioration in a person's condition accompanied by impending loss of capacity to make decisions and/or communicate their wishes to others.

Implicit in this is the need to anticipate both the deterioration in a person's condition requiring end of life care and the loss of capacity to make decisions or communicate choices and preferences for the care. For older people a range of barriers to this process have been identified (29). While the majority of older people with frailty would welcome the chance to discuss end of life care, most do not get this opportunity creating a significant risk of meaningful discussions being left until it is too late. Identified reasons for this have included lack of professional time or suitable precipitating event, family reluctance to discuss end of life care, passive expectations that someone else would make decisions on a person's behalf, and significant uncertainty about future illness and decline (29).

Dealing with uncertainty is inherent in the practice of healthcare and has frequently been cited as a barrier to identifying when treatment goals should be reviewed and care planning refocused on the priorities of maintaining quality of life and a comfortable death. Commentators have noted however that predictions about when a person is likely to die based on clinicians' estimates of prognosis are 'notoriously unreliable' leading to 'prognostic paralysis' (30). Identification of frailty by severity in an older person is likely to assist with prognostication in the presence of multiple long-term conditions.

A number of key enablers have been suggested to support GPs in undertaking routine ACP with older people (31). These include providing practical resources to increase professional confidence such as a 'core' script of words and phrases ensuring focused, brief, and recurrent planning supported by appropriate digital technology to aid decisions and documentation, and a lead coordinating clinician sensitive to the human concerns likely to arise when undertaking difficult conversations routinely. Importantly rigid and unthinking approaches to end of life care planning and delivery can significantly damage the trusting and human relationships older people and their families develop with their care providers (32).

There is evidence that while there are many decision aids widely available to guide ACP, these are either not validated, or disease specific where life trajectories may be more easily predictable (33). One promising approach being tested in the English NHS is to use a guided serious illness conversation (34). This sets out a framework for setting up a guided conversation, which comprises:

- Checking a person's understanding of where they are up to with their condition
- Exploring their preferences for information
- Sharing prognosis as a range, which is tailored to the person's preferences
- Setting goals in the event of deterioration in their condition
- Exploring their fears and worries about the future
- Confirming functional abilities so critical that living life without them cannot be imagined
- Exploring how much medical treatment a person is willing to go through to gain more time
- Confirming how much family members know about a person's priorities and preferences

From this conversation should emerge shared documentation of recommendations, which acknowledge medical realities summarise key goals and priorities and describe the treatment options, which reflect these.

Developing effective and meaningful narratives, which focus ACP on people living with frailty and/or multi-morbidity, could therefore significantly assist with this approach for older people.

## Care homes

Care homes present an environment where there is a high prevalence of older people living with multi-morbidity and frailty (35). They therefore present ideal settings for proactive consideration of ACP for older residents identified to be nearing the end of their life. However current evidence suggests that only a minority of care home residents actively engage in ACP suggesting that its implementation is not optimal (36). This is despite the observation that care homes accommodate a heterogeneous case-mix with frailty prevalence varying between 19 and 76%. With up to 40% residents remaining pre-frail there is opportunity to intervene early to avoid unwanted negative health outcomes.

While care home residents tend to trust their families and care home staff to make important decisions, relatives are in contrast insecure about residents' wishes and find decision making towards the end of life burdensome (37). The deployment of systematic ACP in home settings could therefore help to offset this burden for families and support a more transparent, inclusive, and person-centred approach to end of life care in this setting.

In order for ACP to be deployed successfully in care homes a number of key pre-conditions are required largely centred on professionals and the care home environment (38). These include professionals having adequate skills, knowledge, and willingness to participate in ACP, having good relationships with residents and their families, and access to an administrative system to support the process. In addition, it is important to ensure that ACP in care homes is part of routine practice and adequate time is made available to care home staff and families to participate. Other important contextual factors for successful ACP include community involvement which takes account of local cultural issues and ensuring that there are adequate facilities in place to support palliative and end of life care.

# Dementia

In dementia care the timing of ACP is particularly problematic given the requirement for a person's wishes to be documented while they retain mental capacity for decisions about their future care and treatment (39). There is evidence that professionals in this context believe ACP to be a good idea in theory but remain unconvinced of its true value and lack clarity in respect of their future roles and responsibilities, or the extent to which plans would be legally binding (40). Despite this the deployment of ACP in care homes involving residents with cognitive impairment including dementia is feasible and can shorten length of hospital stay and risk of readmission if they subsequently present to the emergency department when compared with community dwelling older people without an ACP (41).

## Case study

Pete was diagnosed with vascular dementia several years ago and had struggled with employment related hearing loss for 20 years and osteoarthritis for the last ten years. Previously Pete had cared for his wife at home who had Alzheimer's dementia, diabetes, osteoarthritis, and heart failure. Sadly she died just before he was diagnosed with dementia himself.

**Key point**: Pete and his daughter had some prior knowledge of his condition, which can be used to contextualise and make real future ACP discussions.

Pete attended the memory clinic to receive his diagnosis with his daughter Sally. At this appointment they both raised their concerns about how Pete would care for himself in the coming years. His daughter lived and worked some distance away though had been in weekly telephone contact with her parents and visited whenever she could. Pete was worried about being isolated and lonely. He was also worried about falling and injuring himself.

Having cared for his wife until her death, Pete had developed clear views about how he wanted to be cared for in the future. He was adamant that he wanted to live out his life, despite his conditions, at home and that if possible he wanted to receive care at the end of his life in his own home with his daughter present. He was worried about how he would manage his financial affairs as his dementia progressed and also who would make decisions about his care if he could no longer express his wishes. His biggest fear was dying alone.

**Key point**: Pete has begun to form clear views about his future care and treatment based on his own life experiences and values.

Joan, the dementia nurse specialist suggested to Pete and Sally that he think about making Lasting Powers of Attorney to ensure that Sally was able to assist with managing his affairs and legally empowered to assist in making decisions about his health and welfare should he lose the capacity to make decisions for himself.

**Key point**: a new serious illness diagnosis, which is likely to impact on capacity to make decisions has been used to trigger actions to support future care and decision-making.

Following this appointment Pete and Sally visited a solicitor to arrange Lasting Powers of Attorney for his daughter. He also visited his GP who had asked to see him following his dementia diagnosis. His GP explained that given his various health conditions it would be a good time to look at which of Pete's medications were of most benefit to him. Pete did not like taking some of his medications due to side effects and it was agreed to try stopping these.

**Key point**: use of the NICE multi-morbidity guideline has been used to reduce the burden of unwanted health interventions and begun to refocus on care and support planning in the context of a new diagnosis.

A year later Pete's GP asked to see him with Sally again. His memory was deteriorating and he was starting to lose his mobility. The GP explained that a new way of adding up the number of Pete's health conditions called a frailty index, now suggested that Pete had developed something called severe frailty. Neither Pete nor Sally had heard of frailty and did not really understand what it meant. His GP explained that research had discovered that people with severe frailty were at much greater risk of needing hospital care, being admitted to a care home, or reaching the end of their life. His GP provided Pete and Sally with a leaflet explaining more about frailty and explained that one of the practice nurses, Gary had been trained in assessing and caring for people with frailty and dementia.

**Key point**: use of the eFI has triggered a discussion and sharing of information about frailty and the implications of this condition and its known trajectories for future care planning. A key professional has been appointed to build a relationship of trust, coordinate, and administer ACP.

Over the next year Gary visited Pete periodically to assess his various conditions and talk through his wishes and preferences for his care in the future. He had gradually become more bed bound and had become incontinent. Pete explained to Gary that he understood his condition was getting worse and he was worried he was nearing the end of his life. Gary agreed to set up a meeting at Pete's house with his family, the GP and other members of his care team.

**Key point**: in the context of worsening cognitive and physical conditions the care coordinator has precipitated a key decision-making meeting while the older person retains capacity to make important decisions about their future care and treatment.

At this meeting Pete stated his preferences for his care to continue at home, to remain free from distress, and that he wanted to avoid going to hospital 'at all costs'. Gary carefully documented this in a short summary, which the GP entered onto Pete's electronic care record with his permission to be shared with the out of hours GP service, along with completing a 'Do Not Resuscitate' (DNACPR) order which was placed in his home care record.

**Key point**: clear and shared record keeping with permission is essential for successful ACP.

Six months later Pete became very suddenly unwell with breathlessness in the early hours of the morning. The out of hours GP arrived, consulted the electronic records, and identified that Pete had an advanced care plan not to admit to hospital and a hand-held DNACPR order. He phoned Pete's daughter Sally having noted from the care record that she was appointed with Lasting Powers of Attorney for welfare decisions. Since Pete was so distressed they both agreed that he should go to hospital for further assessment and stabilisation.

**Key point**: the ACP was used to guide decisions and signpost a newly involved care professional to the legally appointed advocate and decision maker. Pete's interests in maintained comfort and dignity were kept at the centre of the decision made in difficult circumstances.

The following day assessment in the hospital acute medical unit by a geriatrician was completed who confirmed that Pete had developed bronchopneumonia and delirium. He had nevertheless begun to respond to treatment for this and following discussion with Sally it was agreed to continue treatment in the expectation that Pete would become well enough to return home to be cared for as he was previously in the next few days. Pete's previously agreed DNACPR order was reconfirmed and it was agreed that if he deteriorated further, every effort would be made to provide end-of-life care at his own home with the support of his family, Gary, and the primary care team.

**Key point**: continuous care was maintained with key documentation shared and existing key decisions reviewed in light of previously documented advance care plans.

Fortunately Pete recovered enough to permit discharge back to his own home six days later. His care package was increased and Gary continued to support Pete and his family. A few months later Pete developed a further episode of bronchopneumonia and end of life care was commenced at home without the need to attend hospital again. The preferences for care that Pete had expressed were documented in his advanced care plan and used to guide his end of life care, while his prior decisions not to attend hospital or be subject to cardiopulmonary resuscitation at the end of his life were fully respected.

## Summary

The world population is rapidly changing driven by a decline in fertility and improved life expectancy. This creates new demands for health and social care policy and planning. More people are surviving to later life with multiple long-term conditions (multi-morbidity) and more people are living with disability. Meanwhile current UK government policy response is to focus on healthy ageing and extending disability free life.

The changing shape of societies and families together with their ability and opportunity to be engaged in supporting and delivering successful ACP must be fully considered when initiating discussions with an older person. Frailty is associated with multi-morbidity and the presence of disability in older people. Older people living with frailty have increased risk of acute and unexpected health decline with uncertain, incomplete, and prolonged recovery. The presence of frailty can be recognised and used to inform understanding of an individual's risk of requiring unplanned hospital admission, formal home care, or care-home admission. Severe frailty states are associated with increased mortality risk.

Routine frailty identification by severity can help initiate ACP among people with high potential mortality risk or unmet current need. These people are more likely to be older but not all frail people are old. By understanding disability trajectories in older people living with frailty ACP can be undertaken proactively and with improved understanding of the factors that influence this.

Recognising and acting on potential professional and organisational barriers to ACP for older people could improve its uptake. Guided serious illness conversations could assist with ACP in older people living with frailty by supporting a personalised approach to care for this diverse population group. Explaining the individual and system benefits to professionals and organisations through case reflection or story telling might help support transformational and sustainable change.

## References

1. **The World Bank** (2017). *Population ages 65 and above (% of total)*, The World Bank Group. Available from: http://data.worldbank.org (Accessed 17 January 2017.)

2. **National Institute on Aging, National Institutes of Health** (2011). *Global Health and Aging: Humanity's Aging* [Internet] Available from: https://www.nia.nih.gov/ (Accessed 17 January 2017.)

3. **Murray CJL**, et al. (2012). 'Disability-adjusted life years (DALYs) for 291 diseases and injuries in 21 regions, 1990–2010: a systematic analysis for the Global Burden of Disease Study 2010'. *The Lancet* **380**(9859): 2197–223. doi: 10.1016/S0140-6736(12)61689-4. (Accessed 17 January 2017.)

4. **Brookmeyer R**, et al. (2007). 'Forecasting the global burden of Alzheimer's disease'. *Alzheimer's & Dementia: The Journal of the Alzheimer's Association* **3**(3): 186–91.doi: 10.1016/j.jalz.2007.04.381. (Accessed 17 January 2017.)

5. **United Nations, Department of Economic and Social Affairs, Population Division** (2015). *World population ageing* [report], ST/ESA/SER.A/390, Available from: http://www.un.org (Accessed 17 January 2017.)

6. **Office for National Statistics** (2015). *Population Estimates for UK, England and Wales, Scotland and Northern Ireland: mid-2015* [Internet], Published Online June 2016, Available from: https://www.ons.gov.uk/ (Accessed 17 January 2017.)

7. **Government Office for Science** (2016). *Future of an Ageing Population.* [Internet] Published Online July 2016, Available from: www.gov.uk/go-science (Accessed 17 January 2017.)

8. **Office for National Statistics** (2017). *Labour Force Survey (LFS).* [Internet] Available from: https://www.ons.gov.uk/surveys (Accessed 17 January 2017.)

9. **Stonewall** (2011). *Lesbian, Gay & Bisexual People in later line.* [Internet] Available from: https://www.stonewall.org.uk (Accessed 17 January 2017.)

10. **G-plus** (2009). *The poor relation? Grandparental care.* [Internet] Grandparents Plus. Available from: https://www.grandparentsplus.org.uk. (Accessed 17 January 2017.)

11. **Office for National Statistics** (2011). *Religion in England and Wales.* [Internet] Available from: https://www.ons.gov.uk/peoplepopulationandcommunity (Accessed 17 January 2017.)

12. **Office for National Statistics** (2017). *Life expectancies.* [Internet] Available from: https://www.ons.gov.uk (Accessed 17 January 2017.)

13. **Department for Work & Pensions** (2015). *2010 to 2015 government policy: older people.* [Internet] Available from: https://www.gov.uk/ (Accessed 17 January 2017.)

14. **Department for Work & Pensions** (2012). *DWP Digital Strategy.* [Internet] Published Online December 2012. Available from: https://www.gov.uk/ (Accessed 17 January 2017.)

15. **Holt-Lunstad,** et al. (2015). 'Loneliness and social isolation as risk factors for mortality'. *Perspectives on Psychological Science* **10**(2): 227–37. doi: 10.1177/1745691614568352.

16. **Local Government Association** (2012). *Ageing Well—a whole system approach: A guide to place-based working* [Internet] Available from: http://www.local.gov.uk/ (Accessed 17 January 2017.)

17. **National Institute for Health and Care Excellence** (2016). *Multimorbidity: clinical assessment and management*, NICE guideline [Internet] Published Online September 2016. Available from: https://www.nice.org.uk (Accessed 17 January 2017.)

18. **Violan C,** et al. (2014). 'Prevalence, determinants and patterns of multimorbidity in primary care: a systematic review of observational studies'. *PLoS ONE* **9**(7). doi: 10.1371/journal.pone.0102149.

19. **Clegg A,** et al. (2016). 'Development and validation of an electronic frailty index using routine primary care electronic health record data'. *Age and Ageing* **45**(3): 353–60. doi: 10.1093/ageing/afw039.

20. **Rockwood K,** et al. (2015). 'What are frailty instruments for'? *Age and Ageing* **44**(4): 545–7. doi: 10.1093/ageing/afv043.

21. **Gale CR,** et al. (2015). 'Prevalence of frailty and disability: findings from the English longitudinal study of ageing'. *Age and Ageing* **44**(1): 162–5. doi: 10.1093/ageing/afu148.

22. **Romero-Ortuno R,** et al. (2016). 'Clinical frailty adds to acute illness severity in predicting mortality in hospitalized older adults: An observational study'. *European Journal of Internal Medicine* **35**: 24–34. doi: 10.1016/j.ejim.2016.08.033.

23. **Vernon MJ** (2016). Why is diagnosing frailty important? [Internet] *NHS England Blog*, Available from: https://www.england.nhs.uk/2016/09/martin-vernon-2/ (Accessed 17 January 2017.)

24. **Sylvester KM,** et al. (2014). 'Timely care for frail older people referred to hospital improves efficiency and reduces mortality without the need for extra resources'. *Age and Ageing* **43**: 472–7. doi: 10.1093/ageing/aft170.

25. **Gill TM,** et al. (2015). 'The role of intervening hospital admissions on trajectories of disability in the last year of life: prospective cohort study of older people'. *BMJ* **350**. doi: 10.1136/bmj.h2361.

26. **National Institute for Health and Care Excellencee** (2017). *Making decisions about your care* [Internet] Available from: https://www.nice.org.uk (Accessed 17 January 2017.)

27. **Department for Constitutional Affairs.** (2007) *Mental Capacity Act 2005: Code of Practice* [Internet] Act, Available from: https://www.gov.uk (Accessed 17 January 2017.)

28. **NHS End of Life Care Programme** (2007) *Advance Care Planning: A Guide for Health and Social Care Staff* [Internet] Department of Health, Available from: http://www.ncpc.org.uk (Accessed 17 January 2017.)

29. **Sharp T,** et al. (2013). 'Do the elderly have a voice? Advance care planning discussions with frail and older individuals: a systematic literature review and narrative synthesis'. *British Journal of General Practice* **63** (615): 657–68. doi: 10.3399/bjgp13X673667.

30. **Kimbell B,** et al. (2016). 'Embracing inherent uncertainty in advanced illness'. *BMJ* **354**. doi: 10.1136/bmj.i3802.

31. **Eynon T,** et al. (2013). 'Never the right time: advance care planning with frail and older people'. *British Journal of General Practice* **63**(615): 511–2. doi: 10.3399/bjgp13X673568.

32. **An Independent Review of the Liverpool Care Pathway** (2013) *More Care, Less Pathway* [Internet] Available from: https://www.gov.uk (Accessed 17 January 2017.)

33. **Butler M** et al. (2014). 'Decision aids for advance care planning: an overview of the state of the science'. *Annals of Internal Medicine* **161**(6): 408–18. doi: 10.7326/M14-0644.

34. **Ariadne Labs** (2015) *Serious Illness Conversation Guide* [Internet] Available from: https://www.ariadnelabs.org. (Accessed 17 January 2017.)

35. **Kojima G** (2015). 'Prevalence of frailty in nursing homes: a systematic review and meta-analysis'. *Journal of the American Medical Directors Association* **16**(11): 940–5. doi: 10.1016/j.jamda.2015.06.025.

36. **De Gendt, C** et al. (2013). 'Advance care planning and dying in nursing homes in Flanders, Belgium: A Nationwide Survey'. *Journal of Pain and Symptom Management* **45**(2): 223–34. doi: 10.1016/j.jpainsymman.2012.02.011.

37. **Bollig G,** et al. (2015). 'They know!-Do they? A qualitative study of residents and relatives views on advance care planning, end-of-life care, and decision-making in nursing homes'. *Palliative Medicine* **30**(5): 456–70. doi: 10.1177/0269216315605753.

38. **Gilissen J,** et al. (2017). 'Preconditions for successful advance care planning in nursing homes: A systematic review'. *International Journal of Nursing Studies* **66**: 47–59. doi: 10.1016/j.ijnurstu.2016.12.003.

39. **Sampson EL,** et al. (2011). 'Palliative assessment and advance care planning in severe dementia: An exploratory randomized controlled trial of a complex intervention'. *Palliative Medicine* **25**(3); 197–209. doi: 10.1177/0269216310391691.

40. **Robinson L,** et al. (2013). ' "A qualitative study: professionals" experiences of advance care planning in dementia and palliative care, "a good idea in theory but ..." '. *Palliative Medicine* **27**(5): 401–8. doi: 10.1177/0269216312465651.

41. **Street M,** et al. (2015). 'Advance care planning for older people in Australia presenting to the emergency department from the community or residential aged care facilities'. *Health and Social Care in the Community* **23**(5): 513–22. doi: 10.1111/hsc.12162.

Chapter 6

# Spiritual and ethical aspects of advance care planning

Max Watson and Mark Thomas

'What you are now, we once were; what we are now, you shall be.'
*Plaque in the Capuchean ossary in Rome*

---

**This chapter includes**

- Linking spirituality and Advanced Care Planning (ACP)
- Fear, resilience, and hope and ACP
- Religious views and ACP
- Denial and ACP
- Personal control and ACP
- Ethical principles and ACP
- Spiritual/existential assessment and ACP
- The spiritual work of ACP
- Adaptation and ACP
- Ritual, sacrament, and ACP

---

**Key Points**

- Dying is not primarily a medical event
- The process of thinking about end of life issues can significantly impact on an individuals' attitudes, values, and belief systems. The end (conclusion) of life leads us to think about the end (purpose) of life. It is a time of changing perspectives, important reflections on the past, and a stronger sense of what is most important in people's lives
- Dying patients can challenge the cultural illusion that life is going to last forever. This can be hard for families and professionals to accept and challenges their own fears around mortality
- An ACP can provide some comfort through bestowing a sense of control at a time in life when opportunities to influence events might otherwise not pertain. Care can be tailored to personal needs and preferences and this can be important for patients, their families, and healthcare professionals

- The four ethical principles of autonomy, beneficence, non-maleficence and justice provide a framework within which ACP discussions can take place
- The ACP process can include an objective assessment of the patient's spiritual and existential well-being
- ACP discussions can help in adapting to a new reality for patients and their families. This can bring about a sense of 'realistic hope' and increased resilience leading to better quality of remaining life. It can also trigger discussions with others at a deeper level, voicing unspoken but important truths at this significant time, which can live on in the memory of the bereaved
- The importance and wisdom of religious rituals and religious symbolism cannot be ignored even in the most secular of contexts as they bring comfort to many

**Key Message**

Death is not primarily a medical event. Death is a personal, relational, and spiritual event, yet the majority of professional effort is concerned with the medical aspects of the end of life, often to the neglect of the more pertinent issues facing the dying and their families.

# Linking spirituality and advanced care planning

Over many years and especially in the last two centuries, we have tended towards making the natural dying process a clinical event, in a similar way to the medicalisation of giving birth. Manifestations of the death denying nature of society include:

- The use of euphemisms to describe death
- The hiding of death or references to death from children
- The 'sanitisation' of dying in hospitals and the funeral industry
- The closing of coffins at funerals
- Loss of death and bereavement rituals and practices

It is worth speculating as to how this unbalance became so common in clinical practice. Is it because healthcare professionals have been affected by the same death denying culture that affects the rest of western society? Could some clinical professionals use their ability to 'do' something clinically as a means of avoiding dealing with other issues and the essential demand of end of life care to 'be' with the dying?

Modern medical science describes with increasing accuracy the biological processes of dying, but is usually silent about what dying and death actually is for the individual person.

If healthcare professionals share the same attitudes towards death and dying as the rest of society, it is no surprise when it comes to Advance Care Planning (ACP) that there could be some hesitancy in initiating planning discussions. Discussing death and dignity is inherently 'counter-cultural' and against our societal instincts.

Much attention has been given to the legal and medical implications of ACP and how patients can be enabled to exercise their own choices when they no longer have the capacity to do so. Less attention has been paid to how the process of thinking about your own end of life plans impacts on your emotional, familial, psychological, and spiritual life. Consciously thinking about, and planning around your own end of life has a particularity about it which affects most people. Frequently it causes people to reflect on existential issues and raises questions which they may never have truly faced before. Such a process can challenge our values and impacts on the way we view the world.

ACP has a profoundly spiritual and existential dimension that needs to be acknowledged and supported, regardless of the religious or non-religious background of those involved. For those professionals conducting such discussions it is important to appreciate this for not to do so risks missing important existential cues from the patient and the opportunity to provide support for patients in the final stage of life.

The end (conclusion) of life forces us to think on what is the end (purpose) of life.

## Fear and advance care planning

The sociologist Ernest Becker in his book *The Denial of Death* (2) suggests that the fear of death is a pervasive force which permeates mankind's subconscious. He contends that many of man's heroic, religious, and secular dramas derive from an attempt to overcome death in some way and escape or deny its reality:

The idea of death, the fear of it, haunts the human animal like nothing else; it is a mainspring of human activity—designed largely to avoid the fatality of death, to overcome it by denying in some way that it is the final destiny of man.

Becker's work has been built on by others who decided to assess whether his thesis could be proved. In some fascinating experiments they showed that thinking about death, even if only for a very short time, has the capacity to make people change previously held attitudes and preferences often in favour of more traditional, dualistic, and authoritarian approaches, or regress to paradigms from their formative years.

## How thinking about death changes us

A group of students was asked to fill out a questionnaire. The control group filled out a range of questions about their life experience including a section about their experience of pain, such as a fracture or an operation. The other group of students was asked to answer exactly the same questions but the questions of pain were replaced with questions about death. Where would you like to die? How would you like to die? Etc. (1)

On completion of the questionnaire the students were ushered into a classroom where they had to wait for the certificate of completion. Sitting in the room already were some students. These students were clearly identifiable as being from different and visually distinct racial groups and religions. The control group of students sat down in seats in a completely random fashion. The students who had been made to think about death significantly gravitated towards sitting beside others of their own cultural/religious background.

Such experiments carried out across the world have shown that thinking about death even for only a short time can change voting preferences, as well as your sympathy for more extreme elements within your own tradition. In short, death thoughts for many people can trigger fears and uncertainties at a subconscious level of such strength that they change personal preferences and can promote conservatism.

The process of advanced care planning is primarily concerned with ensuring that life is lived for as long as possible in the way that is preferred—life before death. It is about helping people adapt to a new reality that life is limited and has to be lived out in the context of dying. By their nature these discussions promote facing up to mortality, and as such could cause a significant impact. The process itself can change people's values if mortality is not something he or she has pondered. Indeed, often people who begin the process of ACP end up choosing options which would not have been thought of as obvious for them at the outset. The very process of planning has changed their way of thinking. Because ACP focuses on the quality of life before death, it encourages hope and resilience in those facing the last chapter in their lives.

## Religious views of advance care planning

The truth of this has long been appreciated in spiritual traditions and teaching. Rather than being morbid, or using fear of death to persuade people to change their ways, these practices have been used for thousands of years to help people face reality with a degree of detachment so they are better able to balance their lives in the present and live in the context of their own mortality.

> 'The brothers should contemplate their death each day so that they can be freed from the cloying impact of the cares of the world.'
>
> St. John of the Cross Carmelite friar and priest

> 'The way you live and the way you die are one.'
>
> Montague

> 'Contemplate the dead and the difference between your body and theirs that you may better live in this world.'
>
> Buddha

> And he said: 'You would know the secret of death. But how shall you find it unless you seek it in the heart of life? The owl whose night-bound eyes are blind unto the day cannot unveil the mystery of light.'
>
> Khalil Gibran, The Prophet: On Death

> '. . . when we finally know we are dying, and all other sentient beings are dying with us, we start to have a burning, almost heartbreaking sense of the fragility and preciousness of each moment and each being, and from this can grow a deep, clear, limitless compassion for all beings.'
>
> Sogyal Rinpoche

> 'Real spirituality is all about what you do with your pain—you either transmit it or transform it!'
>
> Richard Rohr

Hundreds of years before Becker the major religions of the world were encouraging their followers to overcome fears of death through facing them and thus being freed from their shadow.

Death awareness and death inevitability have been a more accepted feature of most civilisations until relatively recently. The surfeit of death denial which is a feature of western hubris is actually in stark contrast to what has gone on before. Other societies at different times, be it through the building of a pyramid in Egypt or through the purchase of a Co-op funeral in Manchester have been more pragmatic about death or dying.

## Denial and advance care planning

Death, and all that is associated with it, including ACP, undermines western society's confidence for it clearly implies that modern man is unable to fix everything. From within the cultural bubble that life is going to last forever it can be very hard for an individual to burst the taboo and expose the lie by expressing wishes in relation to their end of life. By so doing they are giving birth to the discomfort of mortality for everyone involved. Our natural and almost automatic response to such expressions is to stifle them, or deem the individuals concerned as being morbid, pessimistic or depressed.

'Mum don't be talking like that, you are going to be fine . . .'

In order to overcome this reticence individuals may have to metaphorically shout to have their voice heard which can make them seem emotionally unbalanced, thus confirming the initial label of instability.

## Case study

MG, a widow of 84 years with advanced chronic obstructive pulmonary disease (COPD), type two diabetes, and angina had been admitted to an acute hospital three times in as many months with chest infections. She had witnessed several people who appeared healthier than her dying on the ward, yet whenever she asked the nurse or doctor about her death she was told not to bother herself thinking like that. The dissonance between what she was seeing and feeling with her own eyes and body and what she was being told by the professionals confused and upset her. She confided in her priest, 'Nobody is telling me the truth, and it makes me feel very frightened and alone'.

Some of such dissonance may be due to the age and life experience of the caring professionals, being younger than the patients they are looking after, younger in years and also in terms of life experience, and maybe in spiritual maturity.

It would be wrong to expect these professionals to not share some of the values of the young society in which they were trained and live. These same professionals and their peers are targeted by youth centred advertising, youth centred music, youth centred media and youth centred entertainments. There is little room on their television schedules for soap operas set in nursing homes or music dealing with old age concerns. Mick Jagger can now draw his old age pension, but our youth centred perspective turns a blind eye to images denoting his old age.

This youth focus leaves our society, with less knowledge and respect than earlier generations for the wisdom that comes through experience and age; wisdom which other cultures and other times have prized and valued highly. This can make cross generational communication difficult, particularly in such a sensitive area as ACP for these conversations benefit from empathy and understanding.

## Personal control and advance care planning

A common concern of many near the end of life is retaining a need for control and self-determination. Seven of the 12 factors for a good death in the Age Concern debate of the age, related to retaining control—control of place, of people present, and other factors (3). At a time when life appears out of control, this can be very important, especially within our more secular society.

'I do not want anybody else to be making my choices for me.'

For such individuals personal autonomy and choice may be understood as essential expressions of their very personhood. An ACP in this context can provide existential comfort through bestowing a sense of control at a time when control is being fundamentally lost at a very deep level. To those for whom control has been very important, the prospect of losing control can cause a very real and deep distress (existential/spiritual pain) because control is so linked to who they perceive themselves to be. If personhood is understood to be the sum and collation of thoughts, preferences and decisions, the loss of this capacity can feel like a loss of their very 'self', or even a loss of everything that is worthwhile in life. This fear, which such a huge loss can signify, is surely one of the motivators for the passion of those wishing to introduce laws on physician assisted suicide in the UK.

The motivations of the individual completing an ACP often influence the nature of the directive created. Where control is crucial the plan may become a very detailed document requiring regular updates and additions to ensure that it is as accurate as possible and conforms with the latest thinking of the individual. The plan itself can become the means by which the individual maintains and expresses their evolving understanding of their identity. In turn this can increase levels of anxiety among professionals who realise that the prospects of fulfilling such detailed objectives will be difficult in the context of real, end of life clinical realities, but from an ethical perspective the completion of an ACP ensures that the care received is more likely to be in accordance with individual preference.

## Ethical principles

There are four bioethical principles that provide the framework for medical decision making and communication with patients, including ACP. These are:

- **Autonomy**: respect the right of an individual to make their own decisions with regard to their own health and future. Respect for autonomy is a component of respect for human dignity
- **Beneficence**: the duty to do the best for the individual or to act in the best interests of the person—i.e. to undertake actions that are intended to benefit the patient (to do good)
- **Non-maleficence**: the duty to do no harm to patients or others
- **Justice**: incorporates the notions of equity and fair distribution. The ethical principle emphasizes that health professionals have responsibility to the wider community as well as to individual patients (4)

These principles support ethical clinical practices including:

- Provision of necessary pain relief based on the patient's individual clinical need
- Withholding or withdrawing life sustaining treatments that are no longer effective or that do not benefit the patient; including any treatment the patient has refused
- Complying with a patient's Advance Decision to Refuse Treatment (ADRT)

These four commonly used bioethical principles can be used to guide a clinician's relationship with their patients, including how they communicate with the patient about their medical condition, their treatment options and planning for future care as they face the end of life.

ACP is based on respect for autonomy; for the person's right to make choices and direct their life. It seeks to enhance the person's exercise of their autonomy because their decisions, preferences and directions are made known in advance, and can be applied at a later point should the person's decision-making capacity become impaired (5).

## Spiritual/existential assessment and advance care planning

It is helpful to make an objective assessment of the person's spiritual/existential well-being as part of any ACP process in order to elicit the individual's state of mind, wishes, values and beliefs, so that care can be given that is in line with their underlying motivations. There are acronyms to help us ask the right questions. One of the most commonly used is FICA:

**F:** Faith. A question might be 'What beliefs sustain you (for example religion, family, nature)'
**I:** Importance. 'How important are those beliefs in your life?'
**C:** Community. 'Who supports you? Who are the important people in your life, around you?'
**A:** Address. 'How can we(as your care providers) address these issues and provide help?' (6)

Source: data from FICA Spiritual History Tool, © Copyright, Christina M. Puchalski, MD, 1996, Available from: https://smhs.gwu.edu/gwish/clinical/fica/spiritual-history-tool

Another similar acronym is HOPE:

**H:** Hope. 'what in your life gives you internal support and provides meaning? What are your sources of hope?'

**O**: Organised religion. 'Is organised religious practice part of your life and how important is that? What aspects of that are particularly important?'

**P:** Personal spirituality. 'What is your personal spirituality independently of organised religion? What aspects of your spirituality do you find most helpful?'

**E:** Effect. 'What have been the effects of your spirituality on end of life care and medical issues? How has being ill effected your ability to cope? What can I as your professional carer do to help?'

Source: data from Anandarajah G and Hight E, 'Spirituality and medical practice: using the HOPE questions as a practical tool for spiritual assessment', *American Family Physician*, Volume 63, pp. 81–9, Copyright © 2001 American Academy of Family Physicians

The overall aim of such questions is to ask how we can best support the person's spiritual well-being and ability to cope, and how we can make best use of their own inner resources as they face the end of life. It is important to stress that such tools are a springboard to human engagement between two people, and should not be used in a formulaic way as a substitute for creating a safe space where people feel free to discuss what is important to them. The aim is to support resilience and to help the person find meaning as they face the end of life.

The carer brings professional expertise and training to the ACP process, but also their human experience and wisdom. Mortality is something we share both as carers and the cared for, and in facing end of life issues, it is good to accept the limitations of expertise no matter how profession-ally skilled we are. The professional carer can bring many gifts to each encounter, but the most important is the ability to be still, to listen and to be fully present for the person in front of you, putting aside both what has come before and what lies ahead. An inner stillness is essential, and many find some sort of regular mindfulness practice a valuable discipline in order to cultivate the skills of presence and active listening.

## The spiritual work of advance care planning

For those who are from a religious or spiritual tradition or who have a yearning for the same, an ACP may include expression of religious or spiritual activities or aspirations that patients would like to complete. Examples of these activities might include a trip to Rome, Mecca or Benares or a particular sacramental act. It might also include the fulfilment of dreams such as swimming with dolphins, seeing an Australian sunset, or climbing the Himalayas.

Less dramatic expressions of spiritual aspects of ACPs might include a desire to reconnect with a previous community, to fulfil particular religious observances, or reconcile a previous differ-ence or conflict, or simply to spend time visiting a favourite place maybe in the countryside or near the sea. Such activities can bring comfort both to patients as well as relatives, and provide a context in which previous family tensions can be reduced, and in which meaning and spiritual assurance grow.

There can be a strong draw to go home, to die in the place of their birth, as is witnessed by many from the UK Asian community going back to Asia—the so called 'Salmon instinct'.

It is not unusual for end of life thoughts to raise the importance of spiritual issues for patients and heighten the search for meaning in life. For the professional listening to such thoughts it is necessary to appreciate their importance and to try to avoid prescribing physical treatments for spiritual discomforts. Conversely it is important not to be so sure that a patient's pains are spiritual that their physical needs are neglected!

An Advance Care Plan provides opportunity for reflection and taking stock on one's life. Not only does it give the chance to plan for the future it also encourages the individual to reflect on the past. ACP without reflecting on the past is building a house without foundations. It can be done but the plans are unlikely to be robust or authentic.

In relation to the reflective component of an ACP there may be personal issues of hurt which come to mind coupled with a desire for reconciliation and resolution of unfinished business. This drive within us exists at a very powerful level as anybody who has worked in a hospice has witnessed.

## Case study

Shortly after Joe was diagnosed with lung cancer he made a promise to his daughter that he would escort her down the aisle on her wedding day. The disease was rapid and Joe's condition deteriorated and within months he was spending most of the day in bed. He refused to let his daughter bring the wedding day forward, despite his deterioration. When he was admitted to hospice the family gave up hope that he would keep his promise. But Joe didn't die. He remained focused on his goal and despite all the physical indicators he fulfilled his promise and accompanied his daughter, albeit in a wheel chair, down the aisle, and then died two days later.

This is a common human drive and relates to an innate desire to complete things where possible, and no more so than in terms of resolving relationship difficulties. The process of ACP can trigger deep emotions and enable important discussions to take place that will live on in the memory of the bereaved.

In his book *The Four Things That Matter Most* Ira Byock (7) suggests that there is a universal generic quality to the nature of this emotional work which is common to many people facing the end of their life. He suggests there is a prime need to sort relationships out before it is too late.

'Please forgive me', 'I forgive you', 'Thank you', and 'I love you', are the outward verbal expressions which Byock gives to these important relational tasks. Tasks which may also be part of an individual's personalACP.

The need for sharing and receiving forgiveness for mistakes that have been made or experienced, for pain given, and pain received is common. As death approaches there is a natural desire to resolve conflict, to pay restitution, and to leave the slate as 'clean' as possible. Such sentiments in our secular world may be viewed with suspicion, but those working regularly in end of life care both with religious and non-religious patients will attest to the power and importance of forgiveness in bringing a sense of peace and restitution in the final stages. Forgiveness is a central part of the faith of many but can also be healing in psychological terms, reducing self-loathing and anger, and encouraging 'wholeness' at a time when a physical cure is not possible.

When tasks of forgiveness and reconciliation have been completed it can have a profound impact on the nature of the last days of a person's life confirming a phrase often quoted from Dame Cicely Saunders, 'The last part of life has an importance out of all proportion to its length'.

Planning for reconciliation is of course, impossible but planning to ensure that there is at least opportunity for such work is important. This work is not just for the patient but also for the individuals who will have to live with the consequences of reconciliation or lack of reconciliation long term.

Bound up in the pain of physical disease is the pain of loss and the pain of suffering. Making sense of this suffering is the journey of a lifetime.

## Adaptation and advance care planning

The discussion of issues related to living out the final stage of life, brings us face to face with the taboo that is death. Gradually there may be an adaptation to this new reality, a coming to terms with the fact that death will happen, so planning for it is perhaps the best we can do in terms of reducing its impact and control. This growing realisation may well come to the dying person before it dawns on their family and loved ones—especially with older people as they face the inevitable with perhaps a degree of relief.

### Case study

A mother, 82 years old, and her 50-year-old daughter were having a discussion about ACP with a nurse in the care home, as a routine part of their ongoing care. The old lady expressed the wish to die in her favourite Victorian lace nightdress, and wished the nurse to write this down specifically. The daughter was horrified and blurted out 'it would be a waste—why on earth do you want that'. Her mother said quite calmly that she wished to wear that nightdress to look nice for her family to see her after she had died. There was a frisson in the room as the realisation dawned on the daughter that her mother was calmly facing her death, whilst she was still fighting it.

## Ritual, sacrament, and advanced care planning

'Now faith is the assurance that what we hope for will come about and the certainty that what we cannot see exists'

*Hebrews 11: 1, The Bible*

'Sacraments are the outward and visible sign of an inward invisible truth'

*Common Prayer Book*

For those who are religious, faith and religious practices may have a profound effect on how they view their dying and on how they plan for their future. Such people may receive great comfort and reassurance from the support of their religious community through sacraments, pastoral visits, prayer and affirmations of their religions' beliefs and hopes. Secular healthcare delivery systems may struggle with creating space where such religious observance can take place but religious support for the dying is still too important to too many people to be excluded from healthcare. The influence of organised religion in ACP has an impact that extends beyond those who society would readily identify as being 'religious'. This is because:

◆ The confirmation of mortality that accompanies worsening health may reconnect people with religious experiences and memories from their past

◆ Many of the texts, icons and teachings of the major religions relate to themes and issues which the dying can readily relate to, and draw comfort from

◆ In the search for meaning at the end of life it is not unusual to look beyond the self to religious references and understandings which can help provide answers to the challenging questions that mortality poses

◆ 'There are no atheists in fox holes', first coined during war, points to the fact that people often turn to God in times of extreme stress when they feel powerless

◆ There is a significant population who find difficulty identifying with or supporting particular religious communities, but who still have strong personal religious beliefs

Asking patients about what is important to them is vital, and this is usually the first step in holding an ACP discussion.

If it is appropriate to introduce religious sacraments and symbols in the most appropriate way these may have a significant impact on how the patient and their family both view the future and plan for the future. A skilled pastoral care approach will discern the best level of religious ritual that is authentic and comfort bringing for the individual and the family involved.

Such activities may include some of the following:

◆ Prayer, meditation, and reading of sacred texts

◆ Worship services

◆ Blessings

◆ Religion-specific sacraments and use of holy objects

◆ Weddings and sacred unions

◆ Observance of holy days

◆ Guided meditation for pain reduction and relaxation

◆ Music, sacred or familiar to the patient/family

◆ Life review and creation of a legacy document or recording for family

◆ Guided meditation for inner guidance or connection to God or a higher power

The beliefs and values of patients and families need to be identified and respected in as much as the healthcare team can ethically and reasonably do so. Such practices should not be assumed just because patients belong to a particular religion, or to no religion but the individual's preferences should always be sought. For example, grieving 'non religious' families may receive seemingly incongruous comfort by knowledge that after-death rituals and practices have been adhered to in accord with religious rites, though they may also be deeply offended by such practices. The only way to find out is to ask and never assume.

The level of religious ritual which is appropriate for each individual and family from their own culture and faith will vary according to the particular situation. A sensitive search by the professional carer for authenticity in religious expression and a non-judgmental and accepting attitude from the professionals involved can be transformational. Even the most hardened sceptic has found comfort and support from specific rituals and prayers in facing and planning for the future. In the multicultural world in which we live there is often a need to refer to an authoritative source for advice on the different rituals linked to different religions. These may vary considerably in different localities, so seeking guidance from the patient, family, and local faith leaders is important (8).

As well as religious rituals, other rituals may be helpful for patients. It can be important for staff to create a sense of ritual security around the dying where, despite the approach of death, there is the support to allow people to feel accepted and given the space and time to complete the tasks of dying—the fulfilment of their Advance Care Plan.

As C Saunders notes in *The Management of terminal malignant disease*,

'The real presence of another person is a place of security. I recall remarking to two psychiatrists that when patients are in a climate of safety they will come to realise what is happening in their own way and not be afraid. One said: 'How can you speak of a climate of safety when death is the most unsafe thing that can happen?' To which the other replied: 'I think you are using the wrong word. I think it should be "security". A child separated from his mother may be quite safe—but he feels very insecure. A child in his mother's arms during an air raid may be very unsafe indeed—but he feels quite secure.' (9)

Ultimately how the individual copes with their pending death and the process of facing up to the responsibilities and realities of this time through ACP is hard to predict. Speaking of his experiences in the concentration camps in world war two Victor Frankl wrote (10):

> 'Even though conditions such as lack of sleep, insufficient food and various mental stresses may suggest that inmates were bound to react in certain ways, in the final analysis it becomes clear that the sort of person the prisoner became was the result of an inner decision and not the result of camp influence alone.'

The capacity to function in the face of mortality relates in part to the quality of resilience which the individual retains. Some aspects of resilience are connected with genetics, some with upbringing, and the remainder are strengthened or weakened through life events (11). In helping people complete ACPs it is often humbling to observe just how resilient some people are to life and all that it has brought them, in contrast to how lacking in resilience others may appear.

Our role as midwives in the birth of ACPs is not to praise or condemn, but as fellow travellers to help deliver the most authentic declaration of future aspirations from the individual as possible and to foster resilience and hope, in the knowledge that one day we too may need the services of just such a 'soul friend'.

## Acknowledgement

The quotation attributed to Saunders was reproduced from Saunders C, *The Management of Terminal Malignant Disease*, Second Edition, London: Edward Arnold, Copyright © 1984 Taylor and Francis, by permission of Taylor and Francis.

## References

1. **Solomon S, Solomon S, Greenberg J**, and **Pyszczynski T** (1991). 'A Terror management theory of social behavior: The psychological functions of self-esteem and cultural worldviews'. In: Zanna M, (ed.) *Advances in experimental social psychology* **24**, 93–159. Oxford: Academic Press.
2. **Becker E** (1973). *The Denial of Death*. New York: Simon & Schuster.
3. *The future of health and care of older people: the best is yet to come* (1999). London: Age Concern.
4. **AHMAC** (2011). Beauchamp et al. (2001), Australian Health Ministers' Advisory Council.
5. **Advance Care Planning Australia** (2017). Care Quality Commission.
6. **Christina M. Puchalski** (1996), *Making Healthcare Whole: Integrating Spirituality into Patient care*. Washington DC: Templeman Press.
7. **Byock I** (2004). *The Four Things That Matter Most: A book about living*. New York: Free Press.
8. **Emmanuel L** and **Neuberger J** (2004). *Caring for Dying People of Different Faiths*. Oxford: Radcliffe Medical Press.
9. **Saunders C** (1984). *The Management of Terminal Malignant Disease* (2nd edn). London: Edward Arnold.
10. **Frankl V** (1963). *Man's Search for Meaning: An Introduction to Logotherapy*. New York: Washington Square Press.
11. **Watson M** (2007). 'Resilience and the psychobiological base'. In: Monroe B, Oliviere D, (eds) *Resilience in Palliative Care—Achievement In Adversity*. Oxford: Oxford University Press. Pp. 29–38.

## Chapter 7

# Advance care planning: a personal view and stories from the frontline

Tony Bonser

'Why can't they understand that I know my own body,
I know what's happening to me, and I know what I want?'
*An ex-nurse, near death, and wanting her own needs recognised
by the medical professionals*

---

**This chapter includes**

- A personal view of ACP from Tony Bonser, whose son, Neil, died aged 35, and who worked for the National Council for Palliative Care

- Examples from others, including those who have undertaken extra training in end of life care, known as GSF (Gold Standards Framework) in primary care, care homes, and hospitals

- The importance and impact of ACP on people nearing the end of life and their families

- Recommendations that ACP should be mainstreamed across health and social care as part of good practice, and become part of the public debate through movements like Dying Matters

---

**Key Points**

- ACP enables a dialogue to be started
- ACP must be centred on patients and enable the implementation of patient wishes
- ACP will centre on giving advice rather than prescribing outcomes.
- ACP has positive effects
- ACP needs high-level communication skills
- ACP helps restore control
- ACP has societal implications

---

**Key Message**

Truly high-level holistic end of life care can only come about as a result of a partnership between professionals, patients and carers, empowering the patients and carers to take their rightful place in an equal relationship.

# What is advance care planning and what does it involve?

## For myself and my wife Dorothy

The concept of Advance Care Planning (ACP) had not entered our minds until March 2009, the year when our son, Neil, died of a sarcoma aged 35. He had to leave his flat in central Preston because he could no longer look after himself, and we cared for him until he was admitted to hospital. One afternoon we were asked to meet the staff on the ward. We thought we had been invited to a case conference to discuss his future treatment, but when we arrived, a nurse asked Neil, 'Neil, what do you want?' This was our first, very last-minute encounter with ACP, though looking at it with the benefit of hindsight, I wonder if there had been previous discussions with Neil that we knew nothing about. His answer, that he wanted to go home to his flat, filled us with apprehension because we knew that we couldn't look after him, but the following day all had been arranged. He was taken to his flat by ambulance and died there very peacefully that evening. He had been given the control to decide where he wanted to be and who he wanted with him at the end.

It has struck me since that time that this contained, in essence, the two vital elements of ACP: **that a dialogue had been started which established his priorities and values, and that moves were then made to implement them.**

The importance of ACP is highlighted for me by a recent Royal College of Physicians Audit of Deaths in Acute Hospitals, 2016 (Royal College of Physicians, 2016) (1), which found that only 4% of those people who died in acute hospitals had any form of ACP, but where it did exist, it was almost invariably taken into consideration. Of course, two important points should be noted: people have the right to change their minds and not all desires can be met.

### Neil: the person-centred approach and ACP

Our experience during Neil's terminal illness led me to consider what the really important needs are for both those with a potentially life-shortening condition, and their families and carers. Obviously, these are highly individual (and sometimes mutually incompatible) but some guiding principles seem to emerge.

The underlying principle behind ACP must be that patients and carers both want to be treated as individuals. This was emphasised by the Neuberger report, on the Liverpool Care Pathway, 'More Care Less Pathway' (2), which stressed the importance of individual care plans, also emerging in the Leadership Alliance's Guidelines, 'One chance to get it right' (3), and the NICE guidelines (4). ACP was embodied for us in the simple question, 'What do you want?' Not only did this allow Neil to have the peaceful death he would otherwise have been denied, (he had a hatred of hospitals almost amounting to a phobia) but it also leaves us, his family, with a feeling that a least at the end he had a good death.

### Tess: choice and empowerment

I'm reminded too of a woman, Tess, whom my wife took to day care at our local hospice. With spreading cancer, she was well aware that her condition was deteriorating, but her relationship with her consultant was so positive that when he gave her the results of a biopsy, after a sudden decline in her quality of life, he was able to give her the alternatives of surgery or altered medication. He also stressed the potential dangers of both but concluded, 'It's your choice'. Knowing him well enough to realise he feared for her survival through surgery, she chose the medication, which allowed her to enjoy a visit from her son living in New Zealand, before her inevitable but peaceful death in the hospice. Effectively, he gave control back to her, at a time when her quality of life was being compromised.

## Carole: professionals have feelings too

The benefits of ACP can extend beyond the patient and family. Because my wife and I are known, as non-professionals, to be concerned about end of life care, and 'safe' to talk to, we are often approached by people with worries.

Carole, a nursing home carer, telephoned me in considerable distress. Two of her residents had died the preceding week, both having been taken to the local acute hospital after a bank nurse had become alarmed at their deterioration. They both died in hospital, frightened and alone in an alien environment, surrounded by people they didn't know and equipment which was of no use to them. We discussed the problem, but I was unable to come up with a solution. The next month she telephoned me again. The same thing had happened. Two residents had died, but this time in the care home as they wished, surrounded by their families, familiar staff and their cherished possessions. The solution had been simple. The care home had invited all residents to complete an ACP, known as a 'Personal Priorities for Care' document, and essential requests were made known to all staff including bank staff. In each case, their wishes were supported. ACP can, through empowering the patient, access the right outcome not just for patient and family, but for professional carer as well.

## Michelle: I want to be heard

It is not enough just to go through the process of ACP. Someone has to take notice of the documentation. The patient must be assured their wishes will be heard.

I used to drive a very determined woman, Michelle, an ex-nurse, to daycare. She had neglected her own health to care for her husband, who also had cancer, but after his death, the disease soon progressed in her. We helped her fill in her Advance Care Plan, not without some discussion. She was strong-minded but reserved the right to change her mind, which she did several times. 'ACP is a process not an event, and of course only comes into play if the patient is unable to take their own decisions at the time.' However, the discussions leading to the written document can inform the family, carers, GP, and consultant as to the patient's wishes. Michelle was well aware of her physical condition, but wanted to reassure herself that the process of dying would leave her some measure of control, so she asked her GP to visit. When she asked what would happen to her, he laughed it off, telling her, 'You're not going to die. You'll live to be 100.'

She called me in great anger. 'Doesn't he realise I don't want to live to be 100? I just want to know if I can be relatively pain free and can have my friends round me.'

In the end she got what she wanted, but not without a struggle. Assumptions were made about how she 'should' feel and what she 'should' want which bore no relationship to her actual wishes. These assumptions effectively prevented her from discussing her own fears and wishes.

As she lay very close to death in a nursing home, the local GP, not her usual one, decided to admit her to the acute hospital. I was at her bedside, and told him of her stated wish not to die in hospital. 'But it's the right place for her,' he told me.

When I asked why, he said, 'Because that's where people should die.'

I told him she had said she wanted to die in the nursing home.

'She might have changed her mind,' he countered.

'But she has an Advance Care Plan.' I said, waving it at him.

'She might have changed her mind.'

At this point, Michelle opened one eye and just said, 'I'm staying here.' And she did. I feel very happy that she was allowed to end her life where she wanted and deserved. Assumptions had been made, including that she didn't have the capacity to make the decision, (because she seemed to be unconscious) and that the GP's view overrode her wishes. ACP restored to her the control which was so important to her at this final stage of her life.

## Neil: giving the patient choices

Empowering people's decision making also implies that there are choices. Fully to empower someone means giving them choices which they are able to make, on the basis of a fair understanding of the reasons behind the choice. At one stage, Neil was told something of the prognosis of his sarcoma, and invited to say what treatment he would choose. Reasonably, he asked what was available. Being told that the main possible routes were via radiotherapy and chemotherapy, he asked which consultant would recommend. The answer, 'Chemotherapy has never proved to be of any use in these circumstances,' left us all wondering what the point of the conversation was. It certainly did not empower Neil.

## Mark: improving quality of life

Mark was another day-care patient at the hospice. Ex-military, his ramrod-straight back showed a determination which was certainly characteristic of him. He enjoyed life, living in sheltered accommodation with his wife, and going out to social events, and the occasional weekend away. When the quality of his life started to deteriorate, he was prescribes chemotherapy. The side effects were disastrous. He became very tired, lost his appetite and also suffered from incontinence—very challenging to his dignity. So when he failed to respond positively, the consultant suggested a further course of chemotherapy. When I took him to the hospice, he was seriously disturbed. He couldn't contemplate the possibility of reverting to the way of life imposed on him by the side effects. I told him that he had the right to decide whether to accept the procedure. He was fully aware that his life wouldn't be long, and had accepted it, but wanted a decent quality of life for as long as possible. Once told he had the right to refuse, he made the decision, and enjoyed an enhanced quality of life for much of the short time left.

## Neil: giving back control

This ability to take control of decisions made about a patient depends on a genuine conversation, couched in a language register fully comprehensible to the patient, and one which gives the patient a large measure of control. Consistently during Neil's last few weeks of life, medical professionals employed euphemisms, medical terminology, and circumlocutions to avoid telling us he was dying. As a result we chased after more and more 'miracle' cures and even took him on long journeys in fruitless attempts to get him on drug trials which could never have helped him and exhausted both him and us. The mis-communication was typified by a GP who told me at one stage, 'It's not looking too good.' I think he was trying to tell me Neil was dying. What I heard was, 'We haven't found a cure yet, but given time we will.' That's what I wanted to hear. What I actually needed to hear was the unvarnished truth. Of course, not everyone wants or can cope with the truth and again, control lies with the patient. However, I believe the patient and on occasions the carers and family also, have the right to be involved in major decision-making regarding their treatment if that is their wish.

## Neil: resuscitation discussions—do not attempt cardiopulmonary resuscitation

Neil was lying in bed in hospital the week before he died. He had his eyes closed. The consultant came up and told us, 'I think you should know that in the event of a heart attack, we have decided not to attempt to resuscitate Neil.' Then he left. We didn't know a heart attack was likely. What I heard was a negative. There is something we can do but we have decided not to do it. We don't know if Neil heard or even if it had been discussed with him. The recent court case, (Tracey, R v Cambridge University Hospitals NHS Foundation Trust & Ors, Court of Appeal—Civil Division, 24 January 2014, [2014] EWCA Civ 33) resulted in some physicians declaring that they would have to attempt resuscitation in all cases to avoid prosecution, but in fact the ruling maintained the decision-making firmly with the professionals, and re-stated best practice, that it should be explained to those intimately concerned, thus empowering them to understand the decisions made concerning the patient's future. The reaction of the consultant in Neil's case has had profound effects on my wife and me from that time, as we can never now discover whether Neil was party to the decision, or indeed heard us being told. Discussions about DNACPR can be complex and very sensitive, and must be held on the basis that all parties know the facts of the situation, but they are an essential and central part of ACP.

## David and Sacha: the improvement for bereaved parents of fulfilling their child's wishes

David was diagnosed with a brain tumour in 2007 at the age of 11. Over the next five years he endured 20 months of chemotherapy, six weeks of radiotherapy, 11 brain operations and a stem cell transplant. In May 2012, after a scan revealed that his cancer had spread everywhere, the family decided to reject any medication that might prolong his life by a very short time. They opted instead to make the very best of his final few weeks—at home. The family were adamant that they wanted to put a stop to the constant toing and froing to hospital.

David's mother Sacha says that the most important factor in ensuring that her son received good care in his final few weeks at home was the existence of an advance care plan.

'When we took the decision to go for palliative care, that's when we had the ACP discussions,' says Sacha. 'They were never called that, but looking back, that's what they were and they provided the basis for the care.

For us, the worst that thing could happen was that he would end up in hospital. But it was arranged that we would have a red flag against our number so that if we called paramedics they would not take him to hospital.'

Sacha adds: 'You wouldn't want to have a baby without talking to another mother. It is painful talking about death but much less painful than an unplanned death. Having a plan is really liberating and in the end it is the fear that gets you and by planning you are confronting your fears. The consolation of my son having a good death was massive, knowing his wishes and having a plan, ensured this was possible. Ask your GP if they are doing GSF and if not, ask them why not.'

ACP is a key part of GSF, used by thousands of GP practices in the UK. Sacha was fortunate that her GP practice had undertaken further GSF training (Going for Gold) and was accredited with the GSF RCGP Quality Hallmark Award.

## Eddie: compassionate care in care homes

Eddie never went anywhere without his flat cap. Two days after his death in April 2014, his son visited Eastleigh Care Home to collect his belongings, including his cap, as he was keen to have it as a keepsake. The nurse he spoke to informed him that they'd dressed Mr Jay in a jacket and tie and sent him to the undertakers with his cap too—just as he would have wanted.

For his daughter-in-law Alice, this was the final demonstration of the compassionate care that all of the staff at Eastleigh had delivered EJ throughout his four and a half year stay at the Minehead home.

Eddie had been living independently with Alzheimer's, albeit with plenty of support from his family, until he suffered a stroke, aged 85. The family had a clear idea of the sort of home they were looking for.

Alice who has worked in care for years herself, was struck on the first visit by the Gold Standards Framework display in the reception area. But, she wondered, would the home really practise what it preached?

'My father-in-law was a real gentleman and deserved the best possible care. I really hoped it wasn't just a tick-box exercise. We quickly realised that it absolutely wasn't. Very early on the nursing staff initiated conversations with us about what we wanted for my father-in-law and acted on our wishes.'

Staff ensured that Eddie received regular visits from the local clergy with whom the home had close ties. They soon had him delivering the newspapers around the home and filling envelopes in the office too, as it was clear that he wanted to keep busy.

Those discussions held between nursing staff and the family early in Eddie's stay also covered the important question of what to do in case he might need to go to hospital.

Alice adds: 'We made it clear that we didn't think he'd want to go to hospital unless it was absolutely necessary. We wanted Eastleigh to feel like his home and the staff made sure that's exactly what happened. He did have to go into hospital with a sepsis at one point, but the nursing staff at the home made it clear to the hospital that he should be discharged as soon as possible and sure enough he was home in 36 hours.'

### Mrs Davidson: advance care planning enabling dignified dying in a care home

Mrs Davidson, 98, a retired nurse, died at a Somerset care home in May 2015 having lived there for three years. Daughter Anne, who lives close to the home, moved her mother there after she had suffered two strokes and could no longer live independently.

Anne says that at a very early stage staff at the home initiated conversations about the care her mother and the family wanted for her. These conversations were open and ongoing and included Mrs D's final wishes.

As a staunch churchgoer she had made it clear to her daughter and staff in the home that she 'didn't want to be kept going' and they agreed a DNR with the nursing team. Anne says that the conversations were handled in such a way that she was made to feel comfortable discussing the potentially difficult subjects of death and dying.

Anne remembers: The matron and reception staff told us about the Gold Standards Framework very early on and encouraged us to read their leaflets about it. I understood GSF to be about the all-round wellbeing of the residents and the best possible standard of care—not just about their clinical needs. The conversations we had were really well handled—listening and leading.

'I remember when my mother was poorly and we were gathered round her bed with the matron and nurses saying to mum—'do you want to go to hospital?' And she said 'no'—because she knew she was being looked after better there than hospital and she regarded it as her home.

So when, near the end of her life, Mrs Davidson was rushed to hospital, she and her daughter were disappointed, although Anne now reflects that it was unavoidable and was dealt with as sensitively as it possibly could have been.

'She'd had a very serious bleed and there really wasn't any alternative but to call an ambulance and take her to hospital,' Anne adds. 'The lovely thing was that the home made it clear that Mum wanted to go back as soon as possible, so they stabilised her and only kept her in for 48 hours. There was no question of her not coming back to the home—which she regarded as her home.'

Anne says that the home took into account all aspects of the person when caring for Mrs D, not just her clinical needs. 'Care in the final days was absolutely fantastic. They would ask if we were happy with how they were caring for at regular intervals and her dignity was absolutely kept to the end. It was exactly how mum would have wanted it.'

## Individual empowerment and the role of society

The empowerment which can be brought about by ACP depends, of course, on a genuinely meaningful and open dialogue between patient and professionals, and often between patient and family. That dialogue must be characterised by an openness which rises above status differences, and a language which is mutually comprehensible. It must be at the behest of the patient and controlled by them, though sometimes it takes the intervention of a professional to initiate the conversation. It can only begin when the patient is ready to start it, and should only take the course and direction they are happy with. It will only come about fully in our society when a societal shift allows both professionals and the public to accept the need for an open dialogue about matters relating to end of life care. It is precisely this shift which the National Council for Palliative Care and the Dying Matters Coalition are seeking to bring about through the Dying Matters Awareness Week agenda, publications, the encouragement of compassionate communities and training for both professionals and the public.

## Acknowledgement

With acknowledgement to Tom Tanner for contributing examples and stories which have been submitted to the GSF Centre, following GSF training or accreditation.

## Further reading

**Royal College of Physicians**. (2016). *End of Life Care Audit—Dying in Hospital*. London, p. 29.

**J Neuberger** (2013) *More Care Less Pathway*. HMG Department of Health. Report on the use and experience of the Liverpool Care Pathway (LCP).

**Leadership Alliance for the Care of Dying People** (June 2014) *One Chance to Get it Right*. Publications Gateway Reference 01509.

NICE guideline [NG31]. *Care of dying adults in the last days of life*. December 2015.

**Tracey, R** v Cambridge University Hospitals NHS Foundation Trust & Ors, Court of Appeal—Civil Division, January 24, 2014, [2014] EWCA Civ 33.

# Context and experience of advance care planning in the UK

# Chapter 8

# Advance care planning in the UK: update on policy and practice

Claire Henry and Keri Thomas

'All people approaching the end of life need to have their needs assessed and their wishes and preferences discussed and an agreed set of actions reflecting the choices they make about their care recorded in a case plan'
*Department of Health End of Life Care Strategy, 2008*

'The Commitment for end of life care puts the creation of a personalised care plan, based on individual needs and preferences, at the centre of our vision of high quality, personalised care.'
*Department of Health England. Our Commitment to you for end of life care, July 2016*

---

**This chapter includes**

- National and international support for advance care planning (ACP), and its importance in the UK
- Background and update on the national policy context of ACP in England and the UK
- Why is ACP important in end of life care?
- Issues surrounding ACP and some practicalities of implementation
- Examples of good practice, demonstrating increasing use in different settings
- Increasing public awareness and Dying Matters
- Conclusion and next steps

---

**Key Points**

- ACP has been strongly recommended as best practice and widely implemented for many years in the UK as a key part of improving care for people nearing the end of their lives with any condition in any setting

- ◆ ACP is supported by national policy, by Government bodies, Royal Colleges, by third sector organisations and as part of many local end of life care strategies
- ◆ The UK Mental Capacity Act 2005 had a major impact in clarifying the importance, practicalities and regulatory framework within which ACP sits (see Chapter 11)
- ◆ ACP was a key part of the 2004 NHS End of Life Care Programme and 2008 EOLC Strategy, recommended in NICE Guidance and England's Ambitions for Palliative and End of Life Care 2015, with many resources available
- ◆ ACP therefore is widely used and adopted in all settings in the UK, as illustrated with some examples in practice at the frontline, including those teams completing GSF Training and accreditation
- ◆ There has been good progress with ACP in the UK, with widespread uptake across many settings, affirmation of its importance and national support from Government, national policy, and regulators (Care Quality Commission, General Medical Council etc.). However there is some evidence that progress in the UK has slipped compared with the degree of national momentum developed in other countries, and there is still much to do etc.

**Key Message**

The UK has made significant progress and was an early adopter of ACP nationally, and with national policy support, ACP has been widely recommended, developed and adopted in all settings. There are numerous examples of good practice across the country and great integration of ACP into standard practice has been made especially in care homes, primary care and through electronic transfer of information. However there is more work to do: despite this central endorsement and support, further work is required to raise the profile and uptake within the general public, with commissioners, regulators and with care providers in all settings, through enhanced training and information transfer, for ACP and person-centred care to become part of normal life and mainstream practice in the UK.

## National and international support for advance care planning—the case for offering advance care planning discussions in every setting

There is a growing international movement sweeping across the world that recognises advance care planning (ACP) as a means of ensuring people receive care aligned to their wishes and preferences as they near the end of their life, whilst also reducing unwanted interventions or the potential for 'too much medicine' in this important last stage of life, (as in the *BMJ* Too Much Medicine comments and citations (1).) This is demonstrated by strong and growing body of research evidence (Chapters 2, 4, 14, 27), by the work of the International Society for Advance Care Planning (ACPEL) launched in 2010 with ongoing biannual international conferences attended by hundreds of delegates from over 40 countries (2) and by the demonstrable progress of growing national movements in other countries, some included in this book (Chapters 18–23).

## Background and update on the national policy context of advance care planning in England and the UK

In England, as in other parts of the world, ACP is becoming increasingly important as a means to improve care for all people nearing the end of life. Back in 2004, the UK NHS End of Life Care

Programme recommended and successfully disseminated use of three 'tools' or 'models of best practice' in end of life care for ACP (e.g. Preferred Priorities of Care or other local ACP models), care in the final year/s of life (e.g. The Gold Standards Framework) and care in the final days of life (e.g. Liverpool Care Pathway) (3). The Department of Health End of Life Care (EoLC) Strategy published in 2008, provided England's first comprehensive framework aimed at promoting high quality care for all adults approaching the end of life in all care settings (4). Since then, the importance of ACP has been reaffirmed by most major policy groups and most recently in England by the cross-system Ambitions for Palliative and End of Life Care (5) and the Government's response to the Choice Review 'Our Commitment to you for end of life care' July 2016 (6) (see Boxes 8.1–2, Table 8.1). Support for the uptake of ACP and development of excellent localised resources is also mirrored in the other nations of Wales, (7) Scotland, (8) and Northern Ireland (9) with considerable progress made in each nation.

Advance Care Planning, initially defined by an ACP subgroup of the End of Life Care Programme (18), is also recommended and supported by many national organisations providing guidance, teaching and resources, as noted and referenced in Box 8.1. These include regulators, Care Quality Commission, General Medical Council, and also Royal Colleges (Royal College of General Practitioners (RCGP) (19), with a recent position paper on palliative and end of life care 2016 (20) Royal College of Physicians (RCP) (21), Royal College of Nursing (22), by third sector organisations (National Council for Palliative Care (23), Dying Matters (24),The Gold Standards Framework Centre (25), Macmillan Cancer Support (26), Marie Curie (27), Compassion in Dying (28), etc.) and as part of many localised end of life care strategies.

Examples of useful resources are suggested at the end of the chapter an in the Appendix, including a guidance leaflet for patients and their families 'Planning your Future Care' (29) and guidance on 'Finding the Words' (30).

**Table 8.1** Our Commitment to you for end of life care The Government Response to the Review of Choice in End of Life Care, Department of Health, July 2016 (5)

| Statement of Commitment | Choice Review advice text | Details of actions in response |
| --- | --- | --- |
| . . . **The Commitment for end of life care puts the creation of a personalised care plan, based on individual needs and preferences, at the centre of our vision of high quality, personalised care.** | Each person who may be in need of end of life care is offered choices in their care focused on what is important to them and that this offer is:<br>◆ Made as soon as is practicable after it is recognised that the person may die in the foreseeable future<br>◆ Based on honest conversations with health and care staff, which supports the person to make informed choices<br>◆ Consistently reviewed through conversations with health and care staff | Our Commitment for end of life care makes clear what every person should expect in their care as they approach the end of life. This means that everyone who wants to have honest discussions and develop a personalised care plan based on their preferences will be supported to do so. This plan will also be shared with others to enable joined up care. The Commitment also makes clear that the people important to the dying person will be involved in their care as much as the person would want and that there will be access to support whenever needed |

## Box 8.1  Policy publications on advance care planning in England

- 2004 National Institute for Health and Clinical Excellence (NICE) *Guidance: Improving supportive and palliative care for adults with cancer* (10)
- 2005 and 2007 Mental Capacity Act 2005 *Code of Practice* (11)
- 2008 NHS *End of Life Care Strategy* (4)
- 2009 National Audit Office *Report on End of Life Care* (12)
- 2009 General Medical Council (GMC) *Guidance, Treatment and care towards the end of life* (13)
- 2011 NICE Guidance—*End of Life Care for adults—quality standards* (14)
- 2015 NICE *Ambitions for Palliative and End of Life care* iv
- 2015 NICE Guidance—*Care of Dying Adults in the last days of life* (15)
- 2016 Care Quality Commission (CQC) *Thematic Review in End of Life care—A different Ending* (16)
- 2016 Department of Health *Our Commitment to you for end of life care The Government Response to the Review of Choice in End of Life Care* v
- 2016 Health Education England *Core Competency Framework for EOLC* (17)

## Why is advance care planning important in end of life care?

About 1% of the population die each year, or half a million people in England with about half of those deaths occurring in NHS hospitals. This contrasts greatly with the situation a century ago when most deaths occurred at home. As a result of these changes, society as a whole is less familiar with the events surrounding death and less open to discussions about death and dying. For many the common factors in attaining a 'good death', have been found to be (31):

- Being treated as an individual, with dignity and respect, with sensitive communication
- Being without pain and other symptoms
- Being in familiar surroundings
- Being in the company of close friends and family
- Being involved in the decision-making process

ACP is a key part of this process if needs and preferences are to be met. The ACP discussion should be recorded and key elements of communicated so that every service involved in supporting the individual will be aware of their priorities, preferences and choices which will be taken into account and accommodated wherever possible. This is now further enhanced with the use of digital records or Electronic Palliative care Coordination Systems or EPACCs (32), ensuring smoother exchange of information across settings and thereby better understanding pf peoples' wishes if they are unable to speak for themselves.

For some the outcome of an ACP discussion may be a general statement of wishes and preferences about what is important to them about how they are cared for or where they wish to die. Others may wish to be more specific about future plans by taking the decision to make an advance decision to refuse treatment or refusal of resuscitation.

# Issues surrounding advance care planning some practicalities of implementation

## Definition

There was a requirement to clarify commonly used terms and agree definitions. This was achieved whilst undertaking a review of the ACP process which then led to the production of a guidance document by the NHS End of Life Care Programme *Advance Care Planning: A Guide for Health and Social Care Staff* (2007) (33). The final definition of ACP—together with other key issues such as an advance decision and statement of wishes and preferences—was agreed by a working party of clinicians and academics. It was emphasised that ACP is a process of discussion between an individual and their care provider and the process is more important than the specific tool used. Outputs include: a statement of wishes and preferences, an advance decision to refuse treatment (ADRT), and a named advocate or LPOA. This can assist decisions in anticipation of loss of mental capacity but this is not the only benefit of these discussions- in addition they can enable the last stage of life to be as fulfilled and aligned to a person's wishes and preferences as possible. However there is still debate amongst some about the significance of ACPs being mainly related to loss of capacity—this was the way that many countries began but many are moving away from this rather medicalised model to the more personal discussion—as explored in Chapters 1, 4, 13, and 14.

The term 'personalised care planning' is also used in some policy documentation to include ACP as a component, or with frail elderly as 'Care and Support Planning' and in other places such as Scotland it can be known as 'anticipatory care planning'. Other additional outputs are possible (e.g. Treatment Escalation Plans/ Ceilings of Care) which can guide the decisions about the limits of medical intervention and are generally considered to be more clinically focussed, rather than seeking a person's broader non-medical wishes and preferences. In other countries however these examples of limits of medical intervention were the basis of the development of ACPs as we know them now (see Chapter 20).

## Principles/process

It is important to remember that this is a voluntary process. No pressure should be brought to bear. In addition the content of any discussion should be determined by the individual concerned. All health and social care professionals should be open to any discussion which may be instigated by an individual and know how to respond to their questions. They should only instigate the discussion if they have made a professional judgment that the ACP process is likely to benefit the individual's care. There is a need to offer regular reviews as part of an ongoing discussion that can change with changing circumstances.

Discussion should focus on the views of the individual although they may wish to invite their carer or another close family member or friend to participate. Some families are likely to have discussed preferences and would welcome an approach to share this discussion. Confidentiality should always be respected.

It should also be borne in mind that ACP requires that the individual has the capacity to understand, discuss options available, and agree to what is then planned (see Chapter 11 on MCA). Health and social care professionals should also be aware of, and give a realistic account of, the support, services, and choices available in the particular circumstances. Should an individual wish to make a decision to refuse treatment (advance decision) this should be documented according to the requirements of the MCA 2005. Finally, professionals need to be aware

> ## Box 8.2  Advance/Personalised Care Planning 'Ambitions for Palliative and End of Life Care: a national framework for local action', 2015–2022 published 2014 (4)
>
> **Personalised care planning** 'Everyone approaching the end of life should be offered the chance to create a personalised care plan. Many people with long term conditions or complex needs will already have a care plan and this should be updated to reflect their changing needs. Although participation must be voluntary, the opportunity for informed discussion and planning should be universal. These discussions should be between the person nearing the end of life, those important to them (as they wish) and their professional carers.
>
> The potential elements of the plan should be broad. It should allow people to express their preferences for care and set personal goals for the time they have left. The offer should include the possibility of recording preferences that might guide others if the person were to lose the mental capacity to make their own decisions (advance care planning). However, the offer should also encompass the chance to appoint a person with lasting powers of attorney or allow the person to trust their professional carers to act in their best interests. Such conversations must be ongoing with options regularly reviewed, revisited and revised.'
>
> Reprinted from National Palliative and End of Life Care Partnership, 'Ambitions for Palliative and End of Life Care: A national framework for local action, 2015–2022', Copyright © 2014 Ambitions for Palliative and End of Life Care, www.endoflifecareambitions.org.uk. Reprinted with permission from Hospice UK, which has now merged with the NCPC.

when they have reached the limits of their knowledge and competence and know when to seek advice.

## Examples of good practice, demonstrating its widespread use in all settings

Many examples of good practice and integration of ACP exist across the country. We conducted a survey at The GSF Centre (Nov 2016) seeking examples of use of ACP from the frontline, those we have come across and some examples from GSF Accredited teams in care homes, primary care and hospitals that have progressed to GSF Accreditation and the Quality Hallmark Award. Offering ACP to every appropriate person (often proactively identified on a database or register or flagged on their notes) by their chosen or usual health or social care provider and integrating this into communication, regular reviews and audits, is a key part of GSF teaching and assessment for accreditation. Many more examples exist no doubt, but this small sample demonstrates the extent of actual implementation in different areas and settings in the UK, though we are also aware that more is needed, especially in the uptake of the public awareness and initiation of ACPs by lay people rather than health or social care professionals (Table 8.2).

## Dying Matters—raising public awareness

Dying Matters is a coalition of thousands of members across England and Wales which aims to help people talk more openly about dying, death and bereavement, and to make plans for the end

**Table 8.2** Examples of good practice of use of ACP at the frontline

| Area | Examples in practice |
|---|---|
| Developing local public awareness | 'We have run about 20 ACP workshops for the public over the past 2 years, free of charge, café style sessions and interactive where we teach them about the importance of having plans in place, and of completing the forms with their GP. We organised an open day in the village hall on 'matters of life and death'—around 150 people attended . . . with 14 stalls, sessions/presentations from funeral directors, solicitors, Age UK, befriending services, hospice, carers OXON, organ donation, bereavement support etc.'<br>*GP Dr EK Oxfordshire* |
| Area-wide— county | 'Use of a County wide ACP document together with clinicians guidance, available on the EPACCs website. www.EPACCs.com, that is being used increasingly in hospitals and the community.'<br>*Dr JB GP and EOLC Lead Nottingham* |
| Area-wide— whole island | 'Jersey has developed an island-wide ACP document approved by all stakeholder groups and led by Jersey Hospice. Following GSF training in all settings (hospital, care homes, primary care etc.) this is offered to identified patients. Increasing numbers of people are completing this and bringing it with them to GP or hospital appointments, enabling their choices and preferences to steer the kind of care provided. A whole-island approach is helping ensure a positive uptake, making a real difference for patients.'<br>*Feedback to GSF team from Facilitators Jersey* |
| Care Homes | 'Every resident is offered the opportunity to complete an ACP within 28 days of admission. These are all reviewed regularly with the resident and we ensure if a resident is admitted to hospital or moved to a new location a copy of their ACP goes with them to ensure continuity of care.<br>We use the GSF ACP tool and have found this beneficial to all the residents.'<br>*CL Milton Keynes GSF Accredited Care Home* |
| Hospital | 'GSF has really helped us ... in improving our coordination and communication. For patients, this means we now engage in more detailed conversations with them about the care they want and where they want to receive it and share these wishes with our health colleagues in the community, which means everyone is working in unison.'<br>*PB Ward Sister Community Hospital Cornwall GSF Accredited Community Hospital*<br>'I think the biggest change has been the culture change ... it's about getting patients and their families to take ownership of their care. GSF is the framework that allows us to make that happen. The best bit is making sure that patients receive the care they want, where they want it, when and how they want it and the satisfaction they and we get from that.'<br>*Dr K, Consultant Royal Lancaster Infirmary GSF Accredited ward* |
| GP Practice | 'GSF training helped us realise that these conversations with our patients were about getting to the heart of what people really want as they approach the end of their lives. Now we view these discussions as very rewarding as they provide the framework for giving patients what they want and deserve.'<br>*Dr LP Birmingham Accredited Practice 2016*<br>'This training has really helped us to have a good structure in place and given everyone in the practice the confidence to initiate what can be difficult conversations with people about where and how they want to be cared for and that means everyone feels more in control.'<br>*Dr SG GP Derbyshire GSF Accredited practice 2014* |
| Hospice | 'We run a 14-week programme for patients with COPD and Heart Failure. We have incorporated a session on advance care planning within the programme.'<br>*TG Lakelands Day Hospice, twice GSF Accredited Corby* |

(continued)

**Table 8.2** Continued

| Area | Examples in practice |
| --- | --- |
| Domiciliary care | 'People might not realise how well Advance Care Planning fits in to the domiciliary care setting and yet it is one of the most natural conversations- our homecare workers become very close to clients over time and can have easy discussions as they do their daily tasks. Now we are able to help them record their wishes and relay this information to others, which gives our clients a louder voice and gives us greater pride in our work.' <br> *Domiciliary Care Trainer following GSF training* |
| Prisons | 'Yes, it's a prison environment but we do what we can to fulfil prisoners' wishes while of course remembering the environment within which we work. The prisoners are given the opportunity to express their preferences in an advance care plan. Most refuse the offer of compassionate release because they know the care here is second to none and they regard this as their home.' <br> *SR Lead Nurse HMP Norwich Prison GSF Accredited 2016* |
| Volunteer groups | 'We train Age UK volunteers/ navigators to go on the wards and have ACP discussions with patients, once they have been identified. The response has been 100% positive so far and more patients are able to have these discussions, which helps us and their GPs know their wishes and choices.' <br> *GSF Lead– Barking Havering and Redbridge Hospital and Local Age UK* |

Reproduced courtesy of the Gold Standards Framework Centre www.goldstandardsframework.org.uk. Source: data from the Gold Standards Framework's National Survey for teams progressing to GSF Accreditation in different settings, run by GSF Centre in November 2016.

of life. The Coalition's Mission is to help people talk more openly about dying, death, and bereavement, and to make plans for the end of life. This will involve a fundamental change in society in which dying, death, and bereavement will be seen and accepted as the natural part of everybody's life cycle.

Changes in the way society views dying and death have impacted on the experience of people who are dying and bereaved. Our lack of openness has affected the quality and range of support and care services available to patients and families. It has also affected our ability to die where or how we would wish. The Dying Matters Coalition is working to address this by encouraging people to talk about their wishes towards the end of their lives, including where they want to die and their funeral plans with friends, family and loved ones. There are numerous freely downloadable resources for the annual Dying Matters week, held in May each year, involving thousands of people taking part in local events. Each year a new theme is launched these have include the big conversation, talk, plan live and what can you do? ACP is always a feature as Dying Matter have found that more people have written and will (35% ComRes survey 2016) than have written down there wishes and preferences (7% ComRes survey 2016). However, the survey has also shown that more people are talking about death dying and bereavement but we now need to see people taking action and writing and then storing their wishes so that they can be shared when needed. Dying Matters members have engaged many practical ways with members of the public from market stalls, death cafes, art exhibitions and plays. Gentle dusk is an example of successful volunteer training in London (34). For further examples see the Dying Matters website www.dyingmatters.org.

However these types of campaigns need funding which can be challenging with all the pressure on health and care services.

# Conclusion and next steps

There is widespread adoption and uptake of ACP in the UK and, supported by national policy initiatives over the last 15 years, it has become part of recognised good practice in many areas. The UK was an early adopter of ACP nationally, and through NHS and Government policy support ACP is widely recommended, developed and adopted, with numerous examples of good practice currently across the country.

However, there has been some are of the opinion that the UK has lost ground in this area over recent years. Much more work is needed in the UK to further raise public awareness and uptake, to mainstream systematically in all settings and to improve effective information transfer to other care providers, so that ACP can be become part of normal mainstream practice throughout the UK.

## Acknowledgements

With acknowledgment and thanks to Prof Bee Wee, England Department of Health Clinical Director for End of Life Care, for her help in checking and making useful suggestions in this chapter.

## References

1. **Godlee F** (2015). 'Too much medicine'. Editor's Choice *BMJ* **350**: h1217. http://www.bmj.com/content/350/bmj.h1217

2. **International Society for Advance Care Planning and End of Life Care (ACPEL)** (2017). Available from: https://www.acpel2017.org/

3. https://www.nottingham.ac.uk/research/groups/ncare/projects/nhs-end-life.aspx

4. **Department of Health** (July 2008). *End of Life Care Strategy: promoting high quality care for all adults at the end of life*, DH, London.

5. **NHS England** (2015). *Ambitions for Palliative and End of life care.* Available from: http://endoflifecareambitions.org.uk/

6. **Department of Health England** (2016). *Our Commitment to you for end of life care.* Available from: https://www.gov.uk/government/uploads/system/uploads/attachment_data/file/536326/choice-response.pdf

7. **IPADS Palliative Care, Wales** (2015). *A Framework for Advance care Planning in Wales.* Available from: http://wales.pallcare.info/index.php?p=sections&sid=68

8. **Good Life Good Death**. *Making an Anticipatory Care Plan Good Life Good Death Good Grief* (2010). Available from: https://www.goodlifedeathgrief.org.uk/content/anticipatory_care_plan/

9. **Transforming your Care Northern Ireland Health and Social care**. Available from: http://www.transformingyourcare.hscni.net/?s=advance+care+planning+

10. **National Institute for Health Clinical Excellence** (March 2004). *Supportive and Palliative Care Guidance*, NICE, London.

11. **Ministry of Justice** (April 2007). *Mental Capacity Act 2005 Code of Practice*, Ministry of Justice, London.

12. **National Audit Office** (November 2008). *End of Life Care*, National Audit Office, London.

13. **General Medical Council** (2016). *Treatment and care towards the end of life.* Available from: http://www.gmc-uk.org/guidance/ethical_guidance/end_of_life_care.asp

14. **National Institute for Health and care Excellence (NICE)** (2015). *End of Life care for Adults.* Available from: https://www.nice.org.uk/guidance/qs13

15. **X1v National Institute for Health and care Excellence (NICE)** (31 Dec 2015). *Care of Dying Adults in the last days of life.* Available from: https://www.nice.org.uk/guidance/ng

16. **Care Quality Commission** (2016). *End of life care: A different Ending.* Available from: http://www.cqc. org.uk/content/different-ending-our-review-looking-end-life-care-published

17. **Health Education England End of life care** (2016). Available from: https://hee.nhs.uk/sites/default/files/ documents/Care%20Navigation%20Competency%20Framework_Final.pdf

18. **NHS National End of Life Care Programme** (revised 2008). *Advance Care Planning: A Guide for Health and Social Care Staff.* London.

19. **Royal College of GPs** (2005). *EOLC Strategy.* Available from: https://www.google.co.uk/ webhp?sourceid=chrome-instant&ion=1&espv=2&ie=UTF-8#q=RCGP+End+of+Life+care+Advance+ care+Planning&*

20. **Royal College of General Practitioners.** *Position Statement on Palliative and End of Life care.* Available from: http://www.rcgp.org.uk/endoflifecare

21. **Royal College of Physicians** (2009). *Advance care Planning Concise Guidance.* Available from: https:// www.rcplondon.ac.uk/guidelines-policy/advance-care-planning

22. **Getting it right every time – advance care planning** (2015). Available from: http://rcnendoflife.org.uk/ the-patient-journey/advanced-care-planning/

23. **National Council for Palliative care** (2015). Available from: http://www.ncpc.org.uk/ planning-and-capacity

24. **NCPC** (2011). *Dying Matters – raising awareness of dying death and bereavement.* Available from: http:// www.dyingmatters.org/

25. **The Gold Standards Framework Centre Advance Care Planning** (2013). Available from: http://www. goldstandardsframework.org.uk/advance-care-planning

26. **Macmillan Cancer Support.** *Advance care Planning.* Available from: http://www.macmillan. org.uk/cancerinformation/livingwithandaftercancer/advancedcancer/advancecareplanning/ advancecareplanning.aspx

27. **Marie Curie** (Oct 2014). *Planning your care in Advance.* Available from: https://www.mariecurie.org.uk/ help/terminal-illness/planning-ahead/advance-care-planning

28. **Compassion in Dying Supporting your choices** (2015). Available from: http://compassionindying.org. uk/

29. **NHS National End of Life Care Programme** (March 2009). *Planning for Your Future Care–a guide,* London. Available from: http://www.ncpc.org.uk/publication/planning-your-future-care

30. **NHS National Health End of Life Care Programme.** Available from: http://endoflifecareambitions.org. uk/wp-content/uploads/2016/09/finding_the_words_workbook_web_1.pdf

31. **NHS England** (June 2014). *One Chance to Get it Right.* Available from: https://www.england.nhs.uk/ ourwork/qual-clin-lead/lac/

32. **Petrova M, Riley J, Abel J,** et al. (2016). 'Crash course in EPACCs (Electronic Palliative Care Coordination Systems): 8 years of successes and failures in patient data sharing to learn from'. *BMJ Supportive & Palliative Care* Published Online First. doi: 10.1136/bmjspcare-2015-001059.

33. **NHS National End of Life Care Programme** (revised 2008). *Advance Care Planning: A Guide for Health and Social Care Staff,* London.

34. **Gentle Dusk.** *Gentle Dusk.* Available from: http://www.gentledusk.org.uk/

## Chapter 9

# Advance decisions to refuse treatment and the impact of wider legislation

Ben Lobo

---

**This chapter includes**

- ◆ Background to advance decisions and care planning for end of life
- ◆ Specific context: English law, society, and culture
  - Mental Capacity Act 2005
- ◆ Explores aspects of the impact of legislation in England and Wales
  - Advance decisions to refuse treatment (ADRTs), Lasting Power of Attorney, and Deprivation of Liberty Safeguards
  - Office of the Public Guardian
  - Court of Protection
    - Capacity and best interests life-sustaining treatment decisions
- ◆ Related topics
  - Advance decisions to refuse treatment and children
  - Decisions relating to cardiopulmonary resuscitation
  - Assisted suicide, legal case challenges and reform
- ◆ Moving forwards

---

**Key Points**

- ◆ The public have increased awareness and expectations of about 'achieving a good death'
- ◆ Advance treatment decisions including refusals can be an important part of an advance care plan (ACP)
- ◆ People in England and Wales can make legally binding refusals of even life sustaining treatment
- ◆ Professionals must ensure that advance decisions exist, be valid and applicable to the circumstances they were intended for.
- ◆ ADRT/ACP must be supported by good clinical practice, professional development, and service redesign

---

**Key Message**

ADRT taken in context of ACP for the end of life is a component of a national strategy to improve services for people to help ensure a good death with dignity and privacy.

## Introduction

People might make a variety of advance decisions that might apply to a range of issues about their health, welfare, finances, or other person matters. This chapter concentrates on the advance refusal of treatment. The chapter describes in part the impact of current legislation and introduces aspects of legal reform.

## Background to advance decisions and care planning for end of life

Most people, especially those living with challenging physical or mental health illnesses, value above all being listened to. It is the first and most important part of the caring relationship and critical to offering personalised care. 'Failure to listen' is one of the most common causes of complaints and errors in healthcare systems.

In the context of advance care planning (ACP) it is paramount we respect the autonomy of the 'Decision Maker' by first listening well and then supporting their preferences and decisions. This must be done using the principles of good clinical practice and professionalism. In the UK the NHS and social care promote personalised care, the offer of choice, the maintenance of privacy and dignity, and they ensuring that services are safe and effective. Our society and the law confirm our right to consent to or refuse treatment and care. Consent for treatment and care cannot be given if the person has lost mental capacity to make that specific decision. Advance decisions to refuse treatment (ADRT) and advance care plans help in such circumstances to ensure the right person-centred outcome.

ACP has already been defined (1). The discussion may help both the person and care providers to have a better and mutual understanding, and lead to:

◆ An advance statement—a record of values and preferences

◆ An advance decision to refuse treatment, ADRT

◆ The appointment of a Lasting Power of Attorney (LPA) (can be a nominated representative for health and welfare)

It must be clearly understood that in English law a patient cannot demand a doctor to give a treatment that is unlawful or futile; especially those treatments that would be considered as assisted suicide and bring about an unnatural death.

## What is an advance decision to refuse treatment?

Some people may decide that they wish to make sure that they do not receive specific treatment(s) at some future time and an ADRT is defined as 'a specific refusal of treatment(s) in a predefined potential future situation'. The MCA enables them to make an advance decision to refuse specific treatment in the future when they have lost capacity to make their own decision.

Such an advance decision will be legally binding on the person's healthcare professionals, if all the requirements of the MCA have been met 'at the time that the decision needs to be taken'. An advance decision to refuse treatment that complies with all the MCA's requirements will be as valid as a refusal of treatment by a competent patient, and must be respected in the same way.

Please note that terms like 'living wills' and 'advance directives' have been superseded in English law and for the rest of the chapter the term advance decisions to refuse treatment (ADRT) is used.

There is growth in the process of ACP in the UK but it still not established in all care settings and performed to the same standard. However, with legislation in the form of the Mental Capacity Act (2), and NHS initiatives aimed at increasing uptake of ACP (1), it is likely that health and social care professionals will be faced more and more frequently with ACP opportunities and challenges. The implementation of ADRT and ACP needs to be contextualised to the health and social care systems and law.

Whilst disputes between patients and clinicians are likely to be rare, the right of a patient or his family to demand or direct treatment should not be regarded as absolute. Instead, the scope for arguing that a patient would have considered a treatment intolerable will be checked by objective consideration as to whether such treatment would be humiliating, debasing, or lacking respect for the patient's dignity so as to breach of Article 3, if permitted (7).

Significantly, the decision in Burke (3) may encourage more patients to express wishes about their medical treatment in advance. Inherently the problem remains that many treatments are not neutral and ideas as to merits and personal best interests clearly shift depending on the type of illness suffered, the prospects of recovery, or perceived closeness to death. There are safeguards in place: the maker can always change or cancel an ADRT if they retain capacity—they may subsequently donate the specific treatment decision powers to an LPA—the ADRT may not be deemed to be valid and applicable by the clinician at the time of the relevant decision, and where there are unresolved concerns and time permits application to the Court of Protection can be made. Some ADRTs may therefore be open to question at the critical moment and may not be legally binding. They should however provide an insight into the maker at the time the ADRT was made and provide some evidence to establish preferences or statements.

US legislation also requires that all individuals admitted to a care home are offered ACP. Preferences are less likely to change if they have been discussed with a doctor (4). Even so, up to one-third of individuals will change their Advance Care Plan over time (months–years), influenced by changes in diagnosis, hospitalisation, mood, health status, social circumstances, and functional ability (5,6).

There is no good evidence that the completion of an ADRT leads to the denial of appropriate healthcare (7,8,9,10,11,12,13) or increases mortality (8,14,15,16).

## Specific context: English law, society, and culture

Healthcare staff must understand and implement the law relating to advance decisions to refuse treatment presented by the Mental Capacity Act (MCA) 2005. The MCA came into force in 2007. It is supported by a Code of Practice: Chapter 9 of the Code relates to advance decisions. Everyone must comply with the requirements of the Act and Code.

The legislative framework for advance decisions to refuse treatment is complex. In 2008 the National Council for Palliative Care and the national End of Life Care Programme published a guide on Advance Decisions to Refuse Treatment. This guidance helps to clarify the law for health and social care professionals and to offer additional practical information to enable them to support people who may choose to consider making an ADRT. An ADRT meets all the requirements of the Act will be legally binding, see (Box 9.1).

The person making an ADRT must take account of the following formalities:

◆ Specify the treatment even if they use layman's language

◆ Specify the circumstances in which they want the refusal to apply, unless they want the refusal to apply in all circumstances. Some people may wish to refuse a particular treatment in all circumstances, for example because of religious or ethical objections, or because of allergy. Many people however will wish to refuse a treatment in some circumstances, but not others. If they specify any circumstances, these must exist at the time the decision for the decision to be legally binding

People should be very careful to be clear about the circumstances in which they want to refuse a particular treatment. For example, a person with Motor Neuron Disease might decide that they

## Box 9.1  A quick summary of the Mental Capacity Act (2005) code of practice: advance decisions to refuse treatment

- An advance decision enables someone aged 18 and over, while still capable, to refuse specified medical treatment for a time in the future when they may lack the capacity to consent to or refuse that treatment

- An advance decision to refuse treatment must be valid and applicable to current circumstances. If it is, it has the same effect as a decision that is made by a person with capacity: healthcare professionals must follow the decision

- Healthcare professionals will be protected from liability if they:
  - Stop or withhold treatment because they reasonably believe that an advance decision exists, and that it is valid and applicable
  - Treat a person because, having taken all practical and appropriate steps to find out if the person has made an advance decision to refuse treatment, they do not know or are not satisfied that a valid and applicable advance decision exists

- People can only make an advance decision under the Act if they are 18 or over and have the capacity to make the decision. They must say what treatment they want to refuse, and they can cancel their decision—or part of it—at any time

- If the advance decision refuses life-sustaining treatment, it must:
  - Be in writing (it can be written by someone else or recorded in healthcare notes)
  - Be signed and witnessed
  - State clearly that the decision applies even if life is at risk

- To establish whether an advance decision is valid and applicable, healthcare professionals must try to find out if the person:
  - Has done anything that clearly goes against their advance decision
  - Has withdrawn their decision
  - Has subsequently conferred the power to make that decision on an attorney, or
  - Would have changed their decision if they had known more about the current circumstances

- Sometimes healthcare professionals will conclude that an advance decision does not exist, is not valid and/or applicable, but that it is an expression of the person's wishes. The healthcare professional must then consider what is set out in the advance decision as an expression of previous wishes when working out the person's best interests (see Code of Practice, Chapter 5)

- Some healthcare professionals may disagree in principle with patients' decisions to refuse life-sustaining treatment. They do not have to act against their beliefs. But they must not simply abandon patients or act in a way that that affects their care

- Advance decisions to refuse treatment for mental disorder may not apply if the person who made the advance decision is or is liable to be detained under the Mental Health Act 1983

wish to refuse antibiotics in the event of a chest infection, but not if they had a urinary tract infection. If so, the advance decision should specify that antibiotics are being refused on one circumstance but not the other. This makes ADRTs quite distinct from other aspects of ACP. The latter may include requests or other statements of wishes about future care and treatment. Such statements of values, wishes, priorities, or preferences about what is to be done should the person lose capacity at some point in the future must be taken into account as part of an overall best interests assessment but are not legally binding.

This guidance states the legal requirements necessary for any advance decision to exist (in an appropriate form) be valid and applicable and provides commentary to help with the sometimes difficult task of assessing whether or not an advance decision is binding. It will often be helpful for the person to discuss their advance decision with a healthcare professional. If necessary this professional may give advice or support during this process about how to make the ADRT. This may also be an opportunity to discuss other aspects of the person's future care and treatment. It is really important that the person who has made an ADRT communicates this to relevant people and organisations to ensure that its existence is known and for professionals to check the validity and applicability when it becomes active (see Table 9.1).

Table 9.1 simplifies the overall process of identifying the need, making, implementing, and evaluating the outcome of an ADRT. This might not be the case for many people involved in making an ADRT. It does, however demonstrate there are number of important factors that can influence the decision. It doesn't however explain that the maker can change their decision as many times as they like, even making unwise decisions. Generating uncertainty does impact on whether the professional will be satisfied that it is binding.

## From statute to choice but what are the realities of this responsibility?

### Personal responsibility

The Act and Code of Practice clearly define that the responsibility for making an advance decision lies with the person making it. The person retains the right to make an advance decision even if

**Table 9.1** The overall process of identifying the need, making, implementing, and evaluating the outcome of an ADRT

| Process | Comment |
| --- | --- |
| Patient/Person ⇩ | Often best supported by a key worker which might include the generalist or a specialist professional either at home/community, in hospital/hospice or another environment e.g. care home |
| Trigger ⇩ | This might be a routine review, new diagnosis, bereavement, admission to hospital, or other assessment |
| Process of preparing ADRT ⇩ | Help and specific resources might be required to write the ADRT to ensure that it is valid and applicable |
| Implementation and Dissemination of ADRT ⇩ | Telling people and organisations might be a challenge. Patients might require support |
| Reviews ⇩ | This might be planned or triggered by an event or change in circumstances (e.g. the advent of a new treatment) |
| Outcomes ⇩ | This is difficult to measure unless there is shared information across care pathways |

it appears unwise and if valid and applicable it must be acted upon. For most people the process that leads up to making the decision requires the careful balance of both benefits and risks. Again it must be stressed that ethical dilemmas, cultural sensitivities, and society can play a significant role. Simple stipulations from patients can bring about tremendous personal and or professional stress, 'This is my (valid and applicable) ADRT. Don't tell the wife!' Confidentiality (and limits placed on it) must be maintained even if the decision might be considered as 'unwise'.

---

### Case study

P has progressive and distressing symptoms because of her motor neuron disease. P understands that her prognosis is poor and she will potentially require help with her breathing and artificial nutrition and may lose capacity at any stage to make such a decision. P has discussed the situation with her husband. P does not want her life to be extended by the use of specific treatments including cardiopulmonary resuscitation or artificial ventilation or feeding. She writes her ADRT with the support of her key worker. She checks that her ADRT meets the legal requirements. She asks her key worker for help to tell local health professionals including the ambulance service.

P was reassured that she has made this decision. Ps husband and family were involved and supported her. P achieved her wish to die with dignity and on her own terms.

**Comment**: For P an ADRT was made in the context of ACP and in expectation of a natural death. Her prognosis was easier to predict. P was very clear what she didn't want and when. For other people with different challenges it might be harder to predict prognosis. Some people might wish to make an ADRT some time in advance of a possible event, illness, or deterioration. Some people make decisions based on values or beliefs we don't share, these can sometimes result in blanket refusals, e.g. because of my religious beliefs I never want to have a blood transfusion even if my life is at risk. Any professional must check that no matter what is implied the ADRT must exist, is valid, and applicable. If it complies with the requirement of the law and there is no evidence to question it, the ADRT must be respected.

---

## Understanding the impact of legislation in England and Wales

Unfortunately there are no national evaluations to measure the direct impact of the Mental Capacity Act or relate legal changes as they apply to ACP and end of life care. An annual report is produced by the Public Guardian but this does not provide the level of detail that would inform the public about the themes or outcomes related to healthcare decisions. The Court of Protection and the High Court as expected publishes only case judgments. Perhaps this challenge should be put to the Public Guardian and the Official Solicitor?

## Advance decisions to refuse treatment, Lasting Power of Attorney and deprivation of liberty and safeguards

It is hoped that most people who engage and make an ACP the plans are followed and have a good outcome. However ADRT's are not commonly seen in UK practice. Not many general health or social care professionals would consider themselves trained and prepared to support such a discussion. A more pragmatic healthcare approach continues to rely on Do Not Attempt Cardio-Pulmonary Resuscitation Decisions and/or Treatment and Escalation Plans. These processes are often driven by healthcare professionals and can happen in a reactive manner during crisis events e.g. an emergency admission to hospital. It is hoped that the anticipated new national guidance from the working party facilitated by the Resuscitation Council UK will incorporate the principles of good palliative care and comply with the MCA and its code which empowers the person as the decision maker.

There is no statutory requirement to register ADRT's with a legal body unlike the system to register a LPA. Therefore it is not known who has made an ADRT, how many have been made, and the outcomes of having made these decisions.

The number of all LPA in this country is increasing significantly every year with 395,000 registered in 2014–15. Where there are problems or complaints cases can proceed to full investigation, in 2014–15 this happened in 743 cases, an increase of 18% from the previous year. These statistics are not broken down into specific themes or categories. Of the cases that reach the Court of Protection many relate to the matters of property and financial affairs.

## Office of the Public Guardian (OPG) England and Wales

The Public Guardian is appointed by the Lord Chancellor as part of the MCA. They are personally responsible to the Lord Chancellor and Secretary of State for Justice. The OPG supports the delivery of the law and its remit is to enable people to plan ahead for both their health and their finances to be looked after should they lose capacity in future, and to safeguard the interests of people who may lack the mental capacity to make certain decisions for themselves. As part of the OPG's core functions they register Lasting Powers of Attorney (LPA) and older Enduring Powers of Attorney (EPA), supervise deputies appointed by the Court of Protection, maintain the registers and investigate complaints or allegations.

## Deprivation of liberty and safeguards (DoLS)

There is a process of local application and authorisation for a DoLS under the Mental Capacity Act, however the court can also make decisions about when someone can be deprived of their liberty. Data from NHS Digital (17) shows that, in 2015/16, DoLS applications received by local authorities rose to the highest levels ever, to 195,840 applications. This statistic is given to demonstrate the scale of the impact of legislation, to explain this can outstrip the capacity to provide formal advocacy and reflect the increasing needs of an ageing population who are most likely to lose capacity from conditions like dementia or delirium. These statistics help to contextualise the need for patients to protect choices and make legal provisions for health and care plans. The secondary consequence to the rise in DoLS authorisations had been the requirement for all of these deaths to be reported to the coroner. In 2015 there were 7637 deaths in all forms of formal detention, 7153 were under a DoLS order. Of these 7153 DoLS deaths 94% of the inquests recorded a conclusion of death by natural causes. In uncontroversial cases, an inquest may be carried out as a 'paper' inquest i.e. decided in open court but on the papers, without witnesses having to attend, and with the relevant medical data being analysed without a post-mortem. This process can add to the time, complexity, extra duties and uncertainty of dealing with a death, in some cases having a negative impact on the bereaved.

To accompany the coming into force on 3 April of the change to the definition of 'state detention' introduced by the Policing and Crime Act 2017, the new Chief Coroner has issued new guidance to accompany (and then supersede) the existing guidance. The guidance, which also addresses the Court of Appeal decision in *Ferreira,* makes clear that 'deaths under DoLS' are not automatically to be considered as being under state detention where the death occurs after 3 April 2017, see (18).

Furthermore the Law Commission (19) published a report setting out recommendations on 13 March 2017, together with a draft Bill. The final report and draft Bill recommends that the Deprivation of Liberty and Safeguards (DoLS) be repealed with pressing urgency and sets out a replacement scheme for the DoLS which they have called the Liberty Protection Safeguards.

ACP can help to reduce the likelihood of the need to make an application to the Court. There are many patients where there have been subject to an unexpected illness and they have made no provision in law for health or financial decisions. It is this superior court which considers the capacity of patients to make life sustaining treatment decisions. This Court's rulings also include what is the actual best interest decision. Some recent examples are given, these help to show how the legislation is used in practical terms (accessed via bailii.org).

## QQ [2016] EWCOP 22

This case consider the mental capacity of QQ (diagnosed with a personality disorder and schizophrenia) to make decisions and advance decisions to refuse anticoagulation for recurrent deep vein thrombosis. COP concluded that a previous advance decision of QQ to refuse anticoagulation was not valid as the patient lacked capacity for this decision primarily because QQ was not able to weigh up and reach a consistent decision. A best interest decision was made after carefully consideration of three treatment options.

## S, Re [2016] EWCOP 32

This related to the decision to withdraw clinically assisted nutrition to a patient in Persistent Vegetative State. The final conclusion in this case reads:
(1) That S lacks capacity to litigate in these proceedings
(2) That she lacks capacity to make decisions about her own medical treatment and, in particular, the provision of artificial nutrition and hydration
(3) That it was no longer in S's best interests to continue to receive artificial nutrition and hydration, and that it is lawful and in her best interests for artificial nutrition and hydration to be withdrawn with the provision of such palliative care, including pain relief, as is considered appropriate to ensure that she suffers the least distress and retains the greatest dignity until such time as her life comes to an end.

## O, Re [2016] EWCOP 24

This was a 58-year-old grandmother of eight grandchildren who suffered a severe hypoxic brain injury. The treating clinicians had concluded that it was no longer in O's interests to continue her life by ventilation, artificially, in the way that was taking place. The Trust made an application to this court seeking an application that their staff might lawfully withdraw and withhold mechanical ventilation and, further, that they might lawfully withhold any escalation of treatment such as cardiopulmonary resuscitation, organ support, antibiotics. Such treatment was, in their evaluation, no longer in O's best interests.

As part of the conclusion the judge remarked, 'The Courts must not pursue the principle of respect for life to the point where life has become empty of real content or to a degree where the principle eclipses or overwhelms other competing rights of the patient i.e. in this case simple respect for her dignity'.

## Cambridge University Hospitals NHS Foundation Trust v BF [2016] EWCOP 26

This case describes a ruling from the court that related to a 36-year-old lady with a diagnosis of paranoid schizophrenia, lacked the capacity to consent to or to refuse medical treatment for ovarian cancer and the operation to cure her, and in the best interest of the patient to undergo the medical treatment the Trust sought to give her.

The judge considered this 'a very grave step indeed to declare lawful medical treatment that a patient has stated she does not wish to undergo, and a graver step still where to make such a declaration will, whatever other benefits may attend that treatment, result in the patient being deprived permanently of her ability to have children. Parliament has conferred upon the court jurisdiction to make a declaration of such gravity *only* where it is satisfied that the patient lacks the capacity to decide whether to undergo the treatment in question *and* where it is satisfied that such treatment is in that patient's best interests'.

## University College London Hospitals NHS Foundation Trust v G [2016] EWCOP 28 (27 May 2016)

'Miss G is very sadly in a permanent vegetative state as a result of a heart attack that caused irreversible hypoxic brain injury. She is being kept alive by means of clinically assisted nutrition and hydration (CANH). The diagnosis of PVS rests on unanimous specialist medical evidence from within and outside the Trust and there is agreement between the doctors and the family and the Official Solicitor that it is not in Miss G's interests for CANH to be continued. On 24 May, I made declarations supporting this course of action'.

## Related topics

### Advance decisions to refuse treatment and children

The Mental Capacity Act 2005 and Code of Practice 2007 describe that only adults (18 and over) have the right in law to make an ADRT. In 2008 in England, Hannah Jones, aged 13 decided that she wanted to refuse a heart transplant. This transplant was essential to maintain her life. The decision to refuse this treatment was challenged by her local health Trust. The High Court ruled that she had been able to make an informed decision and her right to refuse this treatment must be respected. This challenges the age restriction as laid down by the Act and draws parallels about the wider issues of the ability to consent to treatment. There are many children that are expected to die from a variety of 'natural' reasons. Existing practice requires a consensus with the patient, family, and care team. Resuscitation is not performed and the patient is allowed to have a natural death. In circumstances where there is a wider dissemination of the Advance Care Plan which includes allowing such a death a much greater level of scrutiny is brought to bear. Despite the primacy of good clinical practice and medical professionalism the care team must demonstrate they are compliant with the requirements of the law.

### Advance decisions to refuse treatment and decisions relating to cardiopulmonary resuscitation

This subject is addressed in more detail in Chapter 10. It must be emphasised that the MCA and related legislation/policy sets about empowering and enabling many more people to take responsibility and make their own decisions about their lives and welfare. For people who have capacity (or have a nominated proxy decision maker with specific donated powers) good clinical practice would require the professional to have a discussion with this person to explore this type of decision. Further commentary is also contained in the National Council for Palliative Care's publication: *The Mental Capacity Act in Practice: Guidance for End of Life Care*.

## Assisted suicide, legal case challenges and reform

The relevant English law is clear. Section 1 of the Suicide Act 1961 removed criminal liability from the act of suicide itself, but section 2(1) makes it a criminal offence intentionally to encourage or assist (including physician assisted the suicide or attempted suicide of another person. Subsequent attempts to change the law have failed despite a significant amount of public support.

Experiences in other countries including the Netherlands and Switzerland have demonstrated both the benefits as well as the risks in having such legislation. Recent test cases challenging English law have been made. This includes cases where carers/families have helped another member of their family travel to Switzerland for a physician assisted suicide.

Following the instructions of the Law Lords the Director of Public Prosecutions (DPP) for England and Wales stated on the 23 September 2009, 'I am today clarifying those factors of public interest which I believe weigh for or against prosecuting someone for assisting another to take their own life. Assisting suicide has been a criminal offence for nearly fifty years and my interim policy does nothing to change that  . . .. There are also no guarantees against prosecution and it is my job to ensure that the most vulnerable people are protected while at the same time giving enough information to those people, like Ms Purdy, who want to be able to make informed decisions about what actions they may choose to take'. This statement lead to the policy that describes the

# Public interest factors in favour of prosecution

♦ The victim was under 18 years of age
♦ The victim's capacity to reach an informed decision was adversely affected by a recognised mental illness or learning difficulty
♦ The victim did not have a clear, settled, and informed wish to commit suicide; for example, the victim's history suggests that his or her wish to commit suicide was temporary or subject to change
♦ The victim did not indicate unequivocally to the suspect that he or she wished to commit suicide
♦ The victim did not ask personally on his or her own initiative for the assistance of the suspect
♦ The victim did not have a terminal illness; or a severe and incurable physical disability; or a severe degenerative physical condition from which there was no possibility of recovery
♦ The suspect was not wholly motivated by compassion; for example, the suspect was motivated by the prospect that they or a person closely connected to them stood to gain in some way from the death of the victim
♦ The suspect persuaded, pressured, or maliciously encouraged the victim to commit suicide, or exercised improper influence in the victim's decision to do so; and did not take reasonable steps to ensure that any other person did not do so

# Public interest factors tending against prosecution

♦ The victim had reached a voluntary, clear, settled and informed decision to commit suicide
♦ The suspect was wholly motivated by compassion
♦ The actions of the suspect, although sufficient to come within the definition of the offence
♦ Only minor encouragement or assistance

- The suspect had sought to dissuade the victim from taking the course of action which resulted in his or her suicide
- The actions of the suspect may be characterised as reluctant encouragement or assistance in the face of a determined wish on the part of the victim to commit suicide
- The suspect reported the victim's suicide to the police and fully assisted them
- Enquiries into the circumstances of the suicide or the attempt and his or her part in providing encouragement or assistance

The DPP also stated that: 'Each case must be considered on its own facts and its own merits. Prosecutors must decide the importance of each public interest factor in the circumstances of each case and go on to make an overall assessment . . . I also want to make it perfectly clear that this policy does not, in any way, permit euthanasia. The taking of life by another person is murder or manslaughter—which are among the most serious criminal offences'.

High profile UK court cases challenging the law relating to assisted suicide have included and are described in case judgments e.g. Debbie Purdy (Multiple Sclerosis); Dianne Pretty (MND); Tony Nicklinson (Locked in Syndrome).

The DPP in October 2014 clarified the Crown Prosecution Service Policy on cases of encouraging or assisting suicide in light of the outcomes of the Supreme Court. This included the role of healthcare professionals involved in the act.

Paragraph 43.14 of the updated The Policy for Prosecutors in Respect of Cases of Encouraging or Assisting Suicide (20) now reads: A prosecution is more likely to be required if the suspect was acting in his or her capacity as a medical doctor, nurse, other healthcare professional, a professional carer [whether for payment or not], or as a person in authority, such as a prison officer, and the victim was in his or her care.'

There have been specific legal challenges of this policy including Kenwards [2015] (EWHC, 3508) and the General Medical Council [2015] (EWHC, 2096). The GMC which regulates doctors in the UK were instructed in court to ensure that they must investigate doctors that may not comply with the current law and comply with the standards set out in Good Medical Practice (GMC, 2013).

The great public interest and pressure vocalised by people like Debbie Purdy helped lead to the policy and guidelines. These guidelines are supposed to offer some assurances to people that they will not be prosecuted where there are clear cases of need on humane/compassionate grounds e.g. the public interest factors against prosecution. This unfortunately does not remove all doubt as the guidelines do not represent a guarantee preventing prosecution. The person (who wishes to die) may still feel forced into an earlier decision to enact suicide before the need to involve a third party. This would only 'remove life from years' dying on someone else's terms. Legal reform was attempted with the private members bill on Assisted Dying (no 2) but this did not pass its second reading in the English parliament (21).

## Key outcomes to consider

Person/patient and carer related advance decisions outcomes:

- Reassurance that decisions will be respected and acted upon
- Refusal of life sustaining treatment might allow a natural death and maybe influence the preferred place where this is achieved
- Enhanced autonomy through legislative empowerment
- Better communication with healthcare professionals
- Peace of mind knowing that family/friends will not be burdened with decisions
- Anticipate carer/family adjustment to bereavement

Professionals

- Better understanding and promoting of patient choice as part of ACP
- Better informed and clearly documented/communicated patient decisions
- Staff empowered to protect autonomy and support the patient's choice by law and policy of their employing organisation
- Increasing job satisfaction by enabling patient and family centred care and good clinical practice

Organizations

- Clearly defined responsibility to ensure adherence to the Mental Capacity Act and Code of Practice; necessary application to the Court of Protection
- Fulfil Clinical Governance commitment to pursue good clinical practice, ensure patient/carer and professional outcomes whilst correctly managing risk
- Prevent unwanted and possible unnecessary admission to hospital and treatments

## Moving forwards

Advance decisions and related end of life care continue to be real ethical and legal dilemmas often presented in the media. Cases have established new precedents and tested statutory law. This insight has brought into sharp reality the nature of peoples lives, the decisions they would like to and have taken, and the challenges they have to get through to realise these decisions.

It is believed that professional participation in advance decisions has been for many restricted to those with specialist interests in palliative medicine. The medical and wider health and social care profession is being challenged to respond to both the clinical need of the patient and their rights in law. These professionals must demonstrate both the competency and confidence to maintain good clinical practice and comply with the law whether an ADRT or the whole of an ACP.

The requirements in law relate to the content and verification by a witness of an ADRT. The national guide offers information about this process and an example form. As Gold Standards Framework (GSF) or equivalent palliative care and coordination systems are implemented in this country and ACP is better understood, it is expected that decisions including advance decisions will be more openly approached and the outcomes recorded. It is certainly hoped that essential information like an advance decision or DNAR CPR is included in any future electronic records and is shared with multiagency partners in health and social care. There has been widespread 'training' on the Mental Capacity Act as part of the national implementation strategy. Although most programmes reference advance decisions they do not often go into detailed knowledge and skills required to actively participate in the process.

## Conclusion

Health, social care services, and society in general promote and protect personal/patient choice. The law lays down in statute the rights of the person including making an ADRT. With this right comes great personal responsibility and professional accountability to ensure that the right process and outcomes are achieved. ADRT taken in context of ACP for the end of life is a component of a national strategy to improve services for people to help ensure a good death with dignity and privacy. There is a real opportunity to use this legal and societal imperative in the delivery of health and social care services. This legal power can bring significant benefits and when used appropriately minimises (but never removes) risk and when necessary emergency application to the Court of Protection provides the ultimate safeguard (21).

## Acknowledgement

This chapter draws upon the national publication, *Advance Decisions to Refuse Treatment—A Guide for Health and Social Care Professionals*.

## References

1. **NHS End of Life Care Programme** (2007). *Advance Care Planning: A Guide for Health and Social Care Staff*. London.
2. **Department for Constitutional Affairs** (2005). Mental Capacity Act. London. Available from: http://www.opsi.gov.uk/acts/acts2005/ukpga_20050009_en_1
3. R (Burke) v General Medical Council: Queen's Bench Division (Administrative court), (2004).
4. **Emanuel LL, Emanuel EJ, Stoeckle JD, Hummel LR,** and **Barry MJ** (1994). 'Advance directives. Stability of patients' treatment choices'. *Archives of Internal Medicine* **154**(2): 209–17.
5. **Kohut N, Sam M, O'Rourke K** et al. (1997). 'Stability of treatment preferences: although most preferences do not change, most people change some of their preferences'. *Journal of Clinical Ethics* **8**(2): 124–35.
6. **Silverstein MD, Stocking CB,** and **Antel JP** (1991). 'Amyotrophic lateral sclerosis and life-sustaining therapy: patients' desires for information, participation in decision making, and life sustaining therapy'. *Mayo Clinic Proceedings* **66**(9): 906–13.
7. **Froman RD** and **Owen SV** (2005). 'Randomized study of stability and change in patients' advance directives'. *Research in Nursing & Health*, **28**(5): 398–407.
8. **Engelhardt JB, McClive-Reed KP, Toseland RW,** et al. (2006). 'Effects of a program for coordinated care of advanced illness on patients, surrogates, and healthcare costs: a randomized trial'. *American Journal of Managed Care* **12**(2): 93–100.
9. **Connors Jr AF, Dawson NV, Desbiens NA,** et al. (1995). 'A controlled trial to improve care for seriously ill hospitalised patients: The study to understand prognoses and preferences for outcomes and risks of treatments (SUPPORT)'. *The Journal of the American Medical Association* **274**(20): 1591–8.
10. **Lee MA, Brummel-Smith K, Meyer J, Drew N,** and **London MR** (2000). 'Physician orders for lifesustaining treatment (POLST): outcomes in a PACE program. Program of All-Inclusive Care for the Elderly'. *Journal of the American Geriatrics Society* **48**(10): 1219–25.
11. **Hammes BJ** and **Rooney BL** (1998). 'Death and end-of-life planning in one midwestern community'. *Archives of Internal Medicine* **158**(4): 383–90.
12. **Tolle SW, Tilden VP, Nelson CA,** and **Dunn PM** (1998). 'A prospective study of the efficacy of the physician order form for life 14 Advance care planning © Royal College of Physicians, 2009. All rights reserved. sustaining treatment' *Journal of the American Geriatrics Society* **46**(9): 1097–102.
13. **Danis M, Southerland LI, Garrett JM,** et al. (1991). 'A prospective study of advance directives for lifesustaining care' [see Comment]. *The New England Journal of Medicine* **324**(13): 882–8.
14. **Hanson LC, Tulsky JA,** and **Danis M** (1997). 'Can clinical interventions change care at the end of life?'. *Annals of Internal Medicine* **126**(5): 381–8.
15. **Molloy DW, Guyatt GH, Russo R,** et al. (2000). 'Systematic implementation of an advance directive program in nursing homes: a randomized controlled trial'. *The Journal of the American Medical Association* **283**(11): 1437–44.
16. **Goodman MD, Tarnoff M,** and **Slotman GJ** (1998). 'Effect of advance directives on the management of elderly critically ill patients'. *Critical Care Medicine* **26**(4): 701–4.
17. **Office of the Public Guardian** (2017). *What we do*. Available from: https://www.gov.uk/government/organisations/office-of-the-public-guardian

18. **Care Quality Commission** (2016). *The state of health care and adult social care in England 2015/16.* Available from: http://www.cqc.org.uk/

19. **Chief Coroner** (2017). *Deprivation of Liberty Safeguards (DoLS)—3rd April 2017 onwards.* Available from: https://www.judiciary.gov.uk

20. **Law Commission** (2017). *Mental Capacity and Deprivation of Liberty.* Available from: http://www.lawcom.gov.uk

21. **The Director of Public Prosecutions** (2010). *Policy for Prosecutors in Respect of Cases of Encouraging or Assisting Suicide.* Updated October 2014. Available from: https://www.cps.gov.uk

# Chapter 10

# Discussions and decisions about cardiopulmonary resuscitation

David Pitcher

'In any moment of decision the best thing you can do is the right thing, the next best thing is the wrong thing, and the worst thing you can do is nothing.'
*Theodore Roosevelt (1858–1919), 26th President of the USA*

---

**This chapter includes**

- The background to cardiopulmonary resuscitation
- Why do we need to make advance 'decisions' about CPR?
- What is a successful outcome from cardiorespiratory arrest?
- When should CPR be discussed and a recommendation recorded?
- Decisions versus recommendations
- Legal aspects: what must we tell people and discuss with them?
- Important conversations about CPR and other life-sustaining treatments
- Framework for making decisions and recommendations about CPR
- Effective communication and provision of information
- Effective recording of recommendations about CPR and other life-sustaining treatments
- Towards a national approach
- Relationship between CPR and other life-sustaining treatments
- Avoiding discrimination

---

**Key Points**

- CPR is not universally life-sustaining; this is not widely understood
- Making advance recommendations about CPR is part of good clinical practice
- Any decision about CPR must be based on assessment of each individual's situation
- Whenever possible, CPR recommendations should be based on shared decisions
- CPR should be discussed in the context of a person's overall goals of care
- CPR is best discussed alongside other aspects of care and treatment
- A DNACPR recommendation must not compromise other care or treatment

- A consistent and effective format is needed to record recommendations about CPR
- A treatment-escalation-plan style is preferred to a 'DNACPR form'
- Recommendation forms should cross organisational and geographic boundaries

---

**Key Message**

Documents containing recommendations about CPR and other life-sustaining treatment should be widely accepted and made accessible to clinicians who may need to make an immediate decision during a crisis.

---

## Introduction

When a person's heart and breathing stop, those present are faced with making an immediate decision whether or not to start CPR. Explicit recommendations about this, decided on and recorded in advance, can guide those present at the time of a crisis and ensure, as far as possible, that decisions taken are in accordance with the person's needs and wishes.

## Background to cardiopulmonary resuscitation

Modern cardiopulmonary resuscitation (CPR) developed following publication of its efficacy in 1960 (1). Initially, CPR targeted younger people who developed sudden cardiac arrest in ventricular fibrillation during the early stages of acute myocardial infarction. They were described as having hearts that were 'too good to die' (2). It was recognised quickly that the chance of restarting such hearts, and of subsequent survival, was greater if CPR and defibrillation were performed well and without delay. However, training in CPR was not widespread; defibrillators were large, heavy machines and were not widely available. As a result, coronary care units were introduced, primarily to provide prompt access to professionals skilled in CPR and to a defibrillator (3,4).

More healthcare professionals and, increasingly, more members of the public became familiar with CPR, and defibrillators became progressively more portable. Thus, it became possible to attempt CPR, and apply defibrillation in all areas of a hospital, in ambulances, and subsequently in community settings.

## Why do we need to make advance 'decisions' about CPR?

Advance decisions about CPR have been in clinical use since at least the early 1970s (5). Because a major focus of resuscitation training is on minimising delay in starting CPR, there were increasingly frequent examples of people receiving CPR with no realistic prospect of success because they were dying from an advanced and irreversible condition. This led to an undignified death, and for some caused harm by restarting the heart and breathing temporarily, subjecting them and those close to them to a further period of distress or suffering before they died a second time.

To try to achieve maximum success from CPR, many healthcare organisations have policies that require staff to start CPR on a person showing no signs of life, unless there is an explicit recorded recommendation not to attempt CPR. The need for deciding and recording such recommendations is driven by a wish to avoid delivery of CPR to people who do not want it, will not benefit from it, or may be harmed by it.

## What is a successful outcome from cardiorespiratory arrest?

Worldwide efforts to improve outcomes from cardiorespiratory arrest focus on strengthening links in the 'chain of survival' (Figure 10.1).

Whilst this image is invaluable in emphasising the elements needed for CPR to be effective whenever possible, it implies that 'survival' is always the optimal or desired outcome when someone's heart and breathing stop. However, we should step back and consider, for each individual, what a successful outcome might be. Box 10.1 shows some examples.

This spectrum illustrates the importance of basing every recommendation about CPR on each person's individual circumstances, needs and preferences. This is emphasised in detailed national guidance from the British Medical Association, Resuscitation Council (UK), and Royal College of Nursing (6).

Whilst this chapter focuses predominantly on adults, the fundamental principles of ethics and good practice apply equally to children and young people, with the additional need to ensure appropriate involvement in decision-making of those with parental responsibility.

## When should CPR be discussed and a recommendation recorded?

In 2011 the National Confidential Enquiry into Patient Outcome and Death (NCEPOD) published a report on a study of CPR attempts in hospitals (7). Amongst many findings, the study showed that a recommendation about CPR was recorded for one in five or fewer patients, whereas expert advisers considered a recommendation not to attempt CPR appropriate in 196/230 patients (85%) for whom there were sufficient data to assess this. The report recommended that an explicit 'decision' whether or not to attempt CPR be considered and recorded for all acute hospital admissions, ideally during the initial admission process.

However, emergency hospital admission with an acute illness is not an ideal circumstance in which to discuss CPR or make shared decisions and explicit recommendations. Many patients are not well enough to engage fully in informed discussion, and clinicians may not have met the patient before or be fully aware of their medical condition, home situation, beliefs, and wishes. For some people a recommendation about CPR is needed in the setting of an acute illness (e.g. a

## Chain of survival

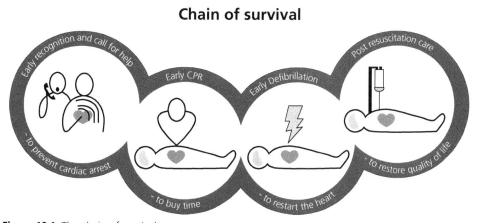

**Figure 10.1** The chain of survival

Reproduced with the kind permission of the Resuscitation Council (UK)

## Box 10.1 Examples illustrating the spectrum of desired outcomes from cardiorespiratory arrest in different individuals

- ◆ **Survival regardless**
  - Even if intervention with CPR carries some risk, this will be the desired outcome for many, especially—but not exclusively and not necessarily—those suffering unexpected, sudden cardiac arrest
- ◆ **Survival with a good quality of life**
  - Some will want survival, but only if there is a good chance that it will be accompanied by a quality of life that they would find acceptable
- ◆ **Avoiding pain and distress**
  - This may be the priority for some people, especially those who may be approaching the end of their life and for whom if survival were possible it would be likely to offer limited quality of life or limited further duration of life
- ◆ **A dignified death**
  - For many people, especially those who know and accept that they are dying, the priority will be ensuring their comfort and dignity

severe head injury, stroke, or acute myocardial infarction). However, for many others it is best to discuss and make a shared decision as part of advance care planning (ACP), when their condition is relatively stable, and they have ample time to consider relevant information, discuss it with people important to them, and make a decision that is right for them when they are ready to do so.

This underlines the importance of 'the link before the chain' (Figure 10.2), promoting many more conversations between people and their clinicians to enhance understanding, encourage more shared decision-making, and advance planning for a future crisis, including death or cardiorespiratory arrest. These conversations should not be limited only to those identified as needing palliative care or end of life care or people admitted to hospital. Many people can benefit from having these conversations and making advance plans. These include those susceptible to abrupt deteriorations in their health, such as older people with frailty (8), and people with advanced disease of one or more major organs (e.g. heart, kidneys, brain, lungs, liver). Others may want to record their care and treatment needs and preferences for some other reason.

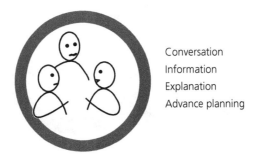

Conversation
Information
Explanation
Advance planning

**Figure 10.2** The link before the chain

## Decisions versus recommendations

When discussing and agreeing advance plans for a person's future care and treatment it is crucial that the people themselves, those close to them, and the clinicians involved all have a clear understanding of what is being agreed and recorded.

What is recorded on a CPR decision form or a treatment escalation plan (TEP) is a **recommendation** about whether or not to attempt CPR or specified types of life-sustaining treatment. The recommendation is recorded to guide immediate decision-making by those present at the time of a life-threatening crisis, including cardiorespiratory arrest. It is those people who have to make an immediate **decision** whether or not to start treatment, based on the circumstances at the time and all the information available to them. Whilst health and care professionals should be familiar with CPR decision forms or equivalent and would be expected to take into account the recommendations, untrained members of the public cannot necessarily be expected to do this.

Therefore, when discussing CPR and other potentially life-sustaining treatments, the shared **decision** that people make with their clinicians is what **recommendations** to record to guide those who respond to a future emergency in which the person has lost capacity to make decisions about their treatment. Those **recommendations** are not 'orders' and are not legally binding, but a clinician who decides to ignore them should have and record a good reason for doing so. The exception to this in England and Wales is an Advance Decision to Refuse Treatment (ADRT), and where one exists and is valid and applicable to the circumstances, it is legally binding (Mental Capacity Act 2005) (9,10). Discussing a person's needs and preferences in relation to CPR and other life-sustaining treatments, as part of advance care planning, provides an opportunity to support them in making an ADRT or appointing a proxy decision-maker for their health and welfare and giving them specific powers to make decisions about life-sustaining treatments.

This distinction between decisions and recommendations emphasises also the subtle matter of exactly what mental capacity a person must have to be fully involved in advance planning about CPR. When making an ADRT, they must be capable of considering and making the decision to refuse the specified potential future treatment. When discussing a recommendation about CPR for recording in another format they must have capacity to participate in deciding what recommendation will be recorded.

There is no formal provision for a person to consent to treatment (that is not currently needed) in advance of a future situation where that treatment may be needed or considered.

A person does not have the right to demand treatment that is not clinically appropriate and therefore is not offered. Some people choose to write an 'advance statement' in which they set out their wishes regarding types of care and treatment they would want to be considered for and those they would not want. Those wishes and preferences may be recorded also on a CPR decision form or TEP. Advance statements, CPR decision forms, and TEPs are not legally binding.

## How have DNACPR recommendations gone wrong?

In the UK, more than half of deaths occur in hospitals. Only about 10% receive attempted CPR, suggesting that most others have a DNACPR recommendation in place. Whilst many of these may have been decided on and documented well, in line with guidelines on good practice, a systematic review (11) highlighted many inconsistencies and failures, as illustrated in Box 10.2.

In April 2000, poor practice in relation to a DNACPR recommendation received media attention, with headlines such as:

◆ **Cancer patient's fury at doctor who 'wrote her off on hospital's death ward'**

◆ **Secret 'not for resuscitation' code on pensioner's notes**

---

### Box 10.2 Some key findings in the systematic review of DNACPR decisions

- Inconsistencies in making and documenting recommendations about CPR at organisational and individual levels
- Unrealistic expectations of the outcome from CPR, particularly by family members and the general public
- Attempted CPR on people with no likely prospect of benefit—sometimes disregarding their wishes, or often when they had been given no prior chance to express them
- Making DNACPR recommendations either without discussion with patients and those close to them, or after inadequate discussion
- Misapplication of DNACPR recommendations by health professionals, leading to withholding or poor-quality delivery of other elements of care and treatment

---

Despite publication of sequential editions of the national guidance *Decisions relating to cardiopulmonary resuscitation* by the BMA, RC (UK), and RCN in 2001 and 2007, examples of poor practice continued. In 2011, media statements such as:

- **A man is suing a hospital trust over his claims doctors put 'do not resuscitate' orders on his wife's medical notes without her consent**
- **Addenbrooke's and Andrew Lansley sued over 'do not resuscitate' rule**

reported the start of a landmark legal case relating to Mrs Janet Tracey (12).

## What must we tell people and discuss with them?

A clinician has no obligation to offer or provide a treatment that they believe would be ineffective or harmful. However, that does not mean that they have no obligation to explain to a person their reasons for recording a recommendation that CPR is not attempted or that other treatments that might be regarded as potentially life-sustaining are not provided. In relation to a DNACPR decision, this was tested and confirmed in the Court of Appeal in 2014 in the 'Tracey case', as summarised in Box 10.3.

What was meant by 'patient involvement'? It cannot mean that a person is entitled to demand receipt of CPR, even when it will not work. When clinicians are as certain as they can reasonably be that CPR would not work, it should not be offered (6). Offering CPR in such circumstances can do harm by giving the person and those close to them a falsely optimistic impression of the seriousness of their condition and prognosis, as well as jeopardising their chance of a dignified death. What is needed is clear, sensitive exploration (and if necessary correction) of their understanding of their condition and prognosis, agreement on their goals of care and then discussion of what treatments may help to achieve those goals. This would include explanation of what CPR is, why it would not work in their situation, and why there is a need to record a recommendation about this in advance. If they do not accept the explanation, they should be offered a second opinion from a suitably senior and experienced clinician. The Tracey judgement did not challenge the clinical decision not to attempt CPR, but stated that the failure to involve the patient and her family deprived her of the opportunity to seek a second opinion. The judgement stated also that

---

### Box 10.3  Some important features of the Tracey case

- Mrs Tracey was in a neurosurgical high-dependency unit after sustaining a fractured neck in a traffic collision

- She had incurable metastatic lung cancer and chronic obstructive pulmonary disease, was on a ventilator, and her condition was not improving

- Despite her request to be involved in decisions about her treatment, a DNACPR form was completed and placed in her records without discussion with her or her family

- The judgement found this to be in breach of Article 8 of the Human Rights Act 1998 (13), the right to a private and family life

- The judgement stated that when considering placing a DNACPR 'notice' in a person's records there should be a presumption in favour of patient involvement, unless that would be likely to cause them physical or psychological harm; there need to be convincing reasons not to involve the patient

---

agreement by a multidisciplinary team on a DNACPR recommendation may reduce the likelihood of needing another opinion.

In situations where there is some possibility of CPR restarting the heart and breathing, the clinical team may feel that the chance of doing harm could outweigh the chance of restoring the person to a worthwhile quality of life. When quality of life is considered, what matters is what the person themselves would want and find acceptable, not the quality of life that the clinicians think may be tolerable by the person or would want for themselves. This underlines the importance of a conversation in which the person's condition, prognosis, and goals of care are agreed, and the relative risks and benefits of CPR in their specific situation are explained accurately and honestly. The discussion that follows should support the person in making an informed choice about whether or not they would want to receive CPR if their heart and breathing were to stop.

## Lessons and 'fallout' from the Tracey case

The detailed judgement in the Court of Appeal in 2014 (12) recognised the complexities and uncertainties involved in discussing and deciding to make DNACPR recommendations. In his judgement, the Master of the Rolls acknowledged: 'It would probably be impossible to devise a scheme which is completely free from difficulty.'

Nevertheless, there are important 'take-home' messages from the Tracey case regarding aspects of good practice needed to both provide high-quality care and minimise the likelihood of complaint or litigation. These are summarised in Box 10.4.

The fear of complaints and litigation influences clinicians' attitudes to making anticipatory recommendations about CPR (14). Sadly, anecdotal reports suggest that, far from encouraging better communication between clinicians and their patients, the Tracey judgement caused some clinicians to make fewer DNACPR recommendations. This left vulnerable people in the 'default position' of potentially receiving a futile CPR attempt. The Tracey case made clear that making a DNACPR recommendation without informing or otherwise involving the person is a breach of their human rights. However, is leaving a person at risk of receiving CPR (when they may not

> **Box 10.4 Key messages from the Tracey judgement: what is needed in CPR decision making**
>
> - More ACP
> - Effective and timely communication
> - High-quality decision making
> - Clear documentation of decisions and reasons for them
> - Clear documentation of discussions about decisions or reasons why discussions were not possible or appropriate

want it, may be harmed by it and have not been given a chance to discuss it) any less a breach of their human rights?

## Who should be involved when the person lacks capacity?

In England and Wales, the Mental Capacity Act (MCA) makes this clear. A person making decisions for someone who lacks capacity to decide for themselves must take into account the views of:

- anyone named by the person as someone to be consulted
- anyone engaged in caring for the person or interested in his welfare
- any donee of a lasting power of attorney granted by the person and
- any deputy appointed for the person by the court

as to what would be in the person's best interests, if it is practicable and appropriate to consult them.

In relation to a DNACPR decision, this was tested and confirmed in the courts in 2015 in the 'Winspear Case' (15), as summarised in Box 10.5.

The Winspear case emphasised a legal requirement to consult people engaged in caring for a person or interested in his welfare. That does not and must not place the burden of making a decision on those people, as it is the duty of the clinical decision-maker to make a decision in the person's best interests, after considering all available information and views. When time and circumstances allow, this is best done by holding a best-interests meeting, at which all those caring for the person or with an interest in their wellbeing can contribute to the decision-making process.

## Making urgent decisions and recommendations

When a person is at high risk of imminent cardiac arrest or death, a decision to recommend CPR or no CPR is needed without delay. Failure to consider and make a decision will leave them at risk of receiving CPR by default, and is poor clinical practice.

If they have capacity to participate in the process they should be involved, regardless of the urgency. The Tracey judgement emphasised that such involvement should not be withheld for fear of causing distress, only if there is a risk of causing harm.

If they lack capacity, it is important to make a considered decision to ensure that the person receives high-quality care, and not to delay this because of immediate lack of availability of a legal proxy, family member or other carer. In the Winspear case, the judge made clear that if a decision was needed at 03:00 hours, contact with the patient's mother would have been neither impracticable nor inappropriate. However, that cannot be assumed to apply in every case. It is hardly ever appropriate to try to hold discussions about CPR and other life-sustaining treatments

## Box 10.5  Some important features of the Winspear case

- Carl Winspear was aged 28 and had cerebral palsy, epilepsy, spinal deformities, and associated conditions. He did not have capacity to make decisions about his treatment
- He was admitted to hospital in mid-afternoon, was hypoxic and febrile, and was treated for a chest infection
- His mother accompanied him and stayed with him into the evening. When she returned home for the night she understood his condition to be stable.
- That night (at about 03:00) the medical registrar signed a DNACPR form, but did not complete all its sections. His entry in the health record stated 'discuss with family in morning', with no indication of who should do that or exactly when
- His mother visited in late morning, discovered that a DNACPR form was in place and objected to it. The DNACPR form was cancelled
- Carl's condition deteriorated despite treatment, and he died a few days later. CPR was not attempted
- The judge ruled that failure to consult Carl's mother before recording a DNACPR recommendation was in breach of Carl's human rights under article 8 of the Act
- The judgement referred also to the MCA and ruled that it was neither impracticable nor inappropriate for Carl's mother to have been contacted and consulted before the DNACPR recommendation was recorded

by telephone. An unexpected telephone call in the middle of the night to summon (for example) a frail, elderly relative of a critically ill person to discuss CPR could place that relative at risk.

When a decision is needed now to ensure that a person receives the best possible care, that decision should be made now. If that decision has to be made without involvement of people who should be involved were the situation less urgent, clear reasons for their involvement being impracticable or inappropriate must be recorded, together with a clear plan for their involvement as soon as is practicable and appropriate.

A common question is how often a recommendation about CPR should be reviewed. Like the recommendation itself, this must be guided by the person's individual circumstances (6). In an acute situation, the person's condition may improve or deteriorate rapidly, so frequent review of a CPR recommendation is needed, involving the person or their representatives whenever possible. It is important also to recognise that capacity for any decision may fluctuate; where capacity is regained, review of a recommendation with the person's involvement will be needed. If the person asks to review an agreed recommendation, that must be respected. However, for some people, especially those with an advanced and irreversible terminal condition, review will not be needed, and involvement of the person in repeated discussion of an agreed DNACPR recommendation would be unnecessarily burdensome to them,

## Important conversations about CPR and other life-sustaining treatments

The principles of ethics and good clinical practice that underpin these conversations are those that apply to all aspects of ACP. Conversations about life-sustaining treatments, including CPR, are referred to often as 'difficult conversations'. Many health professionals and patients feel uncomfortable when talking about dying (16,17). Clinicians may be concerned that they should be striving to keep a person alive, and that discussing a possible DNACPR recommendation is acknowledging failure. When a clinician starts a discussion that focuses specifically on a recommendation to withhold CPR in the event of death some patients express the concern 'you're giving up on me then', or are concerned that they will not receive other treatments that they need.

To avoid such interpretations, the conversation should:

- establish the person's understanding of their condition and prognosis, if necessary correcting any misunderstanding
- establish what expectations and wishes they have
- agree their goals of care
- discuss care and treatments needed to meet those goals
- then discuss treatments that they would not want or that would not be of benefit to them

Having these conversations can be a positive experience in most cases. For a clinician, they are an integral part of good quality care for their patients, but this does need each clinician to have the necessary knowledge and skills to hold such a conversation. Health professionals should ensure that they receive specific training in such communication skills, and healthcare employers should ensure that staff receive that training.

If a patient does not want to have such conversations, discussion should not be forced on them. They should be asked if there is someone that they would like to speak on their behalf in making plans for their treatment, or whether they want to leave all such decisions in the hands of their clinicians. Their wishes should be documented clearly, and they should be assured that they are welcome to have such discussions at any time that they feel able and willing to do so.

There is evidence that both health professionals and the public find a conversation about which treatments to consider and which not to attempt much more acceptable than a conversation that focuses only on withholding a treatment (CPR) that many people regard as universally 'life-saving', even when there are clear circumstances in which it will not be (18). Many members of the public and health professionals have a falsely high expectation of the chance of survival after receiving CPR for a cardiorespiratory arrest (19,20). Quoting the average chance of survival can be highly misleading and should be avoided. Depending on individual circumstances, the chance of survival from cardiorespiratory arrest may range from zero to almost 100%. Clinicians have a duty to provide each person with accurate information about CPR (and any other treatment to be discussed) and its likely success in their individual circumstances.

Figure 10.3 shows a framework to guide decision-making specifically in relation to a recommendation about CPR, to be used in the context of the bullet points already given.

## Effective communication and provision of information

Many people feel tense when discussing sensitive matters such as dying and possible treatment options in a life-threatening emergency. They may not understand fully the information given to them, may not recall the detail afterwards, and sometimes their recollection of what was said can be highly inaccurate. Whilst it is impossible in this chapter to describe all the important elements of effective communication, one important aspect is the checking of understanding. This needs more than just asking the question 'Do you understand?', as many people will tend to answer 'yes', even when they may have misunderstood what was said. Asking them to describe in their own words what has been explained to them can reveal and allow correction of misunderstandings.

As with all aspects of ACP, many people need time to consider what they have been told before deciding their preferences. They may wish to discuss it with others, such as family members,

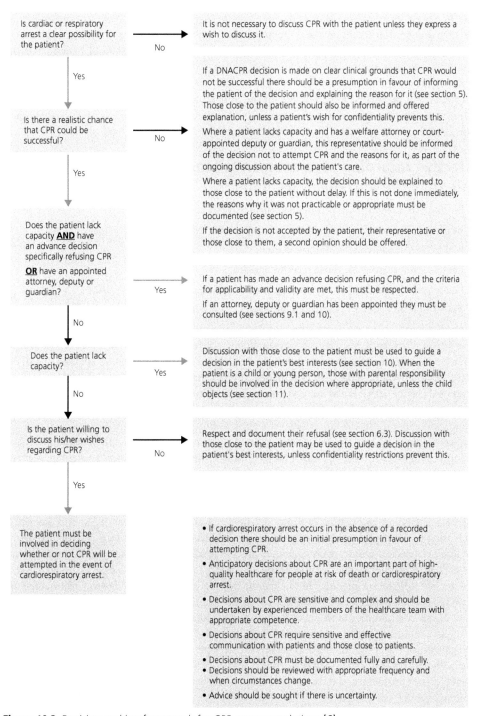

**Figure 10.3** Decision-making framework for CPR recommendations [6]

Reproduced with the kind permission of the Resuscitation Council (UK) and the British Medical Association

and may need further discussion with one or more members of their healthcare team before reaching a shared decision on recommendations about future CPR and other life-sustaining treatments. As it is difficult for people to remember all that they have been told, providing them with information in written or other formats can help to ensure that they have all the information that they need to support the decision-making process. Care must be taken to provide information in the format most suitable for the individual. That may include, but is not limited to, formats that cater for sensory impairments, for limited literacy or for use of languages other than English.

## Effective recording of recommendations about CPR and other life-sustaining treatments

To be effective, a record of recommendations for use in a crisis must:

◆ be accessible immediately, whenever, and wherever needed

◆ make clear, unequivocal recommendations

◆ contain valid reasons for those recommendations

◆ be recognised and accepted by all professionals who may respond in a crisis

◆ have a style and content familiar to those needing to find information rapidly

At one time, most advance decisions about CPR were made in hospital and written in the text of a person's health record. Such entries were often ineffective, being difficult to locate or overlooked when immediate decision making was needed. This led to development of specific DNACPR forms. Although the concept of such a document was accepted widely, many different forms were developed (Figure 10.4). It was not uncommon for a form completed in one healthcare organisation (e.g. a hospital) to be regarded as unacceptable by other organisations (e.g. ambulance services, nursing homes) when they took over a person's care.

Internationally and in the UK, some organisations and health and care communities have adopted TEP-style forms (21,22,18,7). However, inconsistency of style and of acceptance across organisational boundaries persists.

In some communities, a digital format for DNACPR forms or end of life care plans has been introduced. This can allow prompt electronic access to current recommendations by multiple agencies, including ambulance services, out-of-hours services, hospices, GPs, and hospitals. Increasing use of digital technology provides patients with opportunity to access their records, but also presents important governance challenges in relation to data protection. Many people do not have access to digital media, many health and care organisations still use paper-based records, and access to digital records may not be maintained when a person travels away from home, so some reliance on paper forms will continue for the immediate future. Where both formats are used, health communities must have effective policies and governance structures to ensure that recommendations recorded on paper and digital versions are current, and that both formats are recognised as being valid. In order to be effective, a paper form must travel with the person and be readily accessible when needed in a crisis. A well-completed form will only be effective if clinicians explain to patients and those close to them where it should be kept, and the importance of making it readily available.

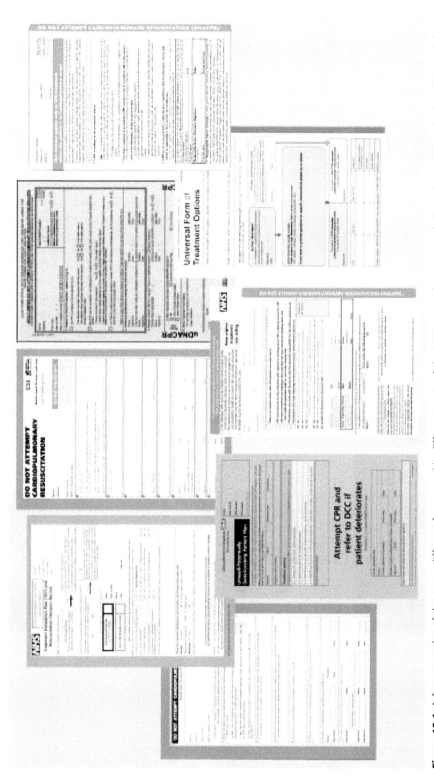

**Figure 10.4** A few examples of the many different forms used in different parts of the UK to record recommendations about CPR and other life-sustaining treatments. These examples use different combinations of colours, including red, white, lilac, and green

## Towards a national approach

In 2014 a meeting at the Royal Society of Medicine discussed the results of the systematic review (10). The participants expressed a strong majority view that advance decisions about CPR should be discussed in the context of a person's broader care and treatment, and that recommendations that arose from those discussions should be recorded on a form that was used and recognised nationally. A Working Group was established, with representation from many stakeholders, including representatives of patients and the public. Using an iterative approach that included public consultation, usability testing, and patient focus groups, the Group has developed the Recommended Summary Plan for Emergency Care and Treatment (ReSPECT), a process and form with the objectives listed in Box 10.6 (23).

The resulting form and materials have been available for adoption by health communities since early 2017 (www.respectprocess.org.uk). ReSPECT is not purely for use in end of life care, as it offers a vehicle also for recommendations that can help to ensure that a person receives active emergency treatment that they should be offered.

For the objectives of the project to be met it is crucial to achieve a change of culture on the part of both clinicians and the public, so that both are willing to have conversations about advance planning for emergencies, and regard these as a worthwhile and expected part of good clinical care. Implementation of ReSPECT in any health community will require good leadership, careful planning, and involvement of all stakeholders, as well as a willingness to recognise that the ultimate goal of achieving a process and document that supports good clinical care across all boundaries should override any personal preferences of style or wording.

The ReSPECT project aims to respond to feedback, so that the form and supporting materials continue to evolve and develop, and remain current and fit for purpose.

## Relationship between CPR and other life-sustaining treatments

This can be a source of confusion from both an ethical and practical perspective, and requires careful consideration in each person's individual circumstances.

It is not appropriate, for example, to make a DNACPR recommendation on the grounds that a person's condition means that they would not be offered organ support in an ICU. Many people, but not all, need a period of ICU support immediately after resuscitation from cardiac arrest. That fact should be taken into account in any shared decision making, but should not compromise the person's access to CPR from which they might recover without organ support.

---

### Box 10.6 Aims and objectives of the ReSPECT process

- To encourage more conversations about advance planning
- To promote effective communication
- To promote identification of person-centred priorities and goals of care
- To promote good decision making
- To promote good recording of decisions and discussions
- To be used across organisational and geographical boundaries
- To be used for individuals of all ages

Another source of confusion is the relationship between a DNACPR recommendation and a decision to deactivate an implanted cardioverter-defibrillator (ICD). ICD deactivation is discussed in detail in guidance from the Resuscitation Council (UK), British Cardiovascular Society, and National Council for Palliative Care (24). Deactivating an ICD can spare a dying person the pain and distress of multiple shocks in their last hours or days. CPR is more intrusive and in many cases less successful than an appropriate ICD shock, so some people choose not to receive CPR before they are ready to have their ICD deactivated. The converse (deactivating an ICD in a dying person without making a DNACPR recommendation) would be highly unusual, but discussion of these as two separate but related decisions will ensure individualised, person-centred care.

## Avoiding discrimination

Decisions about CPR and other life-saving treatments must be made without any discrimination. For example, a person's access to such treatment should not be denied purely on the grounds of age or any disability that they may have. Conversely, a person should not be subjected to CPR with no reasonable likelihood of benefit or without their prior involvement, because they are younger or because of any assumption that they would want this. Involvement of the person or their representatives in the decision-making process remains an important human right. If a person's frailty (e.g. due to advanced age or severe physical disability) reduces their chance of successful CPR, that should be explained as part of their involvement in shared decision making. As already emphasised, when quality of life is considered, what matters is what the person themselves would want and find acceptable.

In 2013 a confidential inquiry into premature deaths of people with learning disabilities (25) reported instances of inappropriate or poorly documented DNACPR recommendations. In a number of cases the decision not to attempt CPR appeared to have been made prematurely in a non-emergency situation, before full assessment of the person and/or before obtaining the views of those who knew them best. People with learning disabilities were more likely than those without to have died from potentially treatable causes.

Care must be taken to ensure that other factors, including socio-economic status, education, religion, and culture, do not lead to discrimination, but also that discussions and decision-making about CPR take into account ways in which culture or religion determine a person's attitudes to all elements of ACP, including CPR.

Discrimination would not only be contrary to good medical practice but would be unlawful (26). Care must be taken to use language in the clinical record that is non-discriminatory and that adheres to human rights and capacity laws.

## Conclusion

For anyone at risk of death or cardiorespiratory arrest, considering and making an advance recommendation whether or not to attempt CPR is part of good clinical practice. It should be discussed in the context of a person's overall goals of care and treatment needs. Recommendations about CPR should be decided on an individual basis as person-centred, shared decisions, and should involve honest, effective communication between clinicians and their patients. Recommendations and valid reasons for them should be recorded clearly on a document that remains with the person and is accessible to any clinician who may need it to guide immediate decision-making in a crisis. Documents containing recommendations about CPR and other life-sustaining treatment should be recognisable and accepted widely, across organisational and geographic boundaries.

## References

1. **Kouwenhoven WB, Jude JR,** and **Knickerbocker GG** (1960). 'Closed chest cardiac massage'. *JAMA* **173**: 1064–7.

2. **Beck CS** (1961). 'Hearts too good to die'. *JAMA* **176**: 141–2.

3. **Julian DG** (1961). 'Treatment of cardiac arrest in acute myocardial ischaemia and infarction'. *Lancet* **ii**: 840–4.

4. **Killip T** and **Kimball JT** (1967). 'Treatment of myocardial infarction in a coronary care unit: a two-year experience with 250 patients'. *Am J Cardiol* **20**: 457–64.

5. **Rabkin MT, Gillerman G,** and **Rice NR** (1976). Orders not to resuscitate. *N Engl J Med*, **295**: 364–6. Available from: http://dx.doi.org/10.1056/NEJM197608122950705.

6. **British Medical Association, Resuscitation Council (UK)** and **Royal College of Nursing** (2016). *Decisions relating to cardiopulmonary resuscitation.* 3rd edition (1st revision). Available from: www.resus.org.uk/dnacpr/decisions-relating-to-cpr/.

7. **National Confidential Enquiry into Patient Outcome and Death (NCEPOD)** (2012). *Time to intervene.* NCEPOD. London. Available from: www.ncepod.org.uk/reports.html.

8. **British Geriatrics Society** (2014). *Fit for frailty—consensus best practice guidance for the care of older people living with frailty in community and outpatient settings.* BGS. Available from: http://www.bgs.org.uk/index.php/component/content/article/295-resources/campaigns/fit-for-frailty/2953-fff-guidance-download

9. **H M Government. Mental Capacity Act 2005.** The Stationery Office. London (2005). Available from: www.legislation.gov.uk/ukpga/2005/9/contents

10. **Department for Constitutional Affairs.** *Mental Capacity Act 2005: Code of Practice.* The Stationery Office. London 2007. Available from: www.gov.uk/government/publications/mental-capacity-act-code-of-practice.

11. **Perkins GD, Griffiths F, Slowther A-M,** et al. (2016). 'Do-not-attemptcardiopulmonary-resuscitation decisions: an evidence synthesis'. *Health Serv Deliv Res* **4**(11). doi: 10.3310/hsdr04110.

12. R (On behalf of David Tracey personally and on behalf of the Estate of Janet Tracey (Deceased)) v (1) Cambridge University Hospitals NHS Foundation Trust (2) Secretary of State for Health [2014] EWCA Civ 822.

13. **H M Government. Human Rights Act** (1998). Avaliable from: www.legislation.gov.uk/ukpga/1998/42/contents.

14. **Myint PK, Miles S, Halliday DA,** and **Bowker LK** (2006). 'Experiences and views of specialist registrars in geriatric medicine on "do not attempt resuscitation" decisions: a sea of uncertainty?' *QJM* **99**: 691–700. http://dx.doi.org/10.1093/qjmed/hcl096

15. Winspear v City Hospitals Sunderland NHS Foundation Trust [2015] EWHC 3250 (QB).

16. **Munday D** and **Petrova M** (2009). 'Exploring preferences for place of death with terminally ill patients: qualitative study of experiences of general practitioners and community nurses in England'. *BMJ* **339**: b2391.

17. **Knauft E, Nielsen EL, Engelberg RA, Patrick DL,** and **Curtis JR** (2005). 'Barriers and facilitators to end-of-life care communication for patients with COPD'. *Chest* **127**: 2188–96.

18. **Fritz Z, Malyon A, Frankau JM** et al. (2013). 'The Universal Form of Treatment Options (UFTO) as an alternative to Do Not Attempt Cardiopulmonary Resuscitation (DNACPR) orders: a mixed methods evaluation of the effects on clinical practice and patient care'. *PLOS ONE* **8**: e70977. Avaliable from: http://dx.doi.org/10.1371/journal.pone.0070977

19. **Jones GK1, Brewer KL,** and **Garrison HG** (2000). 'Public expectations of survival following cardiopulmonary resuscitation'. *Acad Emerg Med* **7**: 48–53.

20. **Ruiz-García J, Alegría-Barrero E,** and **Díez-Villanueva P,** et al. (2016). 'Expectations of survival following cardiopulmonary resuscitation. Predictions and wishes of patients with heart disease'. *Rev Esp Cardiol* **69**: 613–5.

21. **Fritz Z B**, Barclay S. (2014). Patients' resuscitation preferences in context: Lessons from POLST. *Resuscitation* **85**: 444–5.

22. **British Columbia Interior Health Authority**. *Medical Orders for Scope of Treatment (MOST)*. Avaliable from: https://www.interiorhealth.ca/YourCare/PalliativeCare/ToughDecisions/Pages/Medical-Orders-for-Scope-of-Treatment-(MOST).aspx.

23. **Coombes R** (2017). We need to talk about resuscitation. *BMJ* : **356**: j1216.

24. **Pitcher D**, **Soar J**, **Hogg K**, et al. (2016). 'Cardiovascular implanted electronic devices in people towards the end of life, during cardiopulmonary resuscitation and after death: guidance from the Resuscitation Council (UK), British Cardiovascular Society and National Council for Palliative Care'. *Heart* **102**: A1–A17.

25. **Heslop P**, **Blair P**, **Fleming P** et al. (2013). *The Confidential Inquiry into premature deaths of people with learning disabilities* (CIPOLD). Norah Fry Research Centre. Bristol. Avaliable from: www.bristol.ac.uk/cipold/reports/

26. **HM Government**. Equality Act 2010. Avaliable from: http://www.legislation.gov.uk/ukpga/2010/15/contents

# The implications of the Mental Capacity Act (MCA) 2005 for advance care planning and decision making

Simon Chapman and Ben Lobo

---

**This chapter includes**

- An overview of the MCA's impact on end of life care
- Setting the MCA in the context of current policy and practice
- How the MCA can:
  - Be used to improve care
  - Enable and empower people to express and protect choices
  - Support and enable the professional and/or the proxy decision maker
- An introduction and explanation of the role of the IMCA and how it might apply to Advance Care Planning (ACP) and end of life decision making
- An explanation of the legal and ethical process involved in reaching best interest decisions, especially for potentially vulnerable people in care homes and other settings

---

**Key Points**

- Planning ahead: using ACP to identify and protect an individual's preferences and choices should they lose capacity to make a particular decision in the future
- Assessing a person's capacity to make decisions (including making advance care plans)
- Implementing ACP: making decisions on behalf of someone who lacks capacity
- The IMCA is a new provision in English law with a specific role and statutory rights
- IMCAs are not decision makers but ensure the correct process has been followed for a decision to be reached in the best interests of the person who lacks capacity
- There are areas to be tested in case law especially in the interpretation of serious medical treatment that will clarify the role and requirement to involve an IMCA
- Advance care plans which include expressions of preferences and wishes (including treatment decisions) will greatly help both the decision maker and IMCA arrive at reasonable conclusions about what is in the person's best interest

---

**Key Message**

ACP and end of life decisions must follow a robust ethical and legal framework.

# Summary

The Mental Capacity Act (MCA) 2005, which applies in England and Wales, but not Scotland or Northern Ireland, provides the statutory framework within which Advance Care Planning (ACP) must be used, adding to the statutory rights and protection of an individual. The MCA provides a supportive framework within which adults can express and protect their choices and preferences about their future care, should they lose capacity to make their own decisions.

The National End of Life Care Strategy in England (2008) placed great emphasis on introducing ACP, and meeting people's choices and preferences for their end of life care has been a consistent goal of national policy in England since then. The Government Response to the Review of Choice in End of Life Care 2016 described the policy commitments (1). The MCA provides vital legislative support for that policy goal. This Act has been supported by the associated legal administrative and judicial agencies including the Court of Protection.

# Background

## The impact of the Mental Capacity Act

The impact of the Mental Capacity Act on ACP and end of life care can be seen from this list of some of the issues that it covers:

- Statutory frameworks and processes:
  - To assess people's capacity
  - To determine their best interests

- An underlying duty to take all practicable steps to support people so that they can make their own decisions

- An emphasis throughout on person-centred care

- Duty to consult the people who are important to the individual concerned about that person's best interests

- People's preferences and choices about their future care must be taken into account should they lose capacity to make a particular decision

- Advance decisions to refuse treatment

- New types of proxy decision making and advocacy: lasting powers of attorney and independent mental capacity advocates

- It is accompanied by a Code of Practice 2007 to which paid carers must have regard

- It sets up administrative and judicial architecture: the Office of the Public Guardian and Court of Protection

There are still uncertainties as to how well understood and embedded the MCA is in health and social care practice (2). It has a very broad range: it covers every decision made by or on behalf of people with impaired mental capacity, including financial decisions about property or investments, decisions about place of care, day-to-day living, and decisions about medical treatment.

## Planning ahead: using advance care planning to identify and protect people's preferences and choices should they lose capacity to make particular decisions in the future

There are a number of ways that a person with capacity can use MCA provisions to identify and in some cases protect their choices about their future care and treatment, should they lose capacity to decide for themselves as they can:

◆ Nominate people whom they would like to be consulted when decisions are being made

◆ Identify people whom they would not wish to be consulted

◆ Make statements about their preferences and choices to inform and assist people who may later have to make decisions about their care or treatment. These statements must be taken into account when best-interest decisions are made in relation to them

◆ Appoint another person (or more than one person) to consent to or refuse treatment on their behalf, by giving a Personal Welfare Lasting Power of Attorney

◆ Identify specific treatment(s) that they wish to refuse, and any circumstances in which they want that to apply—an advance decision to refuse treatment (ADRT)

A person may do one of these, or any, or all of them in combination. Together they create what is in effect a statutory toolkit for ACP, which an adult with capacity can use at any time of their life. Those who subsequently provide care and treatment to them will need to respond appropriately and in accordance with the MCA.

Some people will do some of these things before they ever become ill. For others, the experience of living with a life-threatening condition may lead them to ask what they can do to control or influence their future care. In all cases it is important for them and everybody concerned to remember that people's wishes and preferences change over time and that any advance care plans they have made should be kept under review. Both they and anybody providing care to them should revisit any advance care plans that have been made on a regular basis.

This section of the chapter considers what people need to do to use ACP in anticipation that they might lose capacity to make particular decisions about their care and treatment, and the factors they should keep in mind. It is written with their perspective foremost. The later section, on implementing people's advance care plans, considers how others should respond to those advance care plans, once the person who made them has lost capacity to make a particular decision.

## Nominating people to be consulted

Under the MCA it is possible for people to nominate others who should be consulted about their best interests, should they lose capacity at a later stage. Those nominees must be consulted if practicable to do so. They will not be decision makers, and this is not the same as creating a proxy decision maker under a Lasting Power of Attorney (LPA). Equally, it is possible to identify people who should not be consulted. One example of this might be a close family member, who in ordinary circumstances might expect to be consulted, but whom the person believes that, for whatever reason, would not be able to give reliable insights into the person's best interests.

### Making statements about preferences and choices

This is the area in which the relationship between legislation (the MCA) and practice (ACP) is most apparent.

The MCA states that a person's wishes, feelings, beliefs, and values, including any written statement that they made whilst they had capacity, must be taken into account when assessing their best interests if they have lost capacity to make a particular decision (3). Compare that with what is included in the following definition of ACP (author's emphasis added):

An ACP discussion might include:

◆ The individual's **concerns**

◆ Their important **values** or **personal goals** for care

◆ Their understanding about their illness and prognosis

- Their **preferences** for types of care or treatment that may be beneficial in the future and the availability of these (4)

So a person can make an advance care plan which includes statements about their choices and preferences, in the knowledge that such statements must be taken into account by anyone who makes a decision about their care or treatment should they lose capacity. Unless they amount to an advance decision to refuse treatment, these statements will not be legally binding. However the person who makes a decision must take them into account and, if they do not follow them, be prepared to explain why not if challenged. This is powerful legislative support for ACP.

The MCA refers in particular to written statements about people's preferences. That is not to say that verbal statements are not valid; they may be very powerful. However it is always wise for people to record their wishes in writing. If they make verbal statements to professional care providers they should be recorded in people's notes and included in Advance Care Plans.

## Lasting Power of Attorney

The change from Enduring Powers of Attorney (EPAs) to LPAs is one of the most significant aspects of the MCA. It had always been possible to appoint a proxy to make decisions about your property and affairs using an EPA. The MCA extends that and makes it possible to appoint people to make decisions about personal welfare, which includes your health and social care. More property and affairs LPAs are being registered than personal welfare LPAs (5). As a result many health and social care professionals have not encountered a personal welfare LPA. However it is likely that their usage will increase.

A Lasting Power of Attorney is a type of agency arrangement. It is formal. Attorneys can only be appointed by using a prescribed form, which can be downloaded via the Office of the Public Guardian website (6). The LPA form must be registered before it takes effect, and a fee is payable (7).

There is some flexibility. An individual can appoint more than one person as an attorney, and can appoint different attorneys to make different kinds of decision. People should only give LPAs to people that they trust. They should not be placed under any pressure to give anybody this power.

Anyone deciding to create an LPA would be well-advised to discuss their wishes with the person to whom they have given the LPA (the 'donee'), to tell them what they would want to happen. This might include making a written statement about their preferences. Like any other decision-maker, the donee will be required to make decisions in the best interests of the person [the donor] who gave them the LPA and this will include taking into account any statements the donor made whilst they had capacity. LPAs are governed by sections 9–14 of the MCA. Further information about LPAs can also be found in Chapter 7 of the Code of Practice.

## Advance decisions to refuse treatment

More information about advance decisions to refuse treatment can be found in Chapter 9. The information in this chapter is intended to describe how advance decisions to refuse treatment fit into the overall range of options available to a person who wishes to do ACP. Of the many important things to understand about advance decisions, the first is that this area of law applies only to decisions to refuse treatment. It does not apply to requests, and it does not apply to non-treatment decisions. People can of course make advance care plans which include requests and which cover issues other than their treatment, for example about their place of care. However, whilst such preferences must always be taken into account, they will not legally binding in the same way that an advance decision to refuse treatment can be (8).

## Relationship between Lasting Powers of Attorney and advance decisions

It is possible both to give an LPA to somebody and to make an advance decision to refuse a specific treatment. If a person does both, the rule is that the one done later is the one that counts. So, if a person gives an LPA to a relative and subsequently makes an advance decision, the advance decision should be followed.

## Offering and recording advance care planning: professionals

Everybody identified as approaching the end of life should be offered the opportunity to participate inACP. They don't need to wait for the offer either; ACP is a right that people can exercise whenever they want to. However it is voluntary. For some it will be a valuable reassurance to know that their preferences and choices have been recorded and will be used in decision making about their care should they lose capacity. Others may find it difficult or distressing to consider their future. People should be offered the opportunity to make advance care plans if they wish to, but they should not be compelled to make them.

Health and care professionals will need training in ACP and communication appropriate to their level (7). Those whose role it is to offer ACP and open discussion about it will need training in how to do this. It should be remembered that some members of staff, such as care assistants, may spend considerable time with a person. The insights and information they gain from conversations with people for whom they are caring may provide very valuable assistance and evidence when it comes to assessing those people's best interests. Their line managers and employers should recognise the potential for this, and support all their staff so that they can contribute to care and decision-making and be ready to record and report significant conversations.

# Implementing advance care planning: making decisions on behalf of someone who lacks capacity

## Capacity

The starting point is assessing the person's capacity. If a person has capacity to make a decision, they should be enabled to make that decision, with appropriate support where necessary. Advance care plans should only be considered when the person is assessed as not having capacity to make a particular decision, even with support. The MCA contains a statutory framework for the assessment of a person's capacity (9), (see Box 11.1).

## Decision-by-decision basis

A person's capacity should not be assessed on a blanket basis so that they are regarded as either having capacity or not (unless they are unconscious, or close to it, or locked-in). Instead, capacity must be assessed on a decision-by-decision basis.

Decisions range enormously in terms of importance and complexity. A person might have the capacity, with support, to make a range of simple decisions which together would have a significant impact on their daily experience of care. For example, a care home resident may be able to decide the following: what to wear; what to eat; where to sit; who to talk with; whether to read, watch television, or go outside. They might not be able to make complicated financial decisions about investments.

## Maximising capacity

This is covered in detail in other chapters. If the decision does not need to be made immediately or in an emergency all reasonable attempts must be made to maximise capacity, for example

## Box 11.1 Mental capacity, the key points

- ◆ A person's capacity should be assessed on a decision by decision basis
- ◆ A person's capacity must not be assessed merely by reference to the person's age, appearance, condition, or an aspect of their behaviour
- ◆ The MCA sets out the following process to be followed when assessing somebody's capacity to make a particular decision:
  - Identify the decision that needs to be made
  - Ask the 'functional' question: does the person have impaired understanding, judgement, memory, or ability to communicate which, even with all practicable support being given, amounts to incapacity to:
    - Understand information about the decision to be made
    - Retain that information in their mind
    - Use or weigh-up the information as part of the decision process; or
    - Communicate their decision?
  - If the answer to the 'functional' question is 'yes':
  - Ask the 'diagnostic question': at the time the decision needs to be made, does the person have an impairment or disturbance of their mind or brain, and is that what is causing their lack of capacity?
- ◆ A person must be supported so that they can make their own decisions so far as possible

treat any reversible medical problem or find and provide specialist communication assistance. This might mean new ways of working, organising ward routine, staffing differently, or learning new methods of communication. There is a duty to support people to make their own decisions, which will mean that anybody who has assessed that a person is unable to make a decision will need to be able to show that they took all practicable steps to support that person, if challenged about it.

## Person-centred assessment: capacity and best interests

The MCA's provisions about assessing both capacity and best interests contain the same prohibition against assessing a person simply by reference to their age, appearance, condition, or any aspect of their behaviour which may lead to the making of unjustified assumptions about them. These are often summed up as 'do not discriminate', and are in the same line as other rights-based legislation; in the care context they emphasise the importance of being person-centred and carefully assessing the individual.

## Legal obligation to act in best interests

If, even with support, the person is assessed as lacking capacity to make a particular decision, then any advance care plans must be considered. In summary this will mean:

- ◆ If it is a decision about treatment, assessing whether there is a legally-binding advance decision to refuse treatment
- ◆ In the absence of that, making a decision in the person's best interests

The MCA sets out a statutory checklist about what must be taken into account when assessing a person's best interests. This will include any advance care plans they made which contain evidence about what they wanted to happen, or not. There is also a duty, where practicable, to consult anybody who is a carer for that person or interested in their welfare, about what their views are about the person's best interests. This will almost always include family members.

## Who is the decision maker?

This is a vital question, and there is potential for considerable misunderstanding, distress, and conflict where this is not clearly addressed. In particular, there is a risk that relatives will carry the burden of making best-interest decisions which are not theirs to make, albeit that they should be consulted about them.

### Where there is no proxy decision maker

Although it is expressed in convoluted language, the result of section 5 of the MCA is that the person who is responsible for the decision is the person who implements it. Section 5 states that a person (D) can do an act in relation to the care or treatment of another person (P) if D reasonably believes both that P did not have capacity to make the decision and that the act was in P's best interests. So for example, where a decision has to be made about the withdrawal of medical treatment at the end of life, the decision maker is the doctor who withdraws the treatment. However, the people who are important to the individual concerned and interested in their care must also be consulted if that is practicable.

### Where there is a proxy decision maker

Where there is a proxy decision maker either under a Lasting Power of Attorney or because the court has appointed a deputy, that person is responsible for making the decision. They must still follow best interests and consult family members and those close to the person where practicable.

Decisions can be challenged if it is felt they cannot be justified by reference to the person's best interests, using the factors identified in the MCA (section 4).

## Decisions by health and social care professionals

In cases where clinical decisions need taken urgently for a person who lacks capacity it is the senior clinicians responsibility to ensure correct treatment and care is delivered. This might include reversing any cause of incapacity and stabilising the patient's condition so that the patient can recover, regain capacity, and then make their own decision. The law makes provision for clinicians to take decisions especially where there is reasonable doubt e.g. the existence, validity, and applicability of an advance decision to refuse treatment. It is important to also understand that there might be decisions that relate to urgent and important social care issues e.g. the safeguarding of a vulnerable adult (who lacks capacity). There are formal mechanisms in England and Wales to achieve this by a partnership agreement with Health, Social Care, and the Local Authority. This is important especially if the vulnerable person requires admission to a care home. The same principles and statutory requirements of the MCA must apply to any decision to protect and offer care to such a person.

The Law Commission published a report setting out recommendations on 13 March 2017, together with a draft Bill. The final report and draft Bill recommends that the Deprivation of Liberty and Safeguards (DoLS) be repealed with pressing urgency and sets out a replacement scheme for the DoLS which they have called the Liberty Protection Safeguards. In addition the draft Bill makes wider reforms to the Mental Capacity Act which ensure greater safeguards for persons before they are deprived of their liberty (10). There is also new Guidance on Mental Capacity Act which can be found on the link provided (11).

## References

1. **Department of Health, NHS England** (2016). *Our commitment to you for end of life care* [Internet], Available from: https://www.gov.uk/.
2. **Select Committee on the Mental Capacity Act 2005**, House of Lords (2014). *Mental Capacity Act 2005: post-legislative scrutiny.* [Internet] Available from: https://www.publications.parliament.uk/
3. Section 4 of the Mental Capacity Act 2005 (MCA).
4. **Henry C** and **Seymour JE** (2007). *Advance Care Planning: a guide for heath and social care professionals.* National End of Life Care Programme, Leicester. (Revised 2008.)
5. **Office of the Public Guardian**, Annual Report 2007–8. Available from: http://www.publicguardian.gov. uk/docs/opg-annuual-report-2007-08.pdf. (Accessed 28 October 2010).
6. **Office of the Public Guardian (OPG).** Available from: www.gov.uk.
7. **Core Skills Training Framework** (2104). Avaialble from: http://www.skillsforhealth.org.uk/services/item/146-core-skills-training-framework
8. **The National End of Life Care Programme and the National Council for Palliative Care** (2008). *Advance Decisions to Refuse Treatment: a guide for health and social care professionals.* Available from: http://www.ncpc.org.uk/ (Accessed 11 September 2017.)
9. **Sections 2 & 3 of the Mental Capacity Act 2005.** See also the National Council for Palliative Care publication: (2017). *Good Decision-making—What you need to know about the Mental Capacity Act and end of life care.* 2nd edition (2017) Available from: www.ncpc.org.uk/publications.
10. **Law Commission** (2017). *Mental Capacity and Deprivation of Liberty* [Internet]. Available from: http://www.lawcom.gov.uk/
11. **New guidance on the Mental Capacity Act** (2016). Available from: https://gallery.mailchimp.com/ea6a78606131cd2a0c50cb52b/files/475fbcf0-2d6c-41b2-995c-ed7f4c4db69c/MCA_Guidance.pdf

Chapter 12

# Experience of use of advance care planning in care homes

Maggie Stobbart-Rowlands and Mandy Thorn

'Focus on the needs of residents'
*GSF Accredited Care Home Manager*

---

**This chapter includes**

- Information about The Care Act (2014)
- Consideration of factors that impact the use of advance care planning (ACP) in care homes
- The Gold Standards Framework in Care Homes (GSFCH) programme
- Discussions about training on ACP within the GSF care homes

---

**Key Points**

- ACP discussions are especially important for residents in care homes ensuring that they are involved in decisions about their care
- Admission to a care home is a key trigger for initiating an ACP discussion.
- ACP should become part of mainstream practice in all care homes
- Care homes lead the way in their extensive use of ACP discussions
- Key challenges for residents include poor means of communication due to dementia/ cognitive impairment or physical deterioration
- Barriers to holding these discussions include staff resistance, communication skills, confidence, and sensitivity of timing
- The Gold Standards Framework in Care Homes (GSFCH) Training Programme supports and recommends that ACP discussions are offered to all residents
- ACP helps to provide a culture of openness within the home and puts the resident at the centre of care provision

---

**Key Message**

Care homes deliver highly personalised care and support to increasingly frail and dependent people. Enabling citizens to have real involvement in shaping their care and support is crucial in delivering high-quality care. How that care is proactively planned, with the involvement of the resident, their family and friends creates the foundation upon which the planning for care at times of serious illness or at the end of life is based (1).

## Introduction

Advance care planning (ACP) is important for all, but is of particular significance for people living in care homes to ensure their choices for care at the end of life are respected.

For many this means having personal choices and preferences for how care is delivered accommodated, and being treated with dignity and respect in familiar surroundings. Many people realise that on entering a care home will be there for the remainder of their life; however, discussions about end of life care are often avoided for fear of upsetting the individual or family, thus missing the opportunity for the person to be involved in planning their future care.

Where ACP has become part of standard practice, as in those care homes using the GSF programme (2), the impact has been considerable.

Staff sometimes struggle when holding ACP discussions, but once they see the difference they can make for the individual and their family, staff grow in confidence and this becomes a natural part of their care. Staff are ideally placed to discuss with those they support what their wishes and preferences are for their future care. Using 'Life Story' work enables staff to explore residents' thoughts and priorities which can be of immense help in understanding the individual and therefore providing improved person-centred care (3).

This chapter highlights the importance of implementing consistent use of ACP; of developing the competence and confidence of staff to impact practice and improve the lives of residents in their care. The context in care homes is explored as are some of the challenges faced. Experiences of staff in care homes are shared while seeking to draw attention to the importance of appropriate training for ACP in care homes. The implementation of the GSFCH training programme (2) is outlined as a vehicle for helping to underpin the principles for ACP in this setting.

## The care home setting

Over the last few years there have been significant changes in the social care sector; the focus has changed to care staff providing most of the care with varying degrees of support (4).

The Care Act (2014) confirmed the importance of providing out of hospital care and support. However, around a third of people in acute hospitals are thought to be in their last year of life (5). Most of those would not wish to be there, but their wishes are often not sought (6).

Many individuals in care homes have multiple co-morbidities with complex health and social care needs, including 80% with dementia (6). This high level of need poses real challenges in ensuring that the appropriate care and support is provided by skilled and confident staff. Planning ahead can be challenging; there is a high turnover of staff and in some areas a reliance on non-indigenous staff which can cause cultural and language difficulties in relating to people with complex conditions and reduced cognitive abilities.

Around 1% of the UK population now live in care homes for older people, this is sure to increase with increasing longevity. Recent figures show that 22% of deaths in the UK occur in a care home (8).

## Aspects that have an impact on the use of ACP in care homes

### Rethinking the excessive use of hospitals

The care home is where the person has chosen to live and would often choose to remain until they die. However, there is evidence that significant numbers of residents are transferred from care homes to acute hospitals in the last days or weeks of life, when this is not necessarily their wish, or in their best interests (7). With lack of, or inadequate ACP discussion, and no plan for proactive care, a crisis can result in an inappropriate hospital admission, see (Figure 12.1). Fifty per cent of frail care homes residents could have died at home. See Chapter 4 on economic benefits.

Hospital admission often becomes the default course of action in a crisis, without consideration of whether the benefits of admission outweigh the negative impacts, especially for people with dementia (7). A greater emphasis towards more proactive planning of care focused on the individual's expressed preferences and wishes is needed.

Some care homes, particularly in urban areas of the UK have a large multicultural component, not only among the staff but also among those who use their services. Many staff have their own pre-conceptions about the benefit of hospital care, and their own cultural norms about death and dying. A lack of acknowledgement of our own and residents' mortality, coupled with a lack of early discussion and planning can result in staff, residents, and their relatives not being prepared for the end of life, resulting in 'unexpected' deaths, many of which could have been anticipated had the signs of deterioration been recognised (9).

## Communication issues

Communication is at the heart of end life care. Talking about death and dying can be difficult for staff as well as for residents and their families, but asking people and noting where and how they would like to be cared for at the earliest available opportunity helps to take the pressure off staff at the time of crisis.

An ACP discussion might include the individual's concerns; their important values or personal goals for care; their understanding about their illness and prognosis; and their preferences for types of care or treatment that may be beneficial in the future. In some instances, with residents who have been living in the care home for many years, approaching a conversation about their wishes towards the end of life can prove more difficult than introducing the topic prior to admission (11).

The most common reason given by care home staff for not wanting to initiate discussion about end of life care is that 'they are afraid of upsetting the person or the family'. In the work of the GSFCH Programme, we have found that staff regularly express three main fears:

- The fear of getting it wrong
- The fear of upsetting residents and families
- The fear of being misunderstood or misquoted

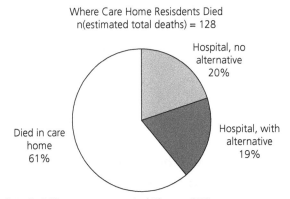

**Figure 12.1** National Audit Office report on end of life care (10)

Source: data from National Audit Office, 'End of Life Care: Survey of Care Homes', Available from: http://www.nao.org.uk/

With considerable turnover of staff both at management level and in the general workforce, there is a constant need to ensure that new staff are fully aware of ACP discussions. Ongoing end of life care and communication skills training is important for all staff.

## Advance care planning: whose role is it?

In our experience of working with over 2600 care homes through the GSFCH Programme, we affirm the importance of every staff member being able to have these discussions, but suggest appropriate people are nominated to lead on this. Whoever undertakes these discussions needs to have formed a good, trusting relationship with the person and their family.

Many prefer to support families to talk with their relative about how they would want their care at the end of life to be delivered before admission to the care home and before further discussion with staff. Residents and relatives are informed that holding such discussions is part of the usual procedure within the home and are given information describing what this might mean for them (12).

Many homes write their own introduction to ACP or use the 'Planning for your future care' leaflet (13). This then helps families feel more at ease in discussing the future care of their relative and can lead to very special and deeper discussions that otherwise might not happen. This helps 'de-medicalise' the topic, making it essentially a discussion about living well now, best care, and preferences for the future.

ACP discussions with an individual resident are intended to make clear their personal wishes, preferences, beliefs, and values about the kind of care they would like to receive and, even more importantly, how they would like to live their life until the end. Timing is important, as is recognising and acknowledging cues from residents. For obvious reasons, it is best to have these discussions when the resident's health is relatively stable, and not when they are in crisis. Discussions should be recorded in such a way that the resident's wishes and priorities can be reviewed and, with permission, shared with key people involved in their care. Of course, this is a voluntary process, and some would prefer not to discuss it at all—and that is completely acceptable.

### Do not attempt cardiopulmonary resuscitation discussions

Recent guidance from the Resuscitation Council, states that for many people anticipatory decisions about CPR are best made in the wider context of ACP, before a crisis necessitates a hurried decision in an emergency setting (14).

This subject does need to be discussed and recorded to prevent inappropriate resuscitation attempts. However, every decision about CPR must be based on a careful assessment of each individual's situation. These decisions should never be dictated by 'blanket' policies.

The guidance goes on to say that although a decision not to attempt CPR that has no realistic prospect of success does not require the consent of the person or those close to them, there should be a presumption in favour of informing them of such a decision. Effective communication is essential to ensure that decisions about CPR are made well and understood clearly by all those involved.

It must be clearly explained to everyone involved, including professionals, that the decision to not attempt CPR relates only to CPR and no other aspect of care will be compromised.

### Case study

An emergency '999' call followed the collapse of an 86-year-old resident of a care home. The home was many miles from the nearest hospital so resulted in air ambulance attendance, the emergency team attempted resuscitation, but this failed and the resident was taken to the nearest hospital classified as 'Brought in Dead'. She had previously stated that she 'didn't want any heroics'—a comment which was not explored further with her, recorded, or communicated to others.

In the circumstances this lack of communication resulted in an undignified death, traumatised family and staff, and led to an inappropriate use of scarce and expensive resources. The multidisciplinary team later reflected on the management and death of this resident, using the Significant Event Analysis template (2) and agreed that. as an action point in future, ACP and DNACPR discussions in the care home would be offered to every resident, recorded, and communicated appropriately to emergency and out of hours services, to prevent a similar catastrophic event occurring again. This later became mainstreamed and adopted through local policy.

# Advance care planning in the The Gold Standards Framework in Care Homes Programme

The theme of ACP is a key element throughout the training programme. It is pivotal in ensuring that the more personalised aspects of care are delivered, and in clarifying how the person wants to live.

A summary of the GSFCH training programme is given in Box 12.1.

'Introducing Advance Care Planning into our home as normal practice has been one of the most important things we have done—it's crucial to helping us focus on the needs of residents, it helps discussions with families and it changes the way we do everything. Even though it may be hard at first, we would very strongly recommend it for every care home.'

(*GSF Accredited Care Home Manager*)

The implementation of the GSF training programme has contributed greatly to the ACP process through teaching, sharing experiences, and examples in practice.

# Training on advance care planning within the Gold Standards Framework in Care Homes training programme

## Topics covered across six workshops

- The 'needs based coding' of all residents related to their trajectory of illness ensures that the right thing happens at the right time and in the right place
- ACP to reduce avoidable hospitalisation
- Communication skills
- Reflective group work with staff from other care homes enables sharing of experiences, challenges, and solutions
- Difficult discussions as people approach the last days of life, the importance of language used
- Care for people with dementia is included in every workshop topic, including 'Best Interest Decisions' for those who lack capacity to make decisions about their future care

## Consolidation leading to the accreditation stage

- The ACP standard for accreditation states 'An Advance Care Planning (ACP) discussion is offered and recorded for all residents'

---

## Box 12.1 The Gold Standards Framework in Care Homes Programme

The programme grew out of the work of GSF in primary care, but is quite independent of it, with a separately evolved training programme tailored specifically to meet the needs of care homes' staff. It is the most widely used training programme in end of life care. Used by care homes across the UK over 2600 care homes are now included, with about 100 being accredited each year. The programme is run by the GSF central team but integrated into local areas with regional centres.

The programme has three aims:

1. To improve the quality of care provided for all residents from admission
2. To improve collaboration with GPs, primary care teams, and specialists
3. To improve outcomes, enabling more to die at home if that is their wish, and reducing inappropriate hospitalisation

Key elements include:

◆ A three-stage quality improvement process with preparation and training in the first year plus consolidation leading to accreditation

◆ The GSFCH accreditation process 'Going for Gold', provides quality assurance using an independent validated process

- It integrates well and leads on to use of other national tools
- The work is strongly peer led and supported, using detailed examples of best practice

The GSFCH Programme can be commissioned from the National GSF Centre—see www. goldstandardsframework.org.uk or email info@goldstandardsframework.co.uk

Source: data from the Gold Standards Framework

---

◆ Accreditation involves self-assessment against twenty standards, a portfolio of evidence, further audits including after death analysis (ADA), and a visit to the care home by a GSF trained assessor.

All findings are reviewed and judged by an independent panel who make the final decision on the award.

> 'Gold Standards Framework and Advance Care Plan discussion information is part of the admission process and is routinely completed at the six-week review. We have found this to be a successful strategy and greatly assists in the provision of good end of life care.'
>
> (*Matron from GSFCH accredited home, 2009*)

A summary of the GSF advance care plan is given in Box 12.2.

## Training the workforce

The level of confidence and skills of the workforce reflects the ability of the staff to fulfil this important role. Some staff expressed a fear of 'communicating a difficult subject' as a reason to hold back. Breaking ACP down into a step by step process can help dispel fears. Whilst teaching communication skills is very important, it cannot be done effectively in isolation of end of life care needs. It is important for both staff and residents to understand what is being communicated, either through the words used or the tone of voice in which it is said, a good understanding of

## Box 12.2 The GSF advance care plan: thinking ahead (2)

1. At this time in your life what is it that makes you happy?
   - What do you hope for? What do you enjoy doing?
   - What or who is important to you?
   - Is there anything you're especially worried about?

2. What elements of care are important to you and what would you like to happen in the future?
   - Statements of wishes and preferences can include personal preferences, such as where one would wish to live, having a shower rather than a bath, or wanting to sleep with the light on. Such statements may also include requests and/or types of medical treatment they would or would not want to receive
   - Discussion should focus on the views of the individual, although they may wish to invite their carer or another close family member or friend to participate
   - Some families are likely to have discussed preferences and would welcome an approach to share this discussion

3. Is there anything that you worry about or fear happening? What would you not want to happen?
   - What worries you most?
   - Can you help me understand a bit better?
   - What else would help you cope?
   - What is helping most now?
   - Do you find yourself thinking about what is going to happen to you?
   - Are there things that bother you that you find yourself dwelling on?

4. Ending difficult conversations but enabling ongoing discussion later
   - Acknowledge emotional intensity of conversation e.g. 'We've talked about a lot of important things today'
   - Help the person to rehearse what they need to do, who to talk to?
   - Try and close the conversation on a positive note
   - End conversation in a safe place for them—refer to everyday, practical topics
   - 'What you have said is very important, can we continue this tomorrow?'
   - 'Is there anything else you want to say?'

Reproduced courtesy of the Gold Standards Framework

non-verbal communication, and picking up on cues is vitally important. Staff do need to understand the concept of the use of 'open' and 'closed' questions, allowing the person time to consider their thoughts, feelings, and opinions.

It is also important to remember the value of opportunistic conversations. Carers who deliver most of the 'hands-on' care are best placed to know the resident's preferences and choices. However, their contribution to ACP can be undervalued. With support and training they recognise the important role they play in the ACP process, and that it is about their relationships with residents and families in everyday practice.

Staff who feel they have communicated well and discussed ACP successfully with residents develop in confidence. Feedback from residents and families appears to have a great effect on staff confidence and morale. Where the death is deemed to be peaceful and comfortable, in the place of choice, with families well supported and informed, staff respond with renewed enthusiasm to continue to develop practice in their home.

## Caring for people with dementia

Staff who care for residents with dementia have difficulty in ascertaining wishes and preferences, especially for those residents who have no family. Staff speak of their own distress and powerlessness at seeing residents with dementia being sent to hospital in the last 48 hours of life because of lack of documentation relating to wishes and preferences (see Chapter 17 on dementia).

People with dementia should be offered the opportunity to have an ACP discussion whilst they still have capacity, however this is much less likely to happen (4) as admission to a care setting normally takes place late in the illness progression, when there has been significant cognitive decline.

Such discussions can take place even though the individual may have quite advanced dementia, if they have capacity—the ability to understand and speculate about the decision to be made. Therefore, we should be more willing to ask people with dementia their views. Families can sometimes be a barrier to these discussions for people who lack capacity, but if staff can develop the confidence to have open and honest discussions, giving clear and comprehensive information about the benefits and burdens of certain actions, e.g. admissions to hospital, working to the principles of the Mental Capacity Act (15), they are more likely to be able to develop partnerships with the families, ensuring that all interventions are in the best interest of the person (16).

## Developing a learning culture in care homes

Learning in care homes requires a multifaceted approach when aiming to change practice in care homes. Staff have a wide variety of learning needs based on age, culture, language, and understanding (17). Role modelling good practice can be effective in developing skills and confidence. A systematic approach to learning that acknowledges and reflects on events should be encouraged in care homes giving the opportunity to reflect on practice and develop further.

Empowering the staff enables them to advocate better for their residents, and helps to build relationships.

Care home staff are often undervalued as a group of workers, and yet we have high expectations of them to provide well-coordinated person-centred care with often limited access to training. The standards of care we expect, particularly for the most vulnerable, are high and investment in the social care workforce development needs to be a high priority.

> 'We are committed to making our residents' stay as perfect as possible, . . .. caring for them in the way we would want to be cared for ourselves. . . . all our staff, feel more confident about having difficult conversations with our residents and their families about the care they want and where they want to be cared for. This, in turn, means we are now always prepared and can avoid crises and unnecessary hospital admissions, making the last months of their lives as valuable as possible.'
>
> (*Accredited Home Manager, 2015*)

## Conclusion

ACP works well in care homes and leads to improved outcomes for residents, relatives, and staff. Many homes have relayed stories of the changes in culture in the home and the increased confidence of staff (2).

'It has provided a culture of openness and realisation'

'. . . completely changed the way we deliver care'

(Comments from accredited homes about ACP)

It is an important part of 'raising the level of care to the level of the best'. Coming together at the GSFCH workshops enables the sharing of challenges, ideas, best practice, and solutions to many of the problems faced daily, enabling care to be of a 'gold standard'. It contributes to developing a culture where these processes become the norm.

ACP is one of the key elements to good end of life care, enabling people to 'live well until they die'. This therefore needs to become part of everyday practice with staff who are confident in having difficult discussions with residents, relatives, and others around end of life care and approaching death. It is important that care home staff are empowered to build the skills that are needed to have effective, meaningful conversations with people approaching the end of their lives, with access to training and development.

The offer of an ACP discussion with all residents is paramount to providing choice of where and how people are cared for and die. As this becomes embedded into everyday practice, we see the benefits that can be achieved for all. The wider context needs to be considered with a greater willingness of all involved to address the needs of improving communication skills, collaborative working, and developing more systematic processes.

'When having the ACP discussion, he expressed the fear of going to an unfamiliar place like hospital and his wish to remain with us for the final days of his life. His wishes were established, communicated to others, and achieved. We all felt satisfied that we had accomplished his wishes for care at the end.'
(*GSFCH Accredited Care Home, 2008*)

---

## Case study

### Transcript of clip from an interview with Peter, a care home resident

Interviewer

'One of the key aspects of GSF is, advance care planning . . . I understand you were very enthusiastic about this.'

Peter

'. . . I think it is very important that whilst you have a clear head . . . you should make sure that how you want to be cared for at the end of your life is in a manner which suits what you feel you need . . ..'

Interviewer

'. . . do you feel that your wishes are known?'

Peter

'It has been exhaustively gone into, so that when the time comes I am totally confident that everything will be done as I would wish. I thought it was important, if only to button up the possibility of over-enthusiastic medical people getting their hands on me and carting me off to hospital, which is the last place I want to be taken to.'

Interviewer

'So, you have on record exactly what you want should you not be able to say it for yourself?'

Peter

'Yes, but I have every confidence that the home will say it all for me.'

Reproduced courtesy of the Gold Standards Framework

---

## Acknowledgements

The quotations attributed to managers and matrons from GSF accredited care homes were reproduced courtesy of the Gold Standards Framework.

## References

1. **Froggatt K**, **Vaughan S**, **Bernard C**, and **Wild D** (2009). 'ACP in care homes for older people: an English perspective'. *Palliative Medicine* **23**: 332–8.

2. *Gold Standards Framework in Care Homes Good Practice Guide* (2015) Available from: www.goldstandardsframework.org.uk

3. Available from: https://www.dementiauk.org/for-healthcare-professionals/free-resources/life-story-work/

4. **St John K** (2015) 'Preventing avoidable hospital admissions for people with advanced dementia'. *End of Life Care Journal* **5**: 1–12.

5. **Hansford P** (2016) 'End of life care is everybody's business'. *End of Life Care Journal* **5**: 1–2.

6. **Clark D**, et al. (2014) 'Imminence of death among a national cohort of hospital inpatients'. *Palliative Medicine* **28**(6). 474–9. doi: 10.1177/0269216314526443.

7. Available from: https://www.alzheimers.org.uk/site/scripts/news_article.php?newsID=1498 Published 26 February 2013.

8. Available from: http://www.endoflifecare-intelligence.org.uk/data_sources/place_of_death

9. DH (2008). *End of Life Care Strategy: promoting high quality of care for all adults at the end of life.* Department of Health. Available from: www.dh.gov.uk/publications

10. **NAO** (2008). **National Audit Office**. *End of life care: care home survey results.* Available from: http://www.nao.org.uk/publications/0708/end_of_life_care.aspx (Accessed May 2009.)

11. **Goodman**, et al. (2015) 'End of life care interventions for people with dementia in care homes: addressing uncertainty within a framework for service delivery and evaluation'. *BMC Palliative Care* **14**(42) doi: 10.1186/s12904-015-0040-0.

12. **Holman D** (2009). Personal communication. St Christopher's Hospice. London. SE 26.

13. *Planning for your future care: a guide.* Available from: http://www.ncpc.org.uk/publication/planning-your-future-care

14. *Decisions relating to cardiopulmonary resuscitation 3rd edition* (2014). Guidance from the British Medical Association, the Resuscitation Council (UK) and the Royal College of Nursing.

15. Mental Capacity Act 2005. London: The Stationary Office.

16. **Dening KH** (2015). 'Advance care planning in dementia'. *Nursing Standard* **29**(51): 41–6.

17. **Froggatt K** (2006). 'Evaluating a palliative care education project in nursing homes'. *International Journal of Palliative Nursing* **6**(3): 140–6.

Chapter 13

# Advance care planning in the community

Peter Nightingale, Scott Murray, and Chris Absolon

'If patient-centred End of Life Care is to become a reality, patients must be empowered to take control of decisions about their treatment. Advance Care Planning is a necessary first step on the road to a fruitful partnership with Healthcare Professionals'
*Tony Bonser, Macmillan volunteer. Trustee for N.C.P. &*
*St Catherine's hospice.*
*Local Champion for Dying Matters*

---

**This chapter includes**

- An overview of issues surrounding Advance Care Planning (ACP) in primary care and in the community
- When should you start ACP in the community?
- Which patients, and who should be involved?
- The barriers to ACP in the community and how to overcome them
- Outcomes and benefits of ACP

---

**Key Points**

- ACP should be used in the community for patients with all serious or progressive illnesses
- ACP should be offered as early as the patient wishes, but certain triggers are suggested
- Various people may initiate ACP discussions in the community
- Participation in ACP conversations is voluntary
- ACP can bring hope, and help patients feel that they have a degree of control
- There are significant barriers to the widespread use of ACP in the community, such as staff resistance, difficulty identifying the appropriate time, time pressures etc., but there is evidence of improvement
- The greatest enabling factor in ACP is a pre-existing relationship between patient and healthcare professional

◆ Patients, family carers, professionals, and the health service, all stand to benefit from earlier and more frequent ACP discussions

---

**Key Message**

ACP is part of good practice within primary care. It is possible to integrate ACP within routine primary care where it will have a significant effect on improving and enabling more to live and die well.

---

## Review of key elements

Advance care planning (ACP) is possible and valuable if it becomes 'everyone's business' in a healthcare community. Community nurses, care administrators, and volunteers as well as GP's can all play a valuable role in supporting the process.

If discussion is wanted by the patient and time is available for the GP or other trained carer, then this could lead to the use of questions such as:

◆ Could you tell me what the most important things are to you in life?

◆ Can you tell me about your current illness and how you are feeling?

◆ Who is the most significant person in your life?

◆ What fears or worries, if any, do you have about the future?

◆ In thinking about the future, have you thought about where you would prefer to be cared for as your illness gets worse?

◆ What would give you the most comfort when you are reaching the end of your life?

## An overview of issues surrounding advance care planning in the community

There have been encouraging and important developments in recent years related to several factors which have driven forward change, these include:

◆ Policy initiatives

◆ Educational opportunities

◆ Information technology (IT)

◆ Professional quality control and regulation

◆ Financial and business incentives

◆ The Compassionate Community movement

## Policy

*A Review of Choice in End of Life Care (2015)* (1) supports the recommendation that by 2020 everyone who is affected by a terminal illness will be offered choices about where and how they are cared for. These and other documents such as the Scottish *Strategic Framework for Action on Palliative Care (2015)* (2) have led to ACP gaining prominence among healthcare professionals. However, despite this, we still know that further policy developments and improvements are needed before ACP is fully integrated into mainstream practice.

---

### Box 13.1 Atul Gawande (Reith Lecture 2014)

♦ People who had a substantive discussion with their doctor about their end of life prefer-ences were far more likely to die in peace and in control of the situation, sparing their family anguish . . .

♦ The process requires as much listening as talking. If you are talking more than half the time you are talking too much . . .

♦ A family meeting requires no less skill than performing an operation . . .

♦ It could be argued that decision making in medicine has failed so spectacularly that we have reached the point of inflicting harm on patients rather than confronting the subject of mortality . . .

Source: data from Gawande A (2014) 'The Problem of Hubris', Episode 3, *Reith Lectures*, BBC Radio 4. Available from: http://www.bbc.co.uk/programmes/b04tjdlj

---

Atul Gawande has had a wide-reaching positive influence in his Reith lecture (see Box 13.1) (3).

## Educational opportunities

The Royal College of GPs, especially in Wales (4); the British Medical Association; the General Medical Council (GMC); and the NHS, as well as health charities, have all produced material to help with primary care education relating to end of life care. Several NHS networks have produced excellent guidance, such as that in the northwest of England (5).

Many of the problems that arise in the community are due to the lack of good quality organisa-tion of care. The Gold Standard Framework (GSF) (6) has at its very core three steps: Identify, Assess and Plan (Figure 13.1). Identification is the first and fundamental step in case planning, and tools such as the GSF Prognostic Indicator Guidance and the Supportive and Palliative Care Indicator Tool (7) are being increasingly used internationally.

In North Lancashire in the UK, all GP practices undertook the GSF 'Going for Gold' training program in 2011. This embedded the use of priority coding in GP practices and helped make sure time was allocated in meetings to discuss those patients who most needed support. It also helped cross boundary care with local hospitals and care homes. In 2014, both the meetings for GSF and the 'Avoiding Unplanned Admissions' Direct Enhanced Service (DES) (8) were com-bined into one longer 'Supportive and Palliative Care Meeting' held monthly for 90 minutes. The use of *GSF Needs-Based Colour Coding* (see Figure 13.2) has made the supportive care meeting manageable.

A typical agenda for this meeting is outlined in Box 13.2. The meetings are designed to cel-ebrate success and build teamwork by personally sharing important patient information with those involved in their care. In Scotland, many practices are similarly combining their palliative care and *anticipatory care* meetings. Naming the meeting 'Supportive Care' and calling our register a 'Supportive and Palliative Care Register' has made it easier to ask patients for consent to share their records on Electronic Palliative Care Coordination Systems (EPaCCs). The 'branding' of support-ive and palliative care is currently a subject of debate (9).

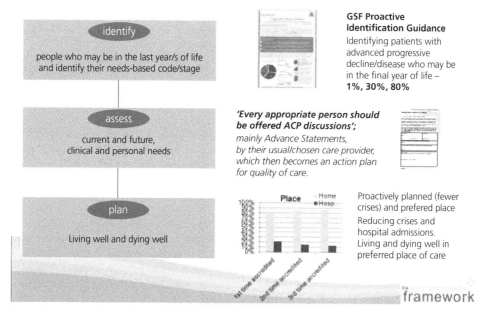

**Improving proactive person-centred care**
GSF 3 Steps Core Summary

**Figure 13.1** Using the Gold Standards Framework (GSF) to improve proactive person-centred care
Reproduced courtesy of the Gold Standards Framework

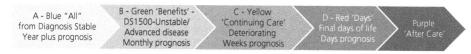

**Figure 13.2** GSF Needs Based Coding
Reproduced courtesy of the Gold Standards Framework

---

## Box 13.2 Typical agenda for a monthly supportive care meeting for a 10,500 patient GP practice

1. Introductions

2. AOB

3. Red Patients (Average approx. three patients—15 mins)

4. Amber Patients (Average approx. 20 patients—30 mins)

5. Review of deaths—celebrating good care and identifying areas to improve

6. Review of relevant admissions/discharges

7. New patients to the register

8. Green/Blue 'changing' patients (81 patients/235patients in Sept 16)

## Case study
### From a UK GP

Doug was a retired electrician, ex-serviceman, aged 81. He had been fit and well until the age of 80 when he had suffered a myocardial infarction due to atherosclerosis—successfully treated with angioplasty.

A year following his myocardial infarction Doug came to see me with symptoms of anaemia. After an urgent referral to our local hospital for diagnosis Doug was found to have cancer in both his bowel and stomach. At the time of his diagnosis Doug made it clear to the consultant that he did not want any active treatment. In his own words, he had had a good life and had faced far worse (a reference to his service days).

Following a phone call from Doug's consultant explaining his diagnosis I arranged to see Doug and his family and talk through his future care. Doug came to the appointment with his wife, Maria, son, and daughter, and together we talked openly about his cancer and prognosis. Doug spoke about his wish not to have active treatment and to be cared for and die at home. With the full support of his family and his permission we recorded this using an ACP document. Doug was willing to be referred to the local hospice team for community support so I made this referral knowing that the team would support his family too.

Over the course of the next 18 months Doug had a number of health issues which needed treating to improve his quality of life. Knowing Doug's wish to remain at home meant that on all but one occasion we treated these in the community avoiding hospital admission. The exception was an episode of unstable angina which Doug agreed to have treated in hospital because it was reversible and he was keen to go to his grandson's wedding in three weeks time. The wedding was a wonderful day for Doug with many happy memories for all his family.

As Doug's condition deteriorated, his needs were discussed with the multidisciplinary team at our monthly GSF meetings. This meant that those of us who were looking after him could make sure his needs were met; his ACP followed and his care well-co-ordinated.

When Doug became too weak to climb the stairs his bed was brought downstairs. Doug had lived in the same house with Maria for 50 years and it was there that he died, peacefully and surrounded by the family he loved.

### Key points for successful ACP

◆ Timely communication from the hospital consultant
◆ Open honest communications throughout between all healthcare professionals, the patient, and their family
◆ Recognising when a health issue (such as unstable angina) is reversible and providing appropriate treatment

A major positive benefit of this process is a shift in focus from the challenge of identifying people based on a prognosis of less than 12 month's life expectancy, towards having conversations about supportive care needs during the last phase of a person's life.

Educational resources and supporting materials have been made more readily available in recent years. Having a well-produced good quality document to hand to people can help start a conversation. Examples of resources and booklets include:

◆ NHS Choices website (10) which has a useful section on planning ahead including 'Planning for your future care', a clear brief booklet produced by NHS Improving Quality
  • 'Your Life, Your Choices: Plan ahead' a booklet produced by Macmillan Cancer Support (11). This is widely used
  • 'Planning Ahead' (12), which is used in Somerset
◆ A communication skills package called SAGE and THYME (13) has also been developed. It has proved popular with many GPs because it builds on prior knowledge of effective person-centred consulting skills, such as the Calgary Cambridge Model (14), and 'bolts on' to techniques that allow sensitive and effective ACP discussions in a time limited environment

Awareness raising campaigns such as the NCPC/Dying matters campaign, 'Find your 1%' have all promoted the development of a positive attitude to ACP.

## Information technology

Electronic Palliative Care Coordination Systems (EPaCCs) have transformed the value of ACP in some localities. They can prove problematic to implement, but when they operate well they have the power to effectively share a patient's expressed wishes with the many health providers involved in their care (15).

Knowing that ACP information can be appropriately shared electronically can be a stimulus to encourage healthcare workers in the community to initiate ACP conversations.

When paper plans are required, it is possible to 'merge' information and produce a document in an attractive format, possibly as an inclusion in a 'passport'. One example of this from Northern Ireland is 'My Healthcare Passport' (16).

## Professional quality control and regulation

The Care Quality Commission, (CQC), identified ACP as a priority area for inspection. They have sought evidence that 'Early and ongoing conversations about end of life care in the last phase of life as part of planning their treatment and care, in a way which responds to their individual communication needs'.

## Financial

Proactive care planning is now more common, and financial incentives, such as the Quality Outcomes Framework Palliative Care points related to GSF bronze/basic level from 2004, or in England a recent scheme to encourage GPs to avoid unplanned admissions with a Direct Enhanced Service (2013–15), can help to mainstream, proactive rather than reactive care. The increase in numbers of patients identified as being suitable for ACP has made it clear that a multidisciplinary approach is required.

### Which patients?

> 'A patient I had known for many years convinced me of the importance of Advance Care Planning (ACP). Ron could so easily have died in hospital, enduring a futile and undignified attempt at resuscitation. He was a retired teacher, with diabetes and heart failure and after a hospital discharge follow up consultation in my surgery had documented his wishes, and these had been shared electronically on our Electronic Palliative Care Co-ordination System (EPaCCS). Ron subsequently died at home with his wife present. After Ron's death, I visited and sat with his wife in the lounge. Ron's Preferred Priorities of Care (PPC) document was on the coffee table. We flicked through it and realised Ron had achieved the death he had wished for those many months before. This was of great comfort to his wife and a professionally satisfying moment for me. Without ACP the bereavement experience of his wife would have been very different. In truth, the family were so grateful they insisted I received a gift for my efforts, (this is a rare event nowadays!) it's a golf club, I try to use it early most Saturday mornings when I get the opportunity!'
> *Dr Peter Nightingale, National GP Lead for End of Life Care*

All people with life-threatening illness are likely to benefit from planning ahead at the end of life (17). Thus, care planning should be considered not only for people with cancer, but also for people with any life-threatening condition.

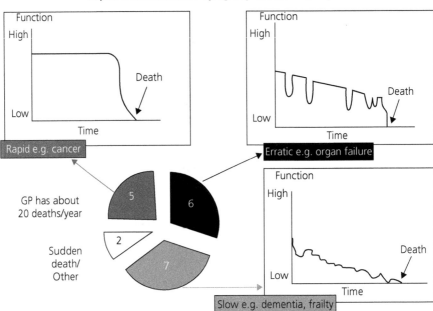

**Figure 13.3** Trajectories of illness related to GP caseload, showing typical numbers of deaths for typical GP with average list size of 2000

Reproduced courtesy of Gold Standards Framework. Source: data from Lunney JR, Lynn J, Foley DJ, Lipson S, Guralnik JM, (2003) 'Patterns of functional decline at the end of life', *JAMA*, Volume 289, Issue 18, pp. 2387-92, doi: 10.1001/jama.289.18.2387

Dying trajectories (18,19) provide a way to identify groups of people with similar service needs for reliably high quality end of life care which ACP can address (Figure 13.3).

The first trajectory or pattern of decline is the maintenance of good function until a short period of relatively predictable acute decline in the last weeks or months of life: progressive cancer typifies this. The second trajectory, with slow decline punctuated by dramatic exacerbations any of which might end in sudden death is seen more typically in organ failure, such as in end-stage chronic obstructive pulmonary disease, heart failure and liver failure. The third trajectory is poor long term functional status with slow decline and elderly patients with dementia, frailty, or multiple co-morbidities fit into this category (20). This proportion is increasing, so frailty and multimorbidity are today's biggest killers. Only one or two per year die following an acute event, so sudden unexpected deaths are rare. Thus, ACP is relevant in possibly 90% of deaths, but predicting and identifying non-malignant patients early for ACP is the greatest challenge, particularly for those with multimorbidity.

In the community, we are well placed with electronic records of patients and routine multidisciplinary meetings to identify patients who will benefit from ACP by considering these three groups, and try to recruit patients from each of these trajectories to practice supportive/palliative care registers. In Scotland GPs are encouraged to use specific computer searches on their practice lists to identify people who might benefit from care planning (21).

The Electronic Frailty Index (eFI) (22) is becoming an increasingly helpful tool embedded into GP record systems.

## When should you start advance care planning in the community?

Research increasingly shows that most patients facing death from cancer and conditions such as renal failure and heart failure value the opportunity to discuss the future, although doctors and nurses often hesitate to raise the subject for fear that the patient might lose hope (23). Relying on waiting for an exact prognosis to share with the patient is futile, as estimating prognosis is difficult in most illnesses. Ideally, care planning may start even before supportive and palliative care is needed, and is encouraged in long-term illnesses and more recently in 'survivorship planning' for cancer patients in England and in 'anticipatory planning' in Scotland.

Initiating conversations can be difficult in the time and resource constrained environment of a modern GP surgery. One option is to make use of trained team members to help the process.

Other General Practices will have access to Health Coaches, or Health Connections workers, and once the need to offer ACP has been established, these are ideal people to have ACP conversations.

It is possible to introduce the benefits of ACP discussions with a statement such as:—'In my job as a GP, I find it much easier to help you to get the type of care you want if we ask you about your preferences, would you like me to do that? . . .I find that if we don't ask, we know you are less likely to get the care you would like. Although clearly, we can never make any guarantees, I can promise we will do our best to provide the type of care you hope for'. The answer may be no, and then the matter can be left until perhaps another opportunity arises—but most people say yes and may have just been waiting for the opportunity.

Triggers for having ACP conversations in the GP surgery include (24):

◆ The patient initiates the conversation

◆ The diagnosis of a progressive life-limiting illness

◆ Taking the opportunity during routine consultations or visits to ask yourself the 'surprise' question and be alert to indicators of frailty. Electronic indicators may help with this

◆ The diagnosis of a condition with a predictable trajectory, which is likely to result in a loss of capacity, such as dementia or motor neurone disease

◆ A change or deterioration in condition which generates feedback from a colleague. For example, a district nurse concerned about a persistent pressure ulcer. Or a discussion with a consultant in secondary care

◆ At discharge after an unplanned hospital admission

◆ Change in a patient's personal circumstances, such as moving into a care home or loss of a family member

◆ Routine clinical review of the patient, such as clinic appointments or home visits

◆ When the previously agreed review interval elapses

◆ Electronic searches for indicators of vulnerability such as eFI, falls or coded elements of GSF Prognostic Indicator Guidance

---

### Case study
### From a UK GP

So, the advantages of ACP . . . of course there are many and I am personally a huge advocate of any care planning.

I had an elderly patient who had never bothered the surgery and sadly was diagnosed with liver cancer following an admission to hospital. She was palliative at discharge and clearly poorly.

During my first visit to her home she mentioned her plans and that she wished to consider euthanasia. I listened and advised I couldn't support her wishes but left the patient and her family with a blank care plan and promised to visit the following week. Leaving the care plan with some simple messages around the patient's wishes and the ethos of an ACP triggered lots of discussions within the family and close friends, which proved to be really helpful.

On my return, she had realised that euthanasia was not the best option and she was looking at alternatives. Over the coming weeks, we completed the plan and left a copy at her home. She deteriorated and was transferred to her preferred place of care and passed away peacefully. So, for me having documentation for reference should an ambulance have been called etc. was really important but I think for the family it was a tool to ignite discussions. I subsequently spoke with the family who were grateful that everything, including open discussions, had gone as smoothly as they could have done.

## Key points for successful advance care planning

◆ Effective listening and open discussions

◆ Providing patients with information about ACP to stimulate discussion

◆ Following an initial ACP conversation with further discussions about ACP

### Who should be involved in advance care planning discussions?

The initiation of an ACP conversation may be most appropriate with the health professional who knows the patient well and this is likely to be someone in primary care.

As GP consultation appointment times are usually short (10–15 minutes), it is often then most practical to provide some written information and arrange a review appointment, sometimes with a trained community nursing professional or trained care administrator/co-ordinator if appropriate.

There have been some encouraging changes in secondary care leading to more ACP conversations being initiated in that setting. This seems to be especially true of respiratory medicine where the 'revolving door' scenario of repeated futile admissions has been avoided for some patients.

The Transforming End of Life Care in Acute Hospital's Programme (25) and the subsequent Building on the Best Programme (26) are good examples of initiatives that have encouraged more cross boundary involvement in ACP.

### Barriers to advance care planning in the community

There can be difficult conversations and situations that arise when trying to introduce ACP. Reasons for problems arising include:

◆ Difficult language and different cultural interpretations of the questions asked

◆ Denial, this is a good form of defence for many people, we have a duty to respect that

◆ There can be a clash of viewpoints within families

◆ The impact of a 'bad news' interview—distress may develop when facing a poor prognosis

◆ A patients desire to 'live for the moment'/'take one day at a time'—a reactive approach to life could conflict with a healthcare professional's desire to be proactive

◆ Staff resistance or even conflict—who is best to do it? It can be time consuming and everyone is busy

◆ When to begin? How to do it? Communication skills confidence and training is not always available

◆ Raising expectations—delivering care in line with wishes may be impossible without hospice beds or 24 hr nursing in an area

◆ And others . . .

It may be necessary, if things are not going well or proving non-productive in a consultation to say something such as: 'thanks very much for helping me to understand your thoughts on this matter, I think it may be best to leave things now and perhaps discuss this again at another time, but only if you want to'. With an open and honest approach, most of these issues can be dealt with. It must always be a voluntary process, and views can change with time, so repeated gentle offers maybe appropriate for some people.

There are other barriers to implementing ACP in the community: from broad socio-cultural issues to the idiosyncrasies of each practice. These include:

## Hope and fear

One of the most frequently mentioned concerns is the fear of 'destroying hope' among patients. Research with patients, however, indicates that patients value the chance to discuss and plan for the future and that ACP can increase not decrease hope by 'normalising' life again so that the fear of the unknown can reduce, and pragmatic plans can be initiated (27).

## Death as a taboo

Discussing death and dying requires confronting deeply held social taboos. Such discussions are assumed to be fraught and emotionally draining for all concerned. Patients report being reluctant to initiate such conversations for fear of upsetting their GP, or simply because they don't know which questions to ask, while GPs fear upsetting their patients by bringing up the issue before the patient is ready.

The current 'national conversation' to encourage the public to talk more about death and dying should greatly facilitate ACP. This will take time to change despite current efforts to raise public awareness, such as the NCPC Dying Matters and the Scottish 'Good life, Good death, Good grief' campaigns.

## Reductionist thinking: box-ticking vs holistic care

There also appears to be a deep, professional distrust against some of the 'formal' or 'structured' ACP among primary healthcare professionals. In particular, there is a concern about palliative care provision becoming a 'tick-box' activity. The common perception among primary healthcare professionals is that palliative care requires the kind of holistic care that they are best placed to provide. Therefore, using the suggested ACP tools to trigger open questions, rather than ticking boxes, but then communicating key factors to others can, in many cases, meet both the needs of holistic care but also systematic communication.

## Time, resources, and coordination

The major concern of GPs is that they lack the time to be able to engage fully in ACP discussions. Some worry that ACP may be used by articulate, well-informed patients in a way that requires so much of the GPs time that their care for patients who are less able to ask for help may be compromised. Further inequalities of care might thus occur unless uptake is promoted especially in the relatively deprived and needy. Also, if this information is not communicated to other relevant agencies, this exercise is futile.

Key areas for further development are therefore:

- Triggers to identify the right time to discuss this area
- Training in communication skills around dealing with uncertainties
- Improved information transfer to appropriate others e.g. EPaCCS, summary care record
- Self-management tools for patients
- Greater public awareness of the need to raise these issues early, and increased knowledge of ACP, Advance Decisions to Refuse Treatment (ADRT), and Power of Attorney (PoA)

## Outcomes and benefits for patients, carers, and practitioners

Secondary analysis of data from the National Survey of Bereaved People in England in 2015 (28) confirmed that ACP was strongly associated with lower rates of hospital death and a range of quality outcomes. Similar strong associations have also been found in Scotland.

ACP in the community may share much with the controversial term 'survivorship planning' (29). The process of planning ahead is an activity that is as relevant to 'fighting' an illness as it is to dealing with that illness's effects on one's life. Understanding ACP in this way opens up the potential to start the process earlier and opens up the possibility for various members of the primary care team to take part in the process.

## The Compassionate Community Movement and advance care planning

The growing Compassionate Community Movement, based on the work of Allan Kellehear and others, includes encouraging community initiated and led ACP.

Compassionate Communities publicly encourage, facilitate, support, and celebrate care for one another during life's most testing moments and experiences, especially those pertaining to life-threatening and life-limiting illness; chronic disability; frailty; ageing and dementia; grief and bereavement, and the trials and burdens of long-term care (30).

The movement acknowledges that professionals cannot meet all the current demands of people with palliative care needs, and this demand is inevitably going to increase as the UK population changes.

ACP can be 'de-medicalised', and brought into the wider community. People who have been carers; village agents; faith groups, and other community volunteers can be very effective in having ACP conversations, and training for this is available through Dying Matters (31).

---

### Case study

### Lay led advance care planning

A retired bank manager has become a passionate advocate of ACP! He became very aware of the importance of Lasting Power of Attorney during his professional life, and has encouraged all his family to arrange one. His mother died two years ago, and he had some concerns about the way she was cared for at the end of her life, and as a result has become a lay member of a Somerset CCG group working to promote ACP. He describes his mother's death as a 'trigger', and having already helped his daughters arrange Lasting Powers of Attorney, gave them both copies of Planning Ahead, the ACP document we use in Somerset and discussed this with them.

He is involved in a voluntary capacity with a number of groups in Somerset, and takes copies of Planning Ahead to give to people!

## Conclusion

There is movement in the right direction regarding ACP in the community, although much more needs to be done.

ACP can and should be used in the community for all progressive illness, not just cancer. To do this, however, requires practitioners to be aware of the different trajectories for each disease, as ACP is not a 'one size fit all' process (32). This requires community health workers to be aware of the potential for ACP and to understand it as a tool for living well.

The most successful interventions seem to be those that can identify a routine, regular trigger point to start ACP, as research on care homes indicated. However, making the process routine may draw resistance from some professionals who see the process as 'an art, not an algorithm' (33). It seems that the greatest facilitator to starting ACP is a pre-existing relationship between the patient and healthcare professionals and it seems also that ACP is a great device for facilitating that relationship; meaning that patients, family, carers, and professionals all stand to benefit. There are great prizes to be won but still much work to be done.

## Acknowledgements

The quotation attributed to Dr Pete Nightingale, National GP Lead for End of Life Care, was reproduced with permission from Macmillan Cancer Support, 'No Regrets: How talking more openly about death could help people die well', April 2017, available from http://www.macmillan.org.uk.

## References

1. **A Review of Choice in End of Life Care**. (2015). *The Choice in End of Life Care Programme Board. What's Important to me.* Available from: https://www.gov.uk/government/publications/choice-in-end-of-life-care Dying Matters. Dr Peter Nightingale: my experience. Available from: http://www.dyingmatters.org/gp_page/dr-peter-nightingale-my-experience

2. **The Scottish Government** (2015). *Strategic Framework for Action on Palliative and End of Life Care 2016–2021.* Available from: http://www.gov.scot/Publications/2015/12/4053
   **Levenstein JH, Belle Brown J, Weston WW** et al. (1989). *Patient-centred clinical interviewing. In Communicating with medical patients* (eds M Stewart and D Roter). Newbury Park, CA: Sage Publications.

3. **Dr Atul Gawande 2014 Reith Lectures.** 'The Problem of Hubris'. BBC Radio 4. Episode 3 of 4. Available from: http://www.bbc.co.uk/programmes/b04tjdlj.

4. **Stewart M** et al. (2003). *Patient-centred medicine: transforming the clinical method.* Abingdon Oxford: Radcliffe Medical Press.

5. **RCGP Wales.** *Advance Care Planning Training Resource.* (2008). Available from: http://rcgpwalestraining.co.uk/rcgp/index.htm

6. **Northwest Advance Care Planning Framework.** (2015). Available from: www.nwcscnsenate.nhs.uk/files/6514/4284/8049/Advance_Care_Planning_Framework_2015-18_FINAL.pdf?PDFPATHWAY=PDF

7. **Gold Standards Framework.** (2012). Available from: www.goldstandardsframework.org.uk

8. **Supportive and Palliative Care Indicator Tool.** (2014). Available from: www.spict.org.uk

9. **Medeconomics.** (2016). *Avoiding unplanned admissions enhanced service 2016/2017.* Available from: http://www.medeconomics.co.uk/article/1390891/avoiding-unplanned-admissions-enhanced-service-2016-17

10. **Caprio AJ.** (2016). 'Palliative care: renaming as supportive care and integration into comprehensive cancer care'. *CMAJ* doi: 10.1503/cmaj.160206.

11. **NHS Choices.** *End of Life Care. Planning Ahead.* Available from: http://www.nhs.uk/Planners/end-of-life-care/Pages/planning-ahead.aspx

12. **Macmillan Cancer Support.** *Your Life and Your Choices. Plan Ahead.* Available from: https://be.macmillan.org.uk/be/p-20337-your-life-and-your-choices-plan-ahead-england-and-wales.aspx

13. **NHS Somerset Clinical Commissioning Group.** *Palliative Care.* Available from: http://somersetccg.nhs.uk/about-us/how-we-do-things/palliative-care/

14. **University of Manchester.** (2017). 'Sage and Thyme'. Available from: http://www.sageandthymetraining.org.uk/

15. **Calgary Cambridge:** *Teaching and learning communication skills in medicine.* Available from: http://gp-training.net/training/communication_skills/calgary/index.htm

16. **Petrova M, Riley J, Abel J,** and **Barclay S** (2016). 'Crash course in EPaCCS (Electronic Palliative Care Coordination Systems): 8 years of successes and failures in patient data sharing to learn from'. *BMJ Supportive & Palliative Care.* doi.org/10.1136/bmjspcare-2015-001059

17. **RCGP Northern Ireland.** *My Healthcare Passport.* Available from: http://www.rcgp.org.uk/rcgp-nations/rcgp-northern-ireland/my-healthcare-passport.aspx

18. **Murray S, Sheikh A,** and **Thomas K** (2006). 'Advanced care planning in primary care'. *BMJ* **333**: 868–69.

19. **Lunney JR, Lynn J, Foley DJ, Lipson S,** and **Guralnik JM** (2003). 'Patterns of functional decline at the end of life'. *JAMA* **289**(18): 2387–92.

20. **Murray SA, Kendall M, Boyd K,** and **Sheikh A** (2005). 'Illness trajectories and palliative care'. *Clinical Review. BMJ* **330**: 1007–11.

21. **Lynn J** (2008). 'Reliable comfort and meaningfulness. Making a difference campaign'. *BMJ* **336**: 958–9.

22. **Mason B, Boyd K, Murray S, Steyn J, Cormie P, Kendall M,** et al. (2015). 'Developing a computerised search to help UK General Practices identify more patients for palliative care planning: a feasibility study'. *BMC Fam Pract* 2015; **16**(1): 99.

23. **Clegg A, Bates C, Young J,** et al. (2016). 'Development and validation of an electronic frailty index using routine primary care electronic health record data'. *Age and ageing* **0**: 1–8. Available from: http://ageing.oxfordjournals.org/content/early/2016/03/03/ageing.afw039

24. **Davison SN** and **Simpson C** (2006). 'Hope and advance care planning in patients with end stage renal disease: qualitative interview study'. *BMJ* Available from: doi: 10.1136/bmj.38965.626250.55.

25. **Mullick A, Martin J,** and **Sallnow L** (2013). 'An introduction to advance care planning in practice'. *BMJ* **347**: f6064. Available from: http://dx.doi.org/10.1136/bmj.f6064

26. **NHS IQ.** *The Transforming End of Life Care in Acute Hospitals Programme.* Available from: http://www.nhsiq.nhs.uk/improvement-programmes/long-term-conditions-and-integrated-care/end-of-life-care/acute-hospital-care.aspx

27. **Murray S, Sheikh A,** and **Thomas K** (2006). 'Advanced care planning in primary care'. *BMJ* **333**: 868–9.

28. **Office of National Statistics England** (2015). *National Survey of Bereaved People (Voices).* Available from: https://www.ons.gov.uk/releases/nationalsurveyofbereavedpeoplevoices2015

29. **National Coalition for Cancer Survivorship.** (1993). *Survivorship Care Planning.* Available from: http://www.canceradvocacy.org/resources/planning-your-care/

30. **Wegleitner K, Heimerl K, Kellehear A** (2016). *Compassionate Communities Case Studies from Britain and Europe.* London: Routledge Taylor and Francis Group.

31. **Dying Matters.** *Advance Care Planning for volunteers.* Available from: http://www.dyingmatters.org/page/advance-care-planning-volunteers

32. **Murray SA, Kendall M, Boyd K,** and **Sheikh A** (2005). 'Illness trajectories and palliative care'. Clinical Review. *BMJ* **330**: 1007–11.

33. **Grossman D** (2009). 'Advance care planning is an art, not an algorithm'. Editorial. *Cleveland Clinic Journal of Medicine* **76**(5): 287–8.

Chapter 14

# Advance care planning in hospices and palliative care

Sarah Russell and Simon Noble

There is no second chance to improve the care of the
dying patient
*Hand written post-it note left by predecessor on hospice office wall*

---

**This chapter includes**

- An overview of the role of the hospice and palliative care approach in advance care planning (ACP)
- Definitions matter: the challenge of overlapping definitions and consensus about what hospice, palliative care, and ACP are
- The changing role of hospice and palliative care and implications for ACP
- New types of conversations e.g. living with dying, managing uncertainty, expectations, ceilings of care and investigations, dying in hospices
- The way forward; collaboration, co-ordination and partnerships with other providers, consistency of approach to conversations

---

**Key Points**

- Increasing population needs and the changing role of hospice and palliative care means that ACP activity takes place in a variety of services and settings
- ACP conversations are also concerned with managing uncertainty, expectations about care, interventions, and investigations
- Co-ordination of information and services as well as a consistency of approach to conversations and is important to ACP

---

**Key Message**

Hospice and palliative care is an approach to care as well as a place, setting or intervention.

---

## Introduction

Globally, there are approximately 16,000 palliative care services with an estimated 204 million people in need of palliative care at the end of life (1). A hospice and palliative care approach is an integral part of these services, with ACP being one part of the activity. Furthermore, there is advocacy for palliative care being appropriate earlier in a persons' illness trajectory (1,2) based upon complexity of need rather than just diagnosis or prognosis (3).

However, there are multiple challenges and opportunities in ACP activity (e.g. discussions, decisions, documents, and dissemination), representing not only unmet need but also the evolving definitions, descriptions, and understanding of both ACP, hospice, and palliative care. In this chapter some of these challenges and opportunities will be explored and examples described of the hospice and palliative care role in ACP.

## Definitions matter

The twentieth-century philosopher Ludwig Wittgenstein (4) argued that the meaning of a word is in its use in the language. Words and definitions facilitate shared meaning. They state and explain something providing a starting point for discussion and agreement (5). There are multiple definitions and understandings of hospice, palliative, terminal, supportive and end of life care with variation in the terminology and definitions (6,7). Some of the challenges for hospice and palliative care are therefore consensuses about e.g. what care it is, level of care, for how long, who provides it, in which disease groups, as well as when in an illness trajectory.

The hospice care approach has its origins in Dame Cicely Saunders' vision of expert pain and symptom control, compassionate care, teaching, and research. Whilst hospices are often seen as just inpatient beds for those dying with cancer, more recently, reports have recommended that hospices need to respond and adapt to an aging population, more people living alone, and dying from non-cancer conditions (7,8). New models of care and partnerships are needed to meet the needs of more people who would benefit from a hospice-care approach, which includes ACP activity.

There are commonalities in description which describe hospice and palliative care as being both an approach to care as well as a service, intervention, place, or building. These include improving quality of life, helping to live as fully as possible, reflecting personal preferences as well as multi-professional teams, medical, psychological, and spiritual support, symptom control, peace, and dignity to both patients and their families. However, there are comments on the wide range of definitions for supportive care, palliative care, and hospice care, as well as dying and actively dying; with significant overlaps and distinguishing features (6,9,10). Whilst supportive, palliative, and hospice care denote inter-professional care which optimise quality of life; the scope of service, patient population, and how each is perceived can differ. This is combined with an increasing call for 'upstream' palliative care earlier in disease trajectories as well as care integrated with curative interventions and oncology (9). Perhaps more significantly for ACP are the associations with the terms 'hospice' and 'palliative care' (i.e. death and dying) as opposed to 'supportive care' (i.e. survivorship and bereavement). This is illustrated by examples in some areas to rename services to supportive rather than palliative care.

ACP definitions experience similar challenges including the plethora of international terms, documents and legal frameworks with varying legislative powers (11). National end of life care strategies and legal frameworks differ widely in terms of definitions, clinical focus, legal requirements, and choice aspects (12). For example, a comparison of palliative care across seven European countries reported significant differences in the presence of legislation and regulations for ACP (13). Despite an increasing interest in ACP a consensus definition remains elusive. Recently, Sudore and colleagues (14) offered a definition from their international Delphi study of

'Advance care planning is a process that supports adults at any age or stage of health in understanding and sharing their personal values, life goals, and preferences regarding future medical care. The goal of advance care planning is to help ensure that people receive medical care that is consistent with their values, goals and preferences during serious and chronic illness.'

Why does the variation in hospice, palliative, and advance care planning definitions and understanding matter? It matters because hospice and palliative care (with ACP being part of it) is widely promoted to make a difference in cancer and non-cancer end of life care. Palliative care improves the quality of life and longevity in patients and increases home deaths (15). However there is a struggle for a common language hampering the development of international standards and norms (11). Some form of consensus is necessary for meaningful clinical or research comparisons (17). Furthermore, the diversity of the terms can be confusing for patients, family members, and healthcare practitioners as well as society in general.

## The changing role of hospice and palliative care

Hospice and palliative care is adapting to the demographic changes of people living longer, with multiple co-morbidities, in a constantly shifting economic, political, and social landscape (18,19). Recent reports have argued that hospice care should be concerned with those with a life-shortening illness not just cancer, as well as dovetail with local health services, authorities, and care homes. Moreover, there is evidence that referral to hospice care is beneficial, with a consequent difference in place of death, time spent in hospital in the last year of life, and hospital care costs (20). Hospice referrals, include those with a non-cancer diagnosis (21) with home-palliative care (including hospice community teams and education interventions) increase the chance of dying at home (15). Among the influences on this are ACP conversations and activity.

## Types of conversations

Communication skills are covered in Chapter 24 of this book as well as within other chapters; so, the detail of conversation tools and models are not covered here. However, the changing role of hospice and palliative care means that ACP conversations are broader than solely decisions and documentation about preferred care or place of death. For example, as hospices support people earlier and for longer in their dying trajectories; what matters most to patients and their families may be concerned with e.g. managing the uncertainty of living with the knowledge of their future death at an uncertain time (22), or managing expectations about ceilings of medical interventions and investigations or availability of nursing and social care. Some of the following examples illustrate how ACP conversations in the hospice setting or palliative care in general are not only changing in terms of topics but also that the timing of conversations are concerned with prognosis, as well as related to the context of how each person lives with, prepares for, and plans for dying (22).

## Conversations about living with dying

ACP conversations in hospice and palliative care settings are concerned with how people live—imagine and contemplate their future death—as well as treatment and care decisions. There is a body of literature regarding this illustrated by e.g. living with the effects of biographical disruption on the body in chronic illness (23) and how dying affects identify (24). Furthermore, there is an on-going discourse about how society constructs and manages the illness, death, and dying experience (25,26). Although there is evidence that e.g. illness narratives affect and shape experiences, thoughts, and fears in the last months of life (27); there are also calls to understand more how daily life is integral to understanding the ways in which people are able to maintain a sense of continuity during the circumstances of impending death as well as understanding more of the actual dying experience (28). For example, the context of a person's life (e.g. relationships with others, previous experience of death, and concerns over being a burden) may influence ACP discussions and decisions (22,29). Furthermore, there is evidence of the need for and value of early conversations about future care, how their condition might affect people in the future as well as treatment preferences (30,31).

There are also examples of hospice services supporting people as they live with dying (rather than just the last days). This provides a forum for ACP conversations which is not only mediated through the medical paradigm of diagnosis, prognosis, and clinical decision making. In other words, it situates conversations within a social space with fellow patients, carers, and community at large. For example, the Spring Centre at the Hospice of St Francis and Starlight Centre at Peace Hospice Care in Hertfordshire (UK) offer a range of wellbeing and resilience programmes. The philosophy of an integrated and holistic approach to wellbeing includes courses at the end of cancer treatment, breathlessness groups, self-management, and independent living groups. This is seen elsewhere in the UK with further examples from Finding Space at St Joseph's Hospice in London, the Coates Centre at Oakhaven Hospice Trust in Hampshire, or the Caritas Centre and Anniversary Centre at St Christopher's Hospice in London and Orpington.

## Living with uncertainty and managing expectations

Contemplating ones' future death involves uncertainty. Glaser and Strauss (32) reported upon critical junctures within a dying trajectory with passages of dying illustrating the complexity of the expectations of death (the uncertainty of timing of death). Other studies have highlighted how clinical uncertainty at the end of life can be distressing for both patients and families (33). Karlsson et al. (34) reported the struggle of living with an uncertain future despite efforts to live in the present. The literature therefore points to the position where living with uncertainty is integral to living with dying. As one of the main objectives of hospice and palliative care is to help people live well until they die, it is not unreasonable to expect ACP conversations to include the uncertainly of living with e.g. prognosis, effect on a persons' life, and the experience of dying, as well as managing symptoms and decisions about future care or interventions.

Policy regularly advocates that people should know what they are entitled to expect as they reach the end of their lives and ACP conversations are often associated with discussions and decisions about preferred place of death. However, they also increasingly include managing expectations about e.g. ceilings of treatment and the extent of investigations as well as available care at the end of life. Studies have shown the importance of clarifying prognostic expectations and end of life care wishes (35) as well as the distinction between services described and those available in practice (36). Examples of types of conversations that might occur in the hospice and palliative care setting are illustrated in Box 14.1.

Some of the recent communication models such as the Serious Illness Conversation Fuide (37) as well as Gwande's 5 key questions (38) are helpful here (see communications chapter for further information).

## Box 14.1  Types of managing uncertainty and expectations conversations

How long do I/they have to live?

When will you know the results or what the plan is?

What are you going to do/why aren't you doing anything?

How long will it take before we know if I/they will get better?

What tests are you going to do/why aren't you doing tests?

Will I/they be as well as I/they were before?

What care can be provided/what do I do if I can't manage?

## Dying in hospices

ACP is often undertaken on the understanding that the most patients would prefer their end of life care to be at home. As such it has historically focussed on preventing unwanted hospital admissions at the end of life or the facilitation of safe discharge home for those who are currently an inpatient. There are a proportion of patients, however who express a wish to have their end of life care in the hospice.

As in other environments, the ability to enable care in the preferred place of death is never guaranteed. This is particularly pertinent to the hospice environment where access to beds is limited and it may not be possible to admit a patient at a chosen or preferred time. There are usually more patients requesting hospice admission than beds available and it is usual for there to be a waiting list. It is important therefore for community teams to be vigilant for signs suggestive of progression into the terminal phase so plans for admission can be made before a crisis arises. Sometimes, additional support in the home will be provided in order to support the patient and family until a bed becomes available.

Where a preference for hospice end of life care has been made, it is should be possible to plan for the finer details of how care will be delivered. Wherever possible patients nearing the end of life will be offered a single room, which has sufficient space for a loved one to stay over. Whilst patients dying at home will be living by their 'own rules', (e.g. patients/carers smoking and drinking alcohol) such social activities may be inconsistent with hospice policies or impact on the care of others. These issues should be discussed before the plan for admission to save any difficulties once admitted. Furthermore, it would be important for staff to know of any visiting restrictions, particularly when there is conflict with potential visitors.

## Coordination of carer and consistency of approach to conversations

Hospice and palliative care is a multi-professional and co-ordinated approach. If ACP is seen as a series of conversations (39) as people live with, prepare for, and plan for their dying (29) rather than a single conversation; then co-ordination and consistency of approach between people and teams is helpful. This is not only between each person-to-person, but also within organisations as well as teams across different care settings.

However, there are challenges. Recent literature identifies patient, practitioner, and system-centred barriers to ACP (40,41). For example, there are arguments that inter-professional clinical settings lack systematic clinical routines to support ACP (42). Boddy et al.'s (40) Australian study reported a lack of a central registry, conflicting state legislation, and questions about roles and responsibilities. Others comment on clinicians' uncertainty of ACP documents and transferability of them across settings (43). This is worrying, especially in light of the evidence that a lack of coordination causes distress and patients and families value coordination of care represented by e.g. shared records, 24 hour/seven-days-a-week services, integrated care and fair access to care (44).

Hospice and palliative care services should respond to the challenges of coordination of services and information. Addressing these issues involves practical solutions. For example, sharing of end of life information through Electronic Palliative Care Coordination Systems (EPaCCS) is reported to reduce hospital admissions and increase dying at home (45,46). Gardiner et al.'s (47) systematic review reported the importance of good communication between providers; clear definition of roles and responsibilities, and appropriate and timely access to specialist-palliative care services. Innovative examples such as telephone and video consultations have been shown to benefit patients (48). The Marie Curie Delivering Choice programme with components such as facilitators, coordination centres, 24 hour/out of hours advice lines, 'discharge in reach' services in hospitals, electronic registers, and key workers increases home deaths with fewer emergency hospital admissions (47). Gold Standards Framework end of life register meetings to discuss and co-ordinate care have also been shown to benefit patients.

In addition to a coordinated and integrated services and care, attention to a consistent and tailored communication skills approach in ACP discussions is of benefit. ACP is a series of conversations (39) involving multiple members of the multi-professional team, not only within e.g. a hospice setting but also across different organisations. Sudore et al. (50) remind us that contemplation as well as decision making is part of ACP with other examples commenting that future care decisions evolve over time (51). ACP is as much situated within the context of a persons' relationship with their family and life and concerns about e.g. being a burden (52) as it is with autonomy and decision making about medical interventions or place of death. As such, patients may desire to have repeated conversations as they consider what is important to them as they live with, prepare and plan for their dying (22).

The tailored approach to ACP conversations recognises not only the value of tailoring honesty, truth telling and information giving to each person (53); but also knowing what is important to a person as well as the way people communicate and make decisions. What this means for hospice and palliative care practitioners is the benefits of a consistent approach (with attendant facilitative skills) to conversations that recognises the different type of discussions that may be held with different practitioners over a period of time.

## Summary

In addition to being a place where end of life care can be provided, the hospice approach plays a key role in ACP for those who wish to receive end of life care in other settings. ACP activity supports people as they live with the knowledge of their death at an uncertain time. The responsibility to be open to discussions is everyone's and hospice staff should see their role as a continuum of work that has already begun in the community. The key to success lies with a consistent approach in all environments not only with the form of the discussions, but also with the communication of ACP discussions with other stakeholder colleagues.

## Acknowledgements

The excerpt attributed to Sudore and colleagues was reprinted from *Journal of Pain and Symptom Management*, Volume 53, Issue 5, Sudore RL et al. 'Defining Advance Care Planning for Adults: A

Consensus Definition From a Multidisciplinary Delphi Panel', pp. 821–32, Copyright © American Academy of Hospice and Palliative Medicine, Published by Elsevier Inc., with permission from Elsevier, http://www.sciencedirect.com/science/article/pii/S0885392416312325.

## References

1. **Connor S, Sepulveda**, and **Bermeda M** (2014). *Global atlas of palliative care at the end of life*. Worldwide Palliative Care Alliance and World Health Organization.

2. **Kaasa S, Knudsen AK, Lundeby T**, and **Loge JH** (Jan 2017). Integration between oncology and palliative care: a plan for the next decade? *Tumori* **103**(1): 1–8.

3. **Higginson IJ** and **Addington-Hall JM** (1999). 'Palliative care needs to be provided on basis of need rather than diagnosis'. *BMJ (Clinical research ed.)* **318**(7176): 123.

4. **Wittgenstein L** (1953). *Philosophical Investigations* Part 1, Section 43. London: Blackwell, Basil.

5. **Russell S** (Apr 2015). 'Do definitions matter in palliative care?' *Int J Palliat Nurs* **21**(4): 160–1.

6. **Hui D, Mori M, Parsons HA, Kim SH, Li Z, Damani S**, et al. (Mar 2012). 'The lack of standard definitions in the supportive and palliative oncology literature'. *J Pain Symptom Manage* **43**(3): 582–92.

7. **Calanzani N, Higginson I**, and **Gomes B** (Jan 2013). 'Current and future needs for hospice care: an evidence-based report'. *London: Commission into the Future of Hospice care*. Hospice UK.

8. **Garber J, Leadbeater C** (2010). *Dying for Change. London, UK Demos*.

9. **Slomka J, Prince-Paul M, Webel A**, and **Daly BJ** (2016). 'Palliative care, hospice, and advance care planning: views of people living with HIV and other chronic conditions'. *J Assoc Nurses AIDS Care* **27**(4): 476–84.

10. **Pastrana T, Junger S, Ostgathe C, Elsner F**, and **Radbruch L** (Apr 2008). 'A matter of definition—key elements identified in a discourse analysis of definitions of palliative care'. *Palliat Med* **22**(3): 222–32.

11. **Russell S** (2014). 'Advance care planning: whose agenda is it anyway?' *Palliat Med* [Internet] **28**(8): 997–9. Available from: http://pmj.sagepub.com/cgi/doi/10.1177/0269216314543426

12. **Sabatino CP** (Jun 2010). 'The evolution of health care advance planning law and policy'. *Milbank Q* **88**(2): 211–39.

13. **Van Beek K, Woitha K, Ahmed N, Menten J, Jaspers B, Engels Y**, et al. (2013). 'Comparison of legislation, regulations and national health strategies for palliative care in seven European countries (Results from the Europall Research Group): a descriptive study'. *BMC Health Serv Res* **13**: 275.

14. **Sudore RL, Lum HD, You JJ, Hanson LC, Meier DE, Pantilat SZ**, et al. (Jan 2017). 'Defining Advance Care Planning for Adults: A Consensus Definition from a Multidisciplinary Delphi Panel' *J Pain Symptom Manage*. doi: 10.1016/j.jpainsymman.2017.08.025.

15. **Gomes B, Calanzani N, Curiale V, McCrone P**, and **Higginson IJ** (2013). 'Effectiveness and cost-effectiveness of home palliative care services for adults with advanced illness and their caregivers' *Cochrane database Syst Rev* **6**: CD007760.

16. **Radbruch L** and **Payne S** (2010). 'White Paper on standards and norms for hospice and palliative care in Europe: Part 2'. *Eur J Palliat Care* **17**(1): 22–33.

17. **Bausewein C** and **Higginson IJ** (Dec 2012). 'Challenges in defining "palliative care" for the purposes of clinical trials'. *Curr Opin Support Palliat Care* **6**(4): 471–82.

18. **Calzini N, Higginson I**, and **Gomes B** (Jan 2013). 'Current and Future needs for hospice care-an evidence based report'. *Help Hospices Comm* [Internet]. Available from: http://cdn.basw.co.uk/upload/basw_103716-5.pdf

19. **Institute of Medicine of the National Academies** (2014). *Dying in America: Improving Quality and Honouring Individual Preferences Near End of Life*. National Academies Press.

20. **Abel J, Pring A, Rich A, Malik T**, and **Verne J** (Jun 2013). 'The impact of advance care planning of place of death, a hospice retrospective cohort study'. *BMJ Support Palliat Care* **3**(2): 168–73.

21. **Cheung WY, Schaefer K, May CW, Glynn RJ, Curtis LH, Stevenson LW**, et al. (Mar 2013). 'Enrollment and events of hospice patients with heart failure vs. cancer'. *J Pain Symptom Manage* **45**(3): 552–60.

22. **Russell S** (2016). *Advance care planning and living with dying: the views of hospice patients* [Internet]. University of Hertfordshire. Available from: http://hdl.handle.net/2299/17474

23. **Reeve J, Lloyd-Williams M, Payne S**, and **Dowrick C** (2010). 'Revisiting biographical disruption: Exploring individual embodied illness experience in people with terminal cancer'. *Health* [Internet]. **14**(2):178–95. Available from: http://hea.sagepub.com/cgi/doi/10.1177/1363459309353298

24. **Hubbard G** and **Forbat L** (2012). 'Cancer as biographical disruption: constructions of living with cancer'. *Support Care Cancer* [Internet]. **20**(9): 2033–40. Available from: http://link.springer.com/10.1007/s00520-011-1311-9

25. **Seale C** and **Addington-Hall J** (Mar 1995). 'Dying at the best time'. *Soc Sci Med* **40**(5): 589–95.

26. **Walter T** (Jul 2003). 'Historical and cultural variants on the good death'. *BMJ* **327**(7408): 218–20.

27. **Kendall M, Carduff E, Lloyd A, Kimbell B, Cavers D, Buckingham S**, et al. (Aug 2015). 'Different experiences and goals in different advanced diseases: comparing serial interviews with patients with cancer, organ failure, or frailty and their family and professional carers'. *J Pain Symptom Manage* **50**(2): 216–24.

28. **Pollock K** and **Wilson E** (Jul 2015). *Care and communication between health professionals and patients affected by severe or chronic illness in community care settings: a qualitative study of care at the end of life*. Southampton UK: Nottingham University Publications.

29. **Russell S** (2016). 'Preparing and Planning for Dying: What's the Difference?' In: *11th Palliative Care Congress* [Internet]. Glasgow: Palliative Care Congress. Available from: http://www.pccongress.org.uk/

30. **Parry R, Land V**, and **Seymour J** (2014). 'How to communicate with patients about future illness progression and end of life: a systematic review'. *BMJ Support Palliat Care* [Internet]. **4**(4): 331–41. Available from: http://spcare.bmj.com/cgi/doi/10.1136/bmjspcare-2014-000649

31. **Barnes S, Gardiner C, Gott M, Payne S, Chady B, Small N**, et al. (Dec 2012). 'Enhancing patient-professional communication about end-of-life issues in life-limiting conditions: a critical review of the literature'. *J Pain Symptom Manage* **44**(6): 866–79.

32. **Glaser, B. G** and **Strauss AL** (1965). 'Temporal aspects of dying as a non-scheduled status passage'. *Am J Sociol* **71**: 48–59.

33. **Bristowe K, Carey I, Hopper A, Shouls S, Prentice W, Caulkin R**, et al. (Oct 2015). 'Patient and carer experiences of clinical uncertainty and deterioration, in the face of limited reversibility: A comparative observational study of the AMBER care bundle'. *Palliat Med* **29**(9): 797–807.

34. **Karlsson M, Friberg F, Wallengren C**, and **Ohlen J** (2014). 'Meanings of existential uncertainty and certainty for people diagnosed with cancer and receiving palliative treatment: a life-world phenomenological study'. *BMC Palliat Care* **13**: 28.

35. **Walczak A, Butow PN, Tattersall MHN, Davidson PM, Young J, Epstein RM**, et al. (Oct 2016). 'Encouraging early discussion of life expectancy and end-of-life care: A randomised controlled trial of a nurse-led communication support program for patients and caregivers'. *Int J Nurs Stud* **67**: 31–40.

36. **Wennman-Larsen A** and **Tishelman C** (Sep 2002). 'Advanced home care for cancer patients at the end of life: a qualitative study of hopes and expectations of family caregivers'. *Scand J Caring Sci* **16**(3): 240–7.

37. **Bernacki RE, Block SD** (Dec 2014). 'Communication about serious illness care goals: a review and synthesis of best practices'. *JAMA Intern Med* **174**(12): 1994–2003.

38. **Gawande A** (2014). *Being Mortal:Medicine and What Matters in the End*. 1st ed. New York: Metropolitian Books, Henery Holt and Company.

39. **Seymour J, Almack K**, and **Kennedy S** (2010). 'Implementing advance care planning: a qualitative study of community nurses' views and experiences'. *BMC Palliat Care* **9**: 4.

40. **Boddy J, Chenoweth L, McLennan V**, and **Daly M** (2013). 'It's just too hard! Australian health care practitioner perspectives on barriers to advance care planning'. *Aust J Prim Health* **19**(1): 38–45.

41. **Lovell A** and **Yates P** (Sep 2014). 'Advance Care Planning in palliative care: a systematic literature review of the contextual factors influencing its uptake 2008–2012'. *Palliat Med* **28**(8): 1026–35.

42. **Arnett K, Sudore RL, Nowels D, Feng CX, Levy CR**, and **Lum HD** (Sep 2016). 'Advance Care Planning: Understanding Clinical Routines and Experiences of Interprofessional Team Members in Diverse Health Care Settings'. *Am J Hosp Palliat Care*. doi: 10.1177/1049909116666358.

43. **Rhee JJ, Zwar NA, Kemp LA** (2013). 'Advance care planning and interpersonal relationships: a two-way street'. *Fam Pract* [Internet]. **30**(2): 219–26. Available from: http://www.fampra.oxfordjournals.org/cgi/doi/10.1093/fampra/cms063.

44. **The Leadership Alliance for the Care of Dying** (2014). *One Chance to Get it Right: Improving people's expereince of care in the last few days and hours of life*. London.

45. **Lindsey K** and **Hayes A** (Feb 2014). 'Supporting care integration with Electronic Palliative Care Coordination Systems (EPaCCS)'. *Int J Palliat Nurs* **20**(2): 60–1.

46. **Ali AA, Adam R, Taylor D**, and **Murchie P** (Dec 2013). 'Use of a structured palliative care summary in patients with established cancer is associated with reduced hospital admissions by out-of-hours general practitioners in Grampian'. *BMJ Support Palliat Care* **3**(4): 452–5.

47. **Gardiner C, Gott M**, and **Ingleton C** (May 2012). 'Factors supporting good partnership working between generalist and specialist palliative care services: a systematic review'. *Br J Gen Pract* **62**(598): e353–62.

48. **Middleton-Green L, Gadoud A, Norris B, Sargeant A, Nair S, Wilson L**, et al. (Feb 2016). 'A Friend in the Corner": supporting people at home in the last year of life via telephone and video consultation-an evaluation'. *BMJ Support Palliat Care*. doi: 10.1136/bmjspcare-2015-001016.

49. **Wye L, Lasseter G, Percival J, Duncan L, Simmonds B**, and **Purdy S** (2014). 'What works in "real life" to facilitate home deaths and fewer hospital admissions for those at end of life?: results from a realist evaluation of new palliative care services in two English counties'. *BMC Palliat Care* **13**: 37.

50. **Sudore RL, Stewart AL, Knight SJ, McMahan RD, Feuz M, Miao Y**, et al. (2013). 'Development and Validation of a Questionnaire to Detect Behavior Change in Multiple Advance Care Planning Behaviors'. *PLoS One* [Internet]. **8**(9): e72465. Available from: http://dx.plos.org/10.1371/journal.pone.0072465

51. **Michael N, O'Callaghan C**, and **Sayers E** (Jan 2017). 'Managing "shades of grey": a focus group study exploring community-dwellers' views on advance care planning in older people'. *BMC Palliat Care* **16**(1): 2.

52. **McPherson CJ, Wilson KG**, and **Murray MA** (Mar 2007). 'Feeling like a burden to others: a systematic review focusing on the end of life'. *Palliat Med* **21**(2): 115–28.

53. **Hancock K, Clayton JM, Parker SM, Wal der S, Butow PN, Carrick S**, et al. (2007). 'Truth-telling in discussing prognosis in advanced life-limiting illnesses: a systematic review'. *Palliat Med* [Internet] **21**(6): 507–17. Available from: http://pmj.sagepub.com/cgi/doi/10.1177/0269216307080823

Chapter 15

# Advance care planning in hospitals

## Clare Marlow, Karen Groves, and Premila Fade

Medical technology provides an arsenal of weapons
to launch against death and the 'war against disease'
has entrenched itself in medical philosophy . . .. The
continued thrust for treatment, wedded with a failure
to recognise the dying process, can rob individuals of
a peaceful, dignified death. Progress being made in
Advance Care Planning and palliative care is limited by
the existing paradigm of death as a 'foe to be conquered'.
It is time for a shift in this paradigm (1).

---

**This chapter includes**
- Advance care planning (ACP) as a key component of good practice in improving end of life care in hospitals
- Identification of appropriate hospital patients with whom to start a conversation about wishes and preferences for future care
- Different approaches to implementing and sustaining ACP in the hospital setting

---

**Key Points**
- ACP has the potential to improve communication between patients and healthcare professionals, increase quality of life and well-being of patients and those important to them, reduce use of futile and often unwanted treatments and unnecessary hospitalisations, and improve patient and family satisfaction with hospital care
- Although the hospital environment may not seem the obvious place for future care planning, the triggers to these conversations may occur during a hospital admission
- Prognostication is crucial to targeting future care planning: evidence suggests that around a third of all patients in general hospitals are likely to be in the last year of life and nearly 90% of people who die are hospitalised in the last year of life
- Up to 40% of patients in hospital over 65 have delirium or dementia and therefore may not be able to engage in ACP, highlighting the need for a clear distinction between ACP and anticipatory clinical management planning

◆ In a national audit of care of the dying in hospitals in England (2015) only 4% of patients had documented evidence of an ACP made prior to admission to hospital; although where there was an ACP, the team took the contents into account when making decisions in 91% of cases

◆ It is important to ensure that appropriate mechanisms are in place to enable access to ACP information by a range of service providers so that it can be taken into account when needed

**Key Message**

There are unique challenges and opportunities surrounding ACP within the hospital setting, but it is recommended as good practice to include offering ACP for all appropriately identified patients, and it is possible to achieve this in busy acute and community hospitals.

## Introduction

The hospital environment, where multiple health and social care professionals, teams, and wards might deal with the care of an individual previously unknown to them and where the main focus of care is on active, short-term input for an acute episode of illness, may not seem the obvious place for future care planning.

Evidence indicates that approximately 30% of all patients in general hospitals will die during the next 12 months; on average, people have 3.5 admissions to hospital in their last year of life, spending almost 30 days in bed in hospital and nearly 90% of people have some hospital care during the final year of life (2,3,4). The large majority of deaths follow a period of chronic illness such as heart disease, cancer, stroke, chronic respiratory disease, neurological disease, or dementia. Almost half (47%) of all deaths take place in hospital (5). Consequently, end of life care is core business for hospitals.

Advance care planning (ACP) is acknowledged as essential to improving choice and care at the end of life and a key component of good practice in improving end of life care in hospitals. An important opportunity may be lost if hospital staff do not consider talking to patients about what they want for their future care during an inpatient admission.

An acute admission to hospital may also serve as a 'wake-up call', a moment of recognition that a condition is no longer reversible, or indeed deteriorating, even with the interventions of an acute team. This recognition could trigger a conversation about 'what if this is as good as it gets?' or 'what if deterioration occurs again?', 'what then are the important things that everyone should know about me?'

## How advance care planning can help improve end of life care in hospital

Good quality end of life care is seen as an essential component of modern healthcare services and there are many examples of good end of life care being provided in different settings. However, the need to improve end of life care in hospitals has been highlighted by several recent publications (6,7,8). Issues raised in these reports include: not recognising that people are dying, poor communication, poor care planning, and lack of co-ordinated services.

It is possible for the patient presenting with acute illness, on a background of advanced disease or multiple co-morbidities, to be treated in exactly the same way as a patient with the same acute illness and no pre-existing advanced disease or co-morbidities, without taking into account the previous deteriorating condition. In this situation the conversations about uncertainty and the reversibility, or not, of the acute illness may not be undertaken appropriately, leaving both patient and those important to them with the sense that they are being undertreated or abandoned.

Several programmes have tried to impact on end of life care in UK hospitals, including the NHS 'Transforming end of life care in acute hospitals' (9), which outlines five enablers, one of which is encouraging ACP in hospitals. The 'Gold Standards Framework in acute hospitals programme' (10) includes early identification of the 30% of patients in their last year of life, needs-based coding to support proactive anticipation of needs at different stages, ACP, living well and dying well through to care after death and in bereavement. There is a growing evidence base of its effectiveness (11) as a comprehensive approach to improving EOLC in hospitals and reducing avoidable hospitalisation, enabling improved collaboration and communication in the community where GSF has been well used for many years and increasing uptake of ACP in all settings (12). GSF accreditation is supported by the British Geriatric Society. In addition the AMBER Care Bundle™ project has sought to address specifically the issue of uncertainty by encouraging conversations about uncertainty of recovery in those with advanced disease, poor prognosis, and acute illness, so that the patient and those important to them are prepared for whichever outcome may ensue (13). Within these programmes, ACP is acknowledged as essential to improving choice and care at the end of life.

It has been shown that ACP is possible in an inpatient setting and has the potential to improve communication between patients and healthcare professionals, increase quality of life and well-being of patients and those important to them, reduce use of futile and often unwanted treatments and unnecessary hospitalisations, and improve patient and family satisfaction with hospital care (14).

## Identifying those with whom to have an advance care planning conversation in hospital

Prognostication is crucial to targeting future care planning, unless this is to be addressed with every individual. Use of the 'Surprise Question'—would you be surprised if the patient were to die in the next year?—may be less helpful than in primary care, in a situation where a person is acutely ill and steady change over time less easy to observe, but the General Medical Council (GMC) definition of end of life care (15) might be of more help to hospital doctors, including deterioration of acute or chronic conditions, uncertainty of prognosis, and indications of imminent dying. However, studies of the use of the surprise question in hospital have suggested that it does have a positive predictive value in this environment (16,17,18,19).

Some acute environments have attempted to use formalised, evidence-based, prognostication tools. The Gold Standards Framework (GSF) original Prognostic Indicator Guidance (PIG), now known as the Proactive Identification Guidance (20) and the Scottish adaptation, known as the Supportive & Palliative Care Indicators Tool (SPICT™), are both generic indicators across all conditions. There is a growing evidence base of the use of the GSF PIG in different settings and with different conditions (21), e.g. it has been used in an acute Australian hospital to help identify those patients who might be in their last year of life and would benefit from ACP discussions (22). It has been shown that it is possible to identify the estimated 30% of patients in hospital who might be in their last year of life in order that earlier proactive care and ACP could be initiated.

Trials of screening interviews used on admission to identify those who would wish to have ACP conversations suggest that patients are more likely to document their wishes, preferences, and decision where the topic is raised in conversation by healthcare staff (23,24). However, the majority of those with advanced disease, even those who state that they have had ACP conversations and documented their wishes, do not have any advance care plans or advance decisions to refuse treatment in their medical records on presentation to acute care (25,26,27). In a national audit of care of the dying in hospitals in England (2015) only 4% of patients had documented evidence of an ACP made prior to admission to hospital; although where there was an ACP, the team took the contents into account when making decisions in 91% of cases (28).

## Who should have the advance care planning conversation?

The conversation may be undertaken by a variety of healthcare professionals involved in the patient's care, e.g. clinical or non-clinical health educators specific to the ACP process. Various education and development programmes exist to support generalist frontline staff who find it difficult to start such conversations (29); it does not require specialist palliative care expertise. Indeed, including future care planning conversations in all appropriate consultations, perhaps at the time of an unplanned admission, can be undertaken earlier than the introduction of specialist palliative care services, may avoid inappropriate readmission to hospital and may benefit those at risk of untimely death. It is, however, essential to have an understanding of disease progression, prognosis, and the risks/benefits of different treatment options—this information may need to be discussed with a senior clinician before initiating an ACP conversation to ensure that realistic options for care are presented.

## The advance care planning process

The success of ACP relies upon staff awareness of the planning possibilities, the enthusiasm of professionals empowering individuals and supporting the process, as well as organisations having the appropriate infrastructure in place (enabling policies, systems, and frameworks).

It is not always possible or even appropriate to have full ACP discussions with every hospital patient nearing the end of life. As part of the GSF programme in all settings the recommendation is that every appropriate individual is offered the chance to have an ACP discussion with their preferred person, and that this becomes part of the action plan for their care (30). Within the GSF acute hospitals programme, it is recognised that not all want or are able to have deeper discussions but it is recommended that ACP includes three levels of discussion (Box 15.1).

Crucially there need to be reliable, functioning, locally developed systems (electronic or manual) in place for the content of future care planning discussions and advance care plans to be available when needed, both within the acute hospital environment and across boundaries into other health and social care settings. Additionally there needs to be some means of knowing that such documented information exists.

## Comprehensive geriatric assessment (CGA)

CGA is a multifactorial, multidisciplinary process used to facilitate holistic care of patients with frailty and multiple co-morbidities. It takes into account the interplay between physical, psychological, social, and cultural aspects of health and disease. It is a process focused on the needs and wishes of the individual which looks to provide the right care for the person not just

---

**Box 15.1 Three levels of advance care planning discussion suggested in the Gold Standards Framework Hospital Programme**

Level 1

◆ Introduce the ACP conversation, providing information/leaflets, e.g. 'Planning Your Future Care' or locally agreed information to support patients and their families to continue discussions with others in future

Level 2—include the above plus:

◆ For each relevant patient clarify the preference for place of care and the nominated proxy decision maker

◆ Have 'do not attempt cardiopulmonary resuscitation' (DNACPR) discussions with each relevant patient/carer, in accordance with hospital policy

◆ With the patient's permission ensure that information is recorded in appropriate documentation and communicated to all involved in care

Level 3

◆ For some patients there may be opportunities to have a more detailed ACP discussion

◆ Ensure that appropriate documentation is completed/updated and, with the patient's permission communicated to all involved in care

Reproduced courtesy of the Gold Standards Framework

---

evidence-based care for the disease. This holistic approach results in less use of intensive medical resources, improves quality of life, and reduces care needs of frail older people.

Treatment escalation planning (TEP) and ACP are an integral part of this process for frail elderly patients, particularly on admission to acute care where interventional medicine is the norm. Older people living with frailty and several chronic diseases benefit less and suffer more from the side effects of medical interventions including hospitalisation itself (which contributes to the development of delirium and loss of function) and medication (use of four or more medicines is a risk factor for falls and delirium). Several tools including the GSF Proactive Identification Guidance (20), the Clinical Frailty Scale (31), and the electronic Frailty Index (32) can be used to predict prognosis and tailor interventions, including ACP, which enable individuals to have a realistic discussion about their future and tailor care to their preferences. Use of ACP in this population reduces hospital admissions but does not adversely affect prognosis.

Up to 40% of patients in hospital over 65 years old have delirium or dementia and therefore may not be able to engage in ACP. Ideally ACP discussions would have been undertaken in the community prior to this time when the person had capacity to make decisions about their future care. Unfortunately this is not often the case. Nevertheless it is vital to ensure that patients receive all the help they need to enable them to participate in the decision-making process and that their wishes are acknowledged even if they lack capacity to make the decision. The best interests framework must be used to make any decisions on behalf of the patient, and consideration of the views of those close to the patient is an integral part of this process. If it is felt that the person may regain capacity and that the decision can wait until this time it should be delayed, and if the person regains capacity after a treatment escalation plan has been made it must be reviewed with them and amended in accordance with their views (see the case study).

## Case study

Mrs Brown, an 88-year-old woman with Parkinson's disease, was admitted to hospital from a nursing home with pneumonia. She was prescribed antibiotics and intravenous fluids by the emergency department doctors in line with national sepsis guidelines and was then referred to the elderly care team for review.

On initial assessment Mrs Brown was delirious and unable to respond to questions, however her vital observations stabilised following emergency treatment. Mrs Brown's daughter, Jackie was present and was able to give more information about her mother. She explained that her mother had been deteriorating for several months and had, on more than one occasion, expressed a wish to die. However at other times she appeared to be happy and enjoyed visits from her grandchildren. These facts were confirmed by the nursing home staff who had in place a DNACPR decision but no other advance care plan.

As part of her comprehensive geriatric assessment a treatment escalation plan was agreed with Jackie: Mrs Brown would be discharged back to her nursing home with intravenous antibiotics administered by the intermediate care team and subcutaneous fluids. Jackie agreed that her mother would be more comfortable in the nursing home but felt her mother was not ready to die yet and would want treatment of the pneumonia including artificial hydration to give her time to improve.

The PEACE template (33), developed specifically to record treatment plans for care home residents, was used.

*PEACE can be used to document ACP with a person who has capacity, or to document an anticipatory treatment plan made using the best interests framework if the person cannot engage in ACP. Possible actions are grouped into 4 different categories: Intensive (all forms of treatment including intensive care if necessary); Hospital (hospital treatment up to ward based ceiling of care); Home (medical treatments including intravenous /subcutaneous treatments which can be provided outside a hospital); Comfort (treatment aimed at control of symptoms). Possible developments are discussed and a plan is made for each scenario. The form used also includes information about the person's underlying medical problems, assessment of capacity, views of those consulted, and advice for care home staff on palliating symptoms.*

Source: data from Hayes N et al., 'Advance Care Planning (PEACE) for care home residents in an acute hospital setting: impact on ongoing advance care planning and readmissions', *BMJ Supportive and Palliative Care*, Volume 1, p. 99, Copyright © 2011 BMJ Publishing Group Ltd.

The initial plan made for Mrs Brown is outlined in Table 15.1.

Mrs Brown was discharged back to her care home and her condition improved, she started to eat and drink and she became more alert. Mrs Brown and Jackie had a long chat about the future, at which time Mrs Brown was able to express her wish to have a peaceful end to her life without further medical intervention except pain relief. The anticipatory care plan was therefore reviewed and amended in line with Mrs Brown's wishes.

Mrs Brown's revised plan is outlined in Table 15.2.

**Table 15.1** Initial care plan for Mrs Brown

| Possible developments | Action category | Comments |
| --- | --- | --- |
| Recurrent infections | Home | Oral or intravenous antibiotics if indicated |
| Dehydration and reduced oral intake | Home | Trial of subcutaneous fluids |
| Acute medical emergency e.g. stroke or heart attack | Comfort | For symptom control |

**Table 15.2** Revised care plan for Mrs Brown

| Possible developments | Action category | Comments |
|---|---|---|
| Recurrent infections | Comfort | Oral antibiotics if indicated for symptom relief only |
| Dehydration and reduced oral intake | Comfort | Offer oral fluids and food, mouth care |
| Any acute medical emergency | Comfort | Prescribe palliative medications to ease symptoms, ensure comfort, dignity, and a peaceful death |

A recent study (34) looked at the role of consultant geriatrician-led anticipatory clinical management plans (ACMP) in association with community palliative care teams (CPCT) in reducing hospital readmissions, improving primary and secondary care communication and upholding patient and family end of life care wishes. Appropriate use of geriatrician-led ACMPs within secondary care for complex elderly frail patients, led to significant reduction in admission and readmission rates. Furthermore this approach improves care quality, facilitates better communication across healthcare sectors, encourages active cross-disciplinary working, and enables implementation of patient's/family's wishes during the end of life period.

**Table 15.3** Overcoming challenges of advance care planning in hospitals

| Challenge | Response |
|---|---|
| Hospital culture—poor recognition that patients are dying or likely to die in near future—emphasis on treatment and cure<br>Lack of knowledge about impact of frailty on prognosis | Education on prognostic indicators leading to earlier identification of patients in their last year of life<br>Involvement of geriatric medicine and specialist palliative care in all areas of acute care |
| Fear of causing distress | Lack of communication and false reassurance are just as likely to cause distress<br>ACP can increase rather than diminish hope (35) |
| Fear of giving up too soon | Talking about death does not make it more likely to happen even if the patient is very unwell |
| Fear of 'unrealistic expectations' from family members | Wider education programme, e.g. linked to 'Dying Matters'<br>ACP may include wish for all possible life-prolonging care but that clinical assessment at the time of deterioration will determine what treatment is offered |
| Lack of knowledge of alternatives | Ensure all hospital staff have access to information about end of life care options and services |
| Poor communication skills | Often linked to fear of causing distress and lack of knowledge—can be addressed with good training programme e.g. GSF programme |
| 'It won't change anything' | A robust process for documentation and dissemination to ensure the ACP information is available when needed at a time of crisis, communicated to all involved in care |
| Up to 40% of patients in hospital over 65 have delirium or dementia and therefore may not be able to engage in ACP | Education around Mental Capacity Act principles<br>If there is a chance that delirium may resolve then ACP should wait until the person is able to engage in the process<br>If it is deemed that capacity for advance care planning has been lost permanently then it is possible to make an anticipatory or end of life care plan in discussion with the person's family/loved ones using best interests |

# Challenges and opportunities surrounding advance care planning in hospitals

There are challenges to ACP in the acute sector. Hospital staff often report lack of time and unfamiliarity with the person as being a barrier to ACP and yet, as has already been identified, hospitalisation also provides an opportunity to discuss the future. The patient and their family are dealing with the worry, fear, and anxiety that admission to hospital and acute illness bring; our instinct is to strive to save life and reassure but burdensome tests and treatments and false reassurance do not reduce suffering, fear, or anxiety.

A realistic assessment of prognosis and benefits/burdens of treatment are required, this necessarily entails some discussion of the future. If resuscitation and treatment escalation for the acute illness need to be discussed, this is clearly the priority and patients and their families may be too distressed by current events to consider discussing the future. However if the patient survives the acute illness and discharge planning is commenced there is an opportunity to broach future care planning. Sometimes patients and relatives have a lot of difficult decisions to make very rapidly regarding future care needs and it is important not to overwhelm people with information.

When we consider the challenges, many of them become opportunities (Table 15.3). Acute illness, as well as causing fear and anxiety, is a time when people re-evaluate their quality of life and their wishes for their future care. This is therefore an ideal opportunity to consider the future and commence ACP discussions, to be continued within the community by GPs and care home staff.

Talking to patients and families about what is important for them grounds staff in the reality of personhood and humanity, helps them to stop, think, consider, and ask whether what they are planning for the person for whom they are caring is really what they would want for themselves. It also helps them to consider the patient's and family's perception of the care they are receiving and brings out in staff the compassion which is at the heart of the care that they give, but which sometimes appears lost in the urgency of the intervention.

## Summary

Recognition that the person could be in the last few months of life, good communication skills, an understanding of the options, and a clear process for documentation and dissemination are key to successful ACP in hospitals. Any member of the clinical team can do ACP as long as they have relevant communication skills and are empowered to do so.

Good integration and communication between primary, secondary, and social care is vital. If an ACP is drawn up but not discussed and understood by the people providing care to the person it is much more likely to fail. Ambulance services, out of hours GP services, intermediate care teams, and emergency departments all need immediate access to advance care plans. It does not matter how comprehensive and detailed the plan, if it cannot be accessed and utilised at the point of crisis it is useless.

ACP is a process which should ideally be completed in stages. Hospitalisation is a good time to start the discussion, however the conversation should be followed up after discharge from hospital usually by the GP or primary care team and any decisions made should be reviewed to allow the person to change their mind.

## Acknowledgements

The epigraph at the beginning of this chapter was originally published in Gellie et al., 'Death: a foe to be conquered? Questioning the paradigm', *Age and Ageing*, Volume 44, Issue 1, pp. 7–10. doi:

## References

1. **Gellie A, Mills A, Levinson M, Stephenson G** and **Flynn E** (2015). 'Death: a foe to be conquered? Questioning the paradigm'. *Age and Ageing* **44**: 7–10.

2. **Clark D, Armstrong M, Allan A, Graham F, Carnon A,** and **Isles C** (2014). 'Imminence of death among hospital inpatients: prevalent cohort study'. *Palliat Med* **28**(6): 474–8.

3. **Lyons P** and **Verne J** (2011). 'Pattern of hospital admission in the final year of life'. *BMJ Support Palliat Care* **1**: 81–2.

4. **Georghiou T, Davies S, Davies A** and **Bardsley M** (2012). *Understanding patterns of health and social care at the end of life.* Nuffield Trust.

5. **National End of Life Care Intelligence Network** (2015).

6. **House of Commons Health Committee** (2015). *End of Life Care.* Available at: http://www.publications.parliamcnt.uk/pa/cm201415/cmselect/cmhealth/805/805.

7. **Independent Review of the Liverpool Care Pathway** (2013). *More Care, Less Pathway.*

8. **Parliamentary and Health Service Ombudsman** (2015). *Dying without dignity.* Investigations by the Parliamentary and Health Service Ombudsman into complaints about end of life care.

9. **National End of Life Care Programme** (2010). *The route to success in end of life care - achieving quality in acute hospitals.*

10. **Corner H** and **Thomas K** (2010). 'The Gold Standards Framework in acute hospitals'. *End of Life Care* **4**(4).

11. http://www.goldstandardsframework.org.uk/evidence

12. **Thomas K, Armstrong Wilson JA,** and **Foulger TT** (2016). *Evidence that use of GSF helps improve Advance Care Planning Discussions in different settings.* National GSF Centre. Available from: http://tinyurl.com/hlvh4bz.

13. **Carey I, Shouls S, Bristowe K, Morris M, Briant L, Robinson C,** et al. (2015). 'Improving care for patients whose recovery is uncertain. The AMBER care bundle: design and implementation'. *BMJ Supportive & Palliative Care* **5**(1): 12–18.

14. **Detering KM, Hancock AD, Reade MC,** and **Silvester W** (2010). 'The impact of advance care planning on end of life care in elderly patients: randomised controlled trial'. *BMJ* **340**: c1345.

15. *Treatment and care towards the end of life: good practice in decision making* (2010). GMC: Available from: www.gmc-uk.org/guidance/ethical_guidance/end_of_life_guidance.asp

16. **Moss AH, Lunney JR, Culp S, Auber M, Kurian S, Rogers J,** et al. (2010). 'Prognostic significance of the "Surprise" question in cancer patients'. *Journal Of Palliative Medicine* **13**(7): 837–40.

17. **Murray S** and **Boyd K** (2011). 'Using the "surprise question" can identify people with advanced heart failure and COPD who would benefit from a palliative care approach'. *Palliative Medicine* **25**(4): 382–2.

18. **Pang W-F, Kwan BC-H, Chow K-M, Leung C-B, Li PK-T,** and **Szeto C-C** (2013). 'Predicting 12-Month mortality for peritoneal dialysis patients using the "Surprise" Question'. *Peritoneal Dialysis International* **33**(1): 60–6.

19. **Da Silva Gane M, Braun A, Stott D, Wellsted D** and **Farrington K** (2013). 'How robust is the 'Surprise Question' in predicting short-term mortality risk in haemodialysis patients'. *Nephron Clin Pract* **123**(3–4): 185–93.

20. http://www.goldstandardsframework.org.uk/pig - http://tinyurl.com/hsfz5zz

21. **Thomas K, Armstrong Wilson JA,** and **Tanner T** (2016). *Evidence that use of GSF improves early identification of patients in different settings.* National GSF Centre. Available from: http://tinyurl.com/h8xvpkz.

22. **Milnes S, Orford NR, Berkeley L, Lambert N, Simpson N, Elderkin T**, et al. (2015). 'A prospective observational study of prevalence and outcomes of patients with Gold Standard Framework criteria in a tertiary regional Australian Hospital'. *BMJ Supportive & Palliative Care.* Published Online First: 21 September 2015. doi: 10.1136/bmjspcare-2015-000864.

23. **Cheang F, Finnegan T, Stewart C, Hession A**, and **Clayton JM** (2014). 'Single-centre cross-sectional analysis of advance care planning among elderly inpatients'. *Intern Med J* **44**(10): 967–74.

24. **Van Scoy LJ, Howrylak J, Nguyen A, Chen M** and **Sherman M** (2014). 'Family structure, experiences with end-of-life decision making, and who asked about advance directives impacts advance directive completion rates'. *Journal Of Palliative Medicine* **17**(10): 1099–106.

25. **Butler J, Binney Z, Kalogeropoulos A**, et al. (2015). 'Advance directives among hospitalized patients with heart failure'. *JCHF. Journal of the American College of Cardiology* **3**(2): 112–21.

26. **Grudzen CR, Buonocore P, Steinberg J**, et al. (2016). 'Concordance of Advance Care Plans With Inpatient Directives in the Electronic Medical Record for Older Patients Admitted From the Emergency Department'. *J Pain Symptom Manage* **51**(4): 647–51.

27. **Shapiro SP** (2015). 'Do Advance Directives Direct?' *Journal of Health Politics Policy and Law.* **40**(3): 487–530.

28. **Royal College of Physicians** (2016). *End of Life Care Audit – Dying in Hospital.* London: RCP.

29. **Davis R** (2015). 'Starting end-of-life conversations in hospital'. *Nursing Times* **111**(4): 18–21

30. **The Gold Standard Framework**. http://www.goldstandardsframework.org.uk/advance-care-planning

31. **Rockwood K, Song X, MacKnight C**, et al. (2005). 'A global clinical measure of fitness and frailty in elderly people'. *CMAJ* **173**(5): 489–95.

32. **Clegg A, Bates C, Young J**, et al. (2016). 'Development and validation of an electronic frailty index using routine primary care electronic health record data. *Age Ageing* **45**(3): 353–60.

33. **Hayes N, Kalsi, T, Steves C**, et al. (2011). 'Advance Care Planning (PEACE) for care home residents in an acute hospital setting: impact on ongoing advance care planning and readmissions'. *BMJ Supportive and Palliative Care* **1**: 99. doi: 10.1136/bmjspcare-2011-000053.114.

34. **Gordon, SF** (2017). 'Dying in the complex frail elderly: Role of multidisciplinary anticipatory clinical management plans in secondary care'. Abstract presented at EAPC Congress 2017 Madrid.

35. **Davison S, Simpson C.** (2006). 'Hope and advance care planning in patients with end stage renal disease: qualitative interview study'. *BMJ* **333**: 866–9.

Chapter 16

# Advance care planning: thinking ahead for parents, carers, children, and young people

Angela Thompson

---

**This chapter includes**

- The spectrum of conditions involved requiring advance care planning (ACP) in paediatrics
- The challenges of ACP in paediatrics
- Advances in tools and pathways to support paediatric ACP
- Maintaining support for the family at the time of and following death
- Messages from special journeys

---

**Key Points**

- Families need care that is transparent and planned in partnership with them
- Care should be well documented, identifiable, communicated, anticipatory, and regularly reviewed
- Families require care that takes account of the whole family's needs—including siblings but especially the child/young person—and enables choice
- Care must encompass parallel planning, provide access to 24/7 expertise in symptom control, and engage in anticipatory bereavement care

---

**Key Message**

ACP in paediatrics applies from the diagnosis of a life-limiting/life-threatening condition onwards. It encompasses the management of intermittent potentially reversible episodes through to end of life care in keeping with the child's best interest. It is an active approach to managing care and acknowledges the child's and family's broader social, emotional, and spiritual needs and keeps the child central and paramount to all planning.

---

## Introduction

Planning for care at the end of life (EOL) in paediatrics poses many challenges and stirs emotions. The range of possibilities to be encompassed is vast and has previously been compounded by a lack of uniformity in approach and documentation of care plans (1). However, more areas are engaging in advance care planning (ACP) as standard and increasing areas of the country utilise the same documentation and processes. The death of a child is any family's worst nightmare.

Families facing these distressing days and years warrant the opportunity for care that is planned in partnership with them, facilitating choice and priority setting, and the best possible care, as the path ahead is anticipated, travelled along, and uncertainties managed.

## Which families are thinking ahead?

Paediatric palliative care covers a broad spectrum of conditions that cause families to live with the threat of death hanging over their child. It is helpful to offer these families both the opportunity and the support to think ahead, to plan to meet their needs from diagnosis through to care at the EOL. Palliative care for families with children with life-limiting or life-threatening conditions is offered to those who broadly sit within the following four groups (2), (see Table 16.1).

The diversity of conditions, time scales, disease trajectory, and the impact upon daily life of both the condition and its management creates a breadth of issues for ACP in paediatrics. These challenges span across many care settings for each child—home, hospital, hospice, school, and short breaks.

It has long been recognised and clearly described by Together for Short Lives, (TfSL) that children's palliative care differs from adult palliative care in several aspects:

◆ The number of children dying is relatively small

◆ Many have rare conditions, some of which are familial, so more than one child within a family may be affected

◆ Palliative care may last only a few days or extend over many years

◆ The whole family are affected

◆ Ongoing cognitive development affects the child's increasing understanding of their disease

◆ Disease management and care provision, including educational provision, is complex

The challenges that each of these points throws into the arena of advanced planning for care at the EOL are significant. They result in one of the key approaches to such planning; that of progressive, step-by-step planning, with the flexibility to change plans and reset priorities as circumstances change.

In addition there are some specific challenges in the implementation of ACP in paediatrics, (see Box 16.1).

**Table 16.1** Life-limiting conditions categories

| | |
|---|---|
| Category 1 | Life-threatening conditions for which curative treatment may be feasible but can fail, where access to palliative care services may be necessary when treatment fails or during an acute crisis, irrespective of the duration of that threat to life. Examples: cancer, irreversible organ failures of heart, liver, kidney |
| Category 2 | Conditions where premature death is inevitable, where there may be long periods of intensive treatment aimed at prolonging life and allowing participation in normal activities. Examples: cystic fibrosis, Duchenne muscular dystrophy |
| Category 3 | Progressive conditions without curative treatment options, where treatment is exclusively palliative and may commonly extend over many years. Examples: Batten disease, mucopolysaccharidoses |
| Category 4 | Irreversible but non-progressive conditions causing severe disability leading to susceptibility to health complications and likelihood of premature death. Examples: severe cerebral palsy, multiple disabilities such as following brain or spinal cord insult |

Reproduced courtesy of Together for Short Lives

## Box 16.1 Challenges to advance care planning and its implementation in paediatrics

- Emotional aspects
- Breadth of conditions managed, many of which are long term
- Prognostic difficulties especially in neonates and in neurological conditions
- Advances in technological support producing ethical dilemmas
- Learning difficulties and developmental progression affecting competency and consent related issues
- Transition to adult services often occurs at a time of deteriorating health
- National uniform approach/format to documentation under development
- Child Death Review Process requirements
- 24/7 access to CCN services variable limiting access to services out of hours

## Securing a firm foundation

How then do we begin to secure a firm foundation upon which we can build good ACP? An early start is essential. Supporting the family along their journey by a multiagency coordinated care-pathway approach brings opportunities for regular reviews, partnership planning, facing early anticipated and unexpected hurdles together, and builds trust between the family and the professionals (2). Opportunities for this foundation setting may be reduced where the disease progression is swift or a sudden onset of a severe complication occurs. Here it is essential for active 'in reach' of community palliative care services into hospital settings to consider choices and wishes with families and the hospital team, set or redefine goals and priorities, and establish appropriate support before potential discharge.

## Meeting the spectrum of challenges

Developing care plans for end of life care (EOLC) in paediatrics holds challenges in its implementation across a spectrum from premature neonates to young people transitioning to adult care (3). Catlin and Carter (4) placed emphasis within their neonatal protocol to communicating palliative care needs to the family as early as possible, including prenatally, in a sensitive and supportive manner, and to plan for and providing appropriate EOLC for their child. BAPM (British Association of Perinatal Medicine) has endorsed multiagency guidance in the UK (5).

## Planning ahead at times of uncertainty and transition

For those transitioning to adult services transitioning often coincides with their most vulnerable health state and end of life phase. Many of these young people and their families will have spent their lives involved in planning to meet their needs in their various care setting such as home, school, and short breaks, with a team they have come to know well (2,6). When their end of life phase coincides with transitioning towards adult services it is crucial that parallel planning continues. Parallel planning looks ahead for the young person to continue to live and need to receive services to support them within the adult sector, whilst at the same time acknowledging the possibility of death occurring and planning together for EOLC. Lack of accurate predictability/prognostication (7) necessitates this if both scenarios are to be well prepared for. The Transition Care Pathway (6) highlights important aspects of care planning for such individuals emphasising the need for planning to commence early and be regularly reviewed and updated. Challenges particularly exist where young people have an ACP in children's services that addresses their wishes around intermittent illnesses as well as around EOLC, where an equivalent opportunity for documentation does not exist in their adult team. The plan agreed in children's services however forms a solid base for discussions, agreements, and their redocumentation and communication within receiving adult services. It is important to recognise that a child/young person's ACP is a plan of care throughout life and will often include active resuscitation, or modified resuscitation, rather than no resuscitation (8). Box 16.2 illustrates some of the core elements of care during transition (6).

It is helpful to keep appropriate options in management open during times of uncertainty since in most cases, especially non-oncological, prognostication will not offer sufficient clarity as to the certain way forward. Hence talking about trialing a course of action to see which benefits the child and reviewing regularly can ease the way forward and enable appropriate care at all stages.

## Tools to engage the family, child, and young person in thinking ahead

Support tools have become increasingly developed to enable difficult discussions around EOLC. The Child and Young Persons Advance Care Plan has been developed following evolution of earlier tools. It now forms the basis for documentation used by the Children and Young People's

---

### Box 16.2 Core elements of end of life care for young people

+ Care in the place of their choice
+ Professionals should be open and honest with young people and families when the approach to end of life care is recognised, with timely open communication and information
+ Joint planning with young people, their families, and relevant professionals should take place, with choices/options in all aspects of care, including complementary therapies
+ Young people and families should be supported in their choices. Goals for quality of life issues should be respected
+ A written plan for care around the time of death should be agreed, taking account of acute or slow deterioration. All professionals who may be involved are informed including emergency services
+ Coordination of services at home where this is a chosen place of care including provision of specialist equipment, should be in place
+ Expert symptom management, including access to 24-hour specialist symptom management advice, and expertise by those suitably qualified and experienced, including access to anticipatorily prescribed out of hours medication
+ Emotional, spiritual, and practical support should be available for all family members
+ Short-break care should be available with medical and nursing input when required
+ Advance care plans including EOLC plans should be regularly reviewed and amended to take into account ongoing changes

Advance Care Plan Collaborative, which covers much of the west and central areas of England. This enables uniformity of documentation, process, and policy across all care settings between which the child may move within these areas allowing both an expectation of, and ready recognition of the coloured purple plans, and with this, peace of mind for families. The collaborative website provides supporting information (http://www.cypacp.nhs.uk). The purple ACPs are held as an original copy by the family and travel with the child/young person at all times. Others who need to be able to access this information quickly have copies on lilac paper to ensure its ready recognition even if not stored as requested at the front of records. Regular agreed reviews are essential.

The ACP supports discussions and documentation of decisions around the child's best interest at that particular point in time. They are developed at the family's pace, in partnership between the family and the child's wider team of professionals. It is essential that the child's lead paediatrician leads these conversations, whilst consulting with the wider clinical team basing agreements upon ethical guidelines and incorporating wishes of the family where these are in keeping with the child's best interest. It will often necessitate several sensitive conversations to come to agreement and completion of the ACP. The ACP can be used to revisit, redefine, and reprioritise plans as circumstances change. They encompass more than management at EOL, allowing crucial clinical information and families' wishes around the management of intermittent illnesses to be clearly documented to enable best-practice care throughout the child's journey by everyone, including e.g. the ambulance team who may need rapid access to succinct, essential information.

## Putting plans into action

Together for Short Lives (TfSL) has comprehensive multiagency pathway guidance (2) specifically for children and young people encompassing all stages from diagnosis, through living with the condition, to moving into EOLC and bereavement. TfSL's pathway work (2) acknowledges the need to respond to the recognition of the move into the end of life phase in a child or young person. This will include open and honest discussions with the family, reviewing their needs and goals and drawing up a plan for this new phase. Holding a multidisciplinary meeting with the involvement of the young person and family where possible, especially where death is likely to occur at home is central to comprehensive care at the EOL.

Important aspects of this meeting are:

◆ To establish and communicate revised care plans

◆ To set out clear guidelines for roles and responsibilities

Holding such meetings at the GP's often enables their participation and provides opportunities to bridge build between professionals. It also helps to:

◆ Develop a unified approach to management

◆ Provide visible evidence of support for primary care teams from the specialist palliative care services

◆ Provide a forum to discuss clinical, social, and psychological issues etc.

◆ Enable the primary care team to become familiar with the 'just in case medicines' placed in the home and the documentation used for symptom management. Examples are the Drug Administration Document used in the UK's West Midlands Paediatric Palliative Care Toolkit (8)

◆ Allow consideration of anticipated complications, based upon:

   • Literature evidence for the underlying condition
   • Knowledge of the complications already experienced specific to the individual's unique disease progression

- Consider the management of related potential complications/scenarios
- Plan the availability of the family's 'virtual team' in and out of hours
- Clarify the family's initial single point of contact

It consequently provides peace of mind to the family that their child's teams are communicating and working together with them at this crucial stage. Anticipation is the central cogwheel around which all will need to be planned for care to be effectively delivered.

A template can be used to assist planning at this stage, outlining key essential information. The meeting will enable a definitive plan for contact in and out of hours, both for family and for front line staff who will require access to 24 hour specialist symptom control support. The template can then be forwarded for information to the out-of-hours services for primary care (Table 16.2).

This template sits alongside and does not replace ACP documentation around resuscitation and symptom-control issues at the EOL. The clear and concise documentation relating to these issues should be provided in relation to the possibilities of both acute, sudden deteriorations and also gradual demise. This in turn should be supplemented by a more detailed care plan of the child's and family's wishes, for example some families wish to confirm who needs to be there at the time of death. These aspects may be included in the children and young people (CYP) advance care plan. (8)

The principle in paediatric ACP is to outline the decisions reached at that point in time for care in the face of either an acute deterioration or a gradual demise in the end of life phase. It empowers children and families in their decision making, allowing as much choice and control as possible within what is both ethical and in the child's best interests and is flexible to accommodate changing circumstances and assists clear communication between families and professionals. It clarifies decisions with detailed practical instructions around the extent of resuscitation, and enables those dealing with an emergency situation to respond appropriately. It is essential that such decisions are in keeping with the Royal College of Paediatrics' and Child Healths' framework for practice (9).

What are young people's views on planning for care at the EOL? A study examining adolescents' wishes around EOLC (10) explored whether differences existed between chronically ill and healthy adolescents with regard to their attitudes to EOL issues. Ninety-six per cent of chronically ill and 88% of healthy teens wanted to share in decision making if they were very ill. At times conflicts of opinions will exist within families, and between families and staff.

**Table 16.2** Template for end of life care multidisciplinary care meeting

| Private and Confidential Medical Information | | | | |
|---|---|---|---|---|
| Planning Meeting re: | Name: | | DoB: | |
| | Address: | | | |
| Meeting held at GP Practice: | | | | |
| Date: | | | | |
| Background Diagnosis: | | | | |
| Medications: | | | | |
| Known and suspected allergies: | | | | |
| Professionals involved: | | | | |
| Name | Role | Address | Contact number | Availability hours |
| Initial point of contact for family: | | | | |
| In hours (8.30 am–5.30 pm): | | | | |
| Out of hours (5.30 pm–8.30 am and weekends): | | | | |

Some high-profile cases have required the court's intervention as the ultimate arbiters to assist in such situations where conflicting opinions exist, so that the best interests of the child can be served (9,11,12). Good care aims to avoid these traumatic conflicts by families and staff walking the journey together over time, developing respect and understanding, crossing barriers together at earlier stages so that care at the EOL can be jointly planned to provide good quality symptom managed days and weeks where life can be lived as fully and preciously as possible. It is also important to consider competence in decision making, and where relevant, address the Mental Capacity Act in young adults as described.

## When death comes: planning to maintain the care

Care around the time of death must be as thorough and professional as before death. Aspects may include (6):

- ◆ Good care of the child's body and the family at the time of death
  - Respecting the need for privacy, time, space, sensitivity of the family's spiritual needs, religious beliefs, and cultural practices
- ◆ Parents should retain their parenting role after the death of their child
  - Respecting their need to retain control of their child's body, to have mementoes and memories. All staff dealing with their child's body treat it with dignity
- ◆ Siblings should be supported and included in all decisions
  - Respecting their need to be supported in decisions around seeing their siblings body, attending the funeral, making a special contribution to the service etc.
- ◆ Parents should have choice regarding place of body after death
  - Respecting the needs of some families to remain close to their child until the funeral either at home or in a special bedroom at the hospice
- ◆ All professionals/agencies should be informed of the death with parents consent
  - Respecting parents' need to give consent and utilising the up-to-date list kept in the child's records of contacts to be made following the child's death
- ◆ Families should receive appropriate written information
  - Respecting that grief exacerbates the need for information about registering the death etc. to be in written format

All these aspects are more likely to be addressed if a bereavement policy is held. Supportive guides can be found in the West Midlands Palliative Care Toolkit (8).

## Supporting the family through grief

When a child dies, it is likely that there will be grandparents and siblings who will be deeply affected besides the parents and other close family members. Siblings warrant particular attention and care before, during, and after their siblings death, and many children's palliative care services place an emphasis upon caring for the siblings, with access to professional support where grief appears complex. Play specialist are increasingly becoming integral members of palliative care teams. Clinical psychology and bereavement services are often closely associated with children's palliative care services. Where grief is less complex, the palliative care team will often provide the main ongoing support to the sibling(s) both in pre-bereavement and post-bereavement work, using tools such as memory boxes, which can be planned for and begun before the death, helping the child to prepare for the anticipated death and to gather items to cement their memories.

Winston's Wish is one organisation which supports children when a significant individual in their life dies. Its role in terms of providing support in relation to the realities for grieving children is outlined in Box 16.3.

## Messages from special journeys

To be able to walk with a family along part of their journey at such a difficult time in their life is a privilege. Each such special journey deserves that we reflect upon it afterwards. Several key aspects are repeatedly raised in discussions with families after their child's death, in relation to aspects which they valued. These include:

◆ Being listened to and heard by professionals, as partners

◆ Being respected and not judged

◆ Feeling as safe and prepared as possible

One family with a child with a terminal solid tumour shared that having an ACP and symptom control plan 'helped us feel safer and less frightened because we knew what might happen next, how we would manage it, and who was there and when to help us. We could reassure our daughter of that. It was as we had discussed and thought through'.

Another family of a boy with a degenerative neurological condition shared that parallel planning had helped them cope through the times of uncertainty—'we knew what was happening; he was getting more ill more quickly, and recovering less well between. We needed to be prepared and have the support we needed either to keep dealing with this emotionally and physically exhausting time or to cope with his death.'

Perhaps the key to family's needs can be summed up as:

◆ Attention to detail within

◆ High quality, timely, responsive, coordinated, transparent care which is effectively planned, documented, and communicated

With this we can take a significant step towards providing families with the best quality of life possible for as long as possible reassured in the knowledge that anticipatory thinking has put plans into place to endeavour to meet their needs and provide high-quality best-practice care. Our children and young people with palliative care needs, and their families deserve nothing less.

---

### Box 16.3 Realities for grieving children and young people (13)

◆ All children and young people grieve

◆ Grieving is a long term process; they revisit their grief and frequently construct a changing relationship with the person who has died

◆ Younger children will need help in retaining memories which facilitate a continuing bond

◆ Children express their grief differently to adults

◆ Children cannot be protected from death

◆ There are clear developmental differences between children and young people in the understanding, experience, and expression of grief

◆ A child's grief occurs within a family and community context and will be influenced by significant adults

Source: data from Stokes J (2004) *Then, Now and Always*, Gloucester: Winston's Wish and Calouste Gulbenkian Foundation.

**Visual summary: End of life care for children and young people**

Diagnosis of life limiting condition

Early stages

Establish how young person and carers want to be involved in decision making

Assemble multidisciplinary support team

Assign named medical specialist to lead and coordinate care

Bereavement

Carry out wishes expressed in ACP

Organ/tissue donation

Care of body

Funeral

Death

Parents/ carers

Advance care plan ACP

Working together, the young person, their carers and support team record important information and decisions.

Help family to prepare   Rituals

Recording memories

Plans for social media

Child / young person

Multidisciplinary support team

Condition specialists

Hospice professionals

Palliative care team

Social care practitioners

Education professionals

Chaplains

Allied health professionals

Record wishes + ambitions

Social activities

Religious/spiritual

Education

Family

End of life

Update treatments

Consider ending treatments

Consider new invasive treatments

Consider non-pharmacological treatments

Other family and important people

Siblings

Grandparents

Boy/girlfriends

Friends

Bereavement support

Team provides ongoing care and support

Social

Practical

Spiritual/ religious

Emotional/ psychological

A living document

ACP is updated as needs change and decisions are made

Agree preferred places for care and death

Care planning

Delivery

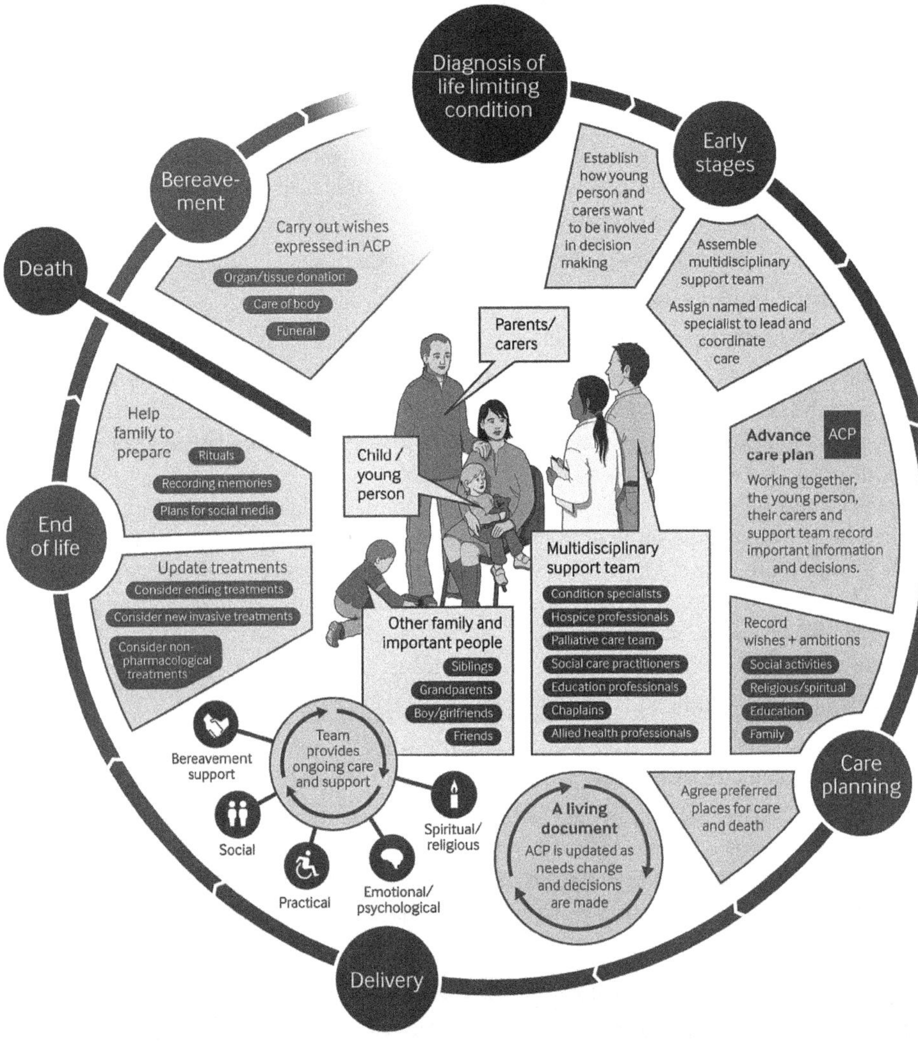

**Figure 16.1** Visual summary: End of life care for children and young people (14,15)

Reproduced from Villanueva G et al., 'End of life care for infants, children and young people with life limiting conditions: summary of NICE guidance', *The British Medical Journal*, Volume 355, pp. 30–2, Copyright © 2016, doi: 10.1136/bmj.i638, with permission from BMJ Publishing Group Ltd

## Journeying further in to the future together

It is never appropriate to remain complacent about developments which need to continue to move forwards to meet demand. Recent emergence of the NICE Guidance for End of Life Care for Children and Young People and summary papers (Dec 2016, 14,15), will support this ongoing development, (see Table 16.1 and Figure 16.1). This reiterates the approaches and philosophy outlined within this chapter, and encourages the utilisation of tools such as the ACP and concepts such as parallel planning described here. It will add to the levers provided by Together for Short Lives, to influence trusts to further develop their service provision according to the NICE guidelines to the benefit of our families (see Box 16.4).

## Box 16.4 Components of an advance care plan for a child or young person with a life limiting condition (14,15)

- Demographic information about the child or young person and their family
- Up to date contact information for:

  The child or young person's parents or carers

  The key professionals involved in care
- A statement about who has responsibility for giving consent
- A summary of the life-limiting condition
- An agreed approach to communicating with and providing information to the child or young person and their parents or carers
- An outline of the child or young person's life ambitions and wishes, such as on:

  Family and other relationships

  Social activities and participation

  Education

  How to incorporate their religious, spiritual, and cultural beliefs and values into their care
- A record of significant discussions with the child or young person and their parents or carers
- Agreed treatment plans and objectives
- Education plans, if relevant
- A record of any discussions and decisions that have taken place on:

  Preferred place of care and place of death

  Organ and tissue donation (see recommendation 1.1.19 in the full NICE guideline 2)

  Management of life-threatening events including plans for resuscitation or life support

  Specific wishes, such as on funeral arrangements and care of the body
- A distribution list for the advance care plan

Source: data from Villanueva G, Murphy M S, Vickers D, Harrop E, & Dworzynski K, End of life care for infants, children and young people with life limiting conditions: summary of NICE guidance', *The British Medical Journal*, Volume 355, pp. 30–32, Copyright © 2016 BMJ Publishing Group Ltd, doi: 10.1136/bmj.i6385

Ongoing development now needs to be firmly underpinned by research to provide the hard facts, rather than anecdotal evidence alone, as, for example, to the use and benefits of ACP for children and young people. Current research around CYP's ACPs that is underway within the West Midlands and reaching out into the ACP Collaborative will provide much-needed hard evidence to enable sensitive and effective planning ahead that is conducted for the benefit of families keeping them and especially their child, central to all we do. We have achieved much, but still have much to do together to offer our families the care they truly merit.

## References

1. **Brook L** (2008). 'A plan for living and a plan for dying: advanced care planning for children'. *Archives of Disease in Childhood* **93**(suppl): A61–66.

2. **Together for Short Lives** (2013). 3rd Edition. *A Core Care Pathway for Children with Life-limiting and Life-threatening Conditions*. Bristol.

3. **Thompson A** (2015). 'Paediatric palliative care'. *Paediatrics and Child Health* **25**(10): 458–62.

4. **Catlin A** and **Carter B** (2002). 'Creation of a neonatal end of life palliative care protocol'. *Journal of Perinatology* **22**(3): 184–95.

5. **Mancini A, Uthaya S, Beardsley C, Wood D,** and **Modi N** (2014). 'Practical guidance for the management of palliative care on neonatal units', *BAPM*. Chelsea and Westminster Hospital.

6. **Together for Short Lives** (2015). *Stepping up*. Bristol.

7. **Shaw K, Brooke L, Cuddeford L,** et al. (2014). 'Prognostic indicators for children and young people at End of Life; a Delphi study'. *Pall Med* 28501–12.

8. **West Midlands Palliative Care Toolkit** (2014). Available from: http://www.togetherforshortlives.org.uk/professionals/external_resources

9. **Larcher V, Craig F, Bhogal K, Wilkinson D,** and **Brierley J** (2015). 'Making decisions to limit treatment in life-limiting and life-threatening conditions in children: a framework for practice'. *RCPCH*. doi: 10.1136/archdischild-2014-306666.

10. **Lyon ME, McCabe MA, Patel KM,** and **Angelo LJ** (2004). 'What do adolescents want? An exploratory study regarding end-of-life decision-making'. *Journal of Adolescent Health* **35**(6): 529.

11. **Larcher V** (2012). 2nd Edition. 'Ethics'. In Goldman A, Hain R, and Liben S (eds) *Oxford Textbook of Palliative Care for Children*, 35–46. Oxford: Oxford University Press.

12. **Dyer C** (2008). 'Trust decides against legal action to force girl to receive heart transplant'. *BMJ* **337**: a2659.

13. **Stokes J** (2004). *Then, now and always*, 1st edition. Cheltenham: Calouste Gulbenkian Foundation.

14. **NICE guideline [NG61] Dec 2016.** *End of Life care for infants, children and young people with life limiting conditions: planning and management.* Available from: https://www.nice.org.uk/guidance/ng61

15. **Villaneueva G, Murphy S, Vickers D, Harrop E,** and **Dworzynski K** (2016). 'End of life care for infants, children and young people with life limiting conditions: summary of NICE guidance'. *BMJ* **355**: i6385; 30–32.

# Chapter 17

# Advance care planning and people with dementia

Karen Harrison Dening

"Even when the experts agree, they may well be mistaken"
*Bertrand Russell* (1872–1970)

---

**This chapter includes**

- Contextual discussions on 'ageing and dementia', 'what is dementia?', 'dementia and multi-morbidity', and 'dementia: a life-limiting condition'
- Topics of autonomy, decision making, family, and personhood for those with dementia
- Guidance on communication with people with dementia
- Illustrative case studies

---

**Key Points**

- Introduce advance care planning (ACP) and support discussions as early after the diagnosis as possible to give people with dementia the opportunity to explore their wishes and preferences for future care
- There are various care transitions and triggers for the conversation along the trajectory of dementia
- Good communication skills and knowledge of dementia is essential
- Do not assume family members know the wishes and preferences of the person with dementia
- People with dementia and their families require support and information throughout the process of ACP. Family members may feel loss and require bereavement support prior to the persons death

---

**Key Message**

ACP is beginning to demonstrate many advantages to individuals and their ability to extend autonomy and control at a time when these are compromised. In dementia this may be experienced very early on in the disease process so it is essential that people with dementia are offered the option to consider and record their wishes and preferences for end of life whilst they have the cognition and capacity to do so. Whilst family members often become very involved in their care as time passes, they may not always be able to accurately reflect an understanding and knowledge of a persons wishes yet may be placed in a decision-making situation.

## Setting the context

Advance care planning (ACP) is a voluntary process of discussion and review to help an individual who has capacity to anticipate how their condition may affect them in the future. The mechanisms of ACP are given focused attention in other sections of this book so this chapter will consider ACP in the context of dementia; a progressive and life-limiting illness, where the mental capacity to make decisions can be lost fairly early on in the illness. There is a small growing literature on ACP and its application in dementia in the UK highlighting that its uptake is small and patchy due to several factors.

People with a life-limiting illness, especially dementia, are not routinely consulted about their wishes and preferences for future care. There are potential barriers that may contribute to this (1), see (Box 17.1).

However, in dementia, there are several additional barriers to initiating ACP:

◆ Acknowledgement that dementia is a terminal/life-limiting illness

◆ The potential for loss of decision making capacity early on in the disease trajectory

◆ Care professionals might lack confidence in starting discussions due to lack of knowledge of the condition

◆ Care professionals might not recognise or know how to manage factors that influence the prognosis

◆ Lack of prospective care management as the illness progresses

## Ageing and dementia

More people are living longer into old age (2). In the UK alone, the percentage of older people (aged 65 years and over) has grown by 47% since 1974, and has therefore increased to make up nearly 18% of the total population in 2014 (3). The numbers of those reaching the oldest ages are increasing the fastest: in 2008 there were 1.3 million people in the UK aged 85 and over, with this expected to increase to 1.8 million by 2018 and to 3.3 million by 2033 (4). These changes to the age

---

### Box 17.1 Barriers to completing an advance care plan

◆ Procrastination, or waiting to do it later

◆ Dependence on family for decision making

◆ Lack of knowledge about ACP

◆ Difficulty in talking about the subject

◆ Waiting for the healthcare professional to initiate a discussion by the patient

◆ Waiting for the patient to initiate discussion by the health professional

◆ Believing a lawyer is needed to fill out the forms

◆ Fatalism, or acceptance of the 'will of God'

◆ Fear of 'signing my life away'

◆ Fear of not being treated

Reproduced courtesy of Karen Harrison Dening (1)

structure of the population influence both the prevalence and incidence of age-related conditions such as dementia (5).

## What is dementia?

Dementia is a term used to describe a syndrome; a collection of symptoms including a decline in memory, reasoning, and communication skills, and a gradual loss of skills needed to carry out daily living activities. These symptoms are caused by structural and chemical changes within the brain as a result of neurodegenerative changes. The cognitive changes arising in dementia are determined to a large extent by the areas of the brain that are affected by the underlying pathological processes. In other words, the process of dementia is the end-stage manifestation of numerous brain disorders (6,7). This syndrome may result from Alzheimer's disease, cerebral vascular disease, and from other conditions primarily or secondarily affecting the brain. (See Figure 17.1 for the most common types of dementia.)

## How many people are affected by dementia?

In the UK it has been estimated that as many as 25 million people (42% of the UK population) will know a close friend or family member affected by dementia (9). Estimates are that the number of people in the UK with dementia (both diagnosed and undiagnosed) is currently around 820,000. Despite the potential improvements in health promotion that have reduced the incidence of vascular disease (10), we know that increasing age appears to be the strongest risk factor for developing dementia and that these numbers are forecast to rise.

## Dementia: a life-limiting condition

As life expectancy increases so people often develop a range of conditions and disabilities in the years before death (11). Frail older people (including those with dementia) are the greatest users

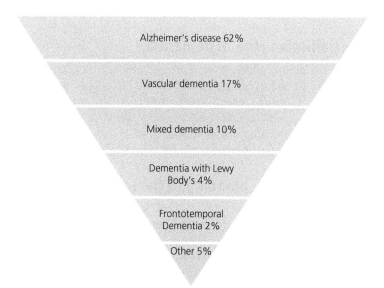

**Figure 17.1** The most common forms of dementia diagnosed in over 65 year olds in the UK

of health and social care (12). Despite this, dementia and frailty have not traditionally been seen as 'terminal' or 'life limiting' syndromes (13). In one study of carers and physicians at nursing home admission, only 1.1% of residents were perceived to have life expectancy of less than six months. However, 71% died within that period (14). Acute physical illness, such as pneumonia or urinary tract infection may be an indicator of imminent death in people with advanced dementia (15,16,17). Dementia is a progressive, irreversible, neurodegenerative condition (18), and once diagnosed people will die with dementia regardless of the primary cause of death (19). Xie et al. (18) in an analysis of a longitudinal population-based cohort study, reported a median survival time from symptom onset of dementia to death was 4.5 years concluding that one in three people (30%) will die with or from dementia. Although dementia has been identified as one of the leading causes of death (20), the exact numbers of deaths where dementia is a primary or secondary cause remains uncertain and this is thought to be due to under-reporting on death certificates (21).

## Dementia and multimorbidity

As dementia is largely a disease of old age, many people with dementia will also have other illnesses or disabilities. Multimorbidity is where two or more chronic conditions exist, where one is not necessarily more central than the others (22). Multimorbidity represents the most common 'disease pattern' found among the elderly and is characterised by complex interactions of co-existing diseases where a medical approach focused on a single disease does not suffice. People with dementia show high levels of multi-morbidity (23), common conditions including cardiovascular disease, diabetes, and musculoskeletal disorders such as fractures.

Whilst many people with dementia die of a medical complication, such as pneumonia or another infection, dementia itself and the ensuing frailty can be the cause of death. Frailty with generalised wasting, dehydration, malnutrition, and more specifically sarcopaenia can be seen with dementia and, especially with advanced disease, immobility and dependency on care. However, the lack of recognition of dementia as a life-limiting illness has led to neglect in the need for ACP to address the end of life care for this group of people (24). The professionals can pursue multi-disease management and fuel polypharmacy whilst missing the need to understand the holistic needs and priorities of patient and those close to them.

## The case for palliative care in dementia

ACP is a prominent of element palliative care, developed originally in cancer care. Data from a retrospective population-based survey of nearly 4,000 deaths (25,26) was analysed to explore people's experience of dying from causes other than cancer. Results suggested that nearly 20% of people with non-malignant disease were as much in need of specialist palliative care services as those with cancer, specifically in promoting autonomy through ACP. However, equitable access to palliative care services for people affected by dementia, and specifically ACP, should be offered (27).

## Drivers for advance care planning in dementia

The End of Life Care Strategy (28) stated that *all* people should be offered ACP to explore their wishes and preferences for end of life care, and that these should be respected and acted upon wherever possible. The National Dementia Strategy (29) stated that people with dementia and their carers should be involved in planning end of life care. But ACP for people with dementia in reality is still not a mainstream intervention (30,31). The European Association of Palliative Care white paper makes 57 recommendations for effective palliative care in dementia (32); domain three focuses on ACP (see Box 17.2).

---

## Box 17.2 Domain 3. Setting care goals and advance planning

3.1 Prioritising of explicit global care goals helps guide care and evaluate its appropriateness

3.2 Anticipating progression of the disease, ACP is proactive. This implies it should start as soon as the diagnosis is made, when the patient can still be actively involved and patient preferences, values, needs, and beliefs can be elicited

3.3 Formats of advance care plans may vary in terms of preferences, the amount of detail required, and what is available in the specific setting for the individual

3.4 In mild dementia, people need support in planning for the future

3.5 In more severe dementia and when death approaches, the patient's best interest may be increasingly served with a primary goal of maximisation of comfort

3.6 ACP is a process, and plans should be revisited with patient and family on a regular basis and following any significant change in health condition

3.7 Care plans should be documented and stored in a way that permits access to all disciplines involved in any stage and through transfers

Source: data from EAPC Dementia White Paper, 'Recommendations on palliative care and treatment of older people with Alzheimer's disease and other progressive dementias', Copyright © 2013 European Association for Palliative Care, Available from http://www.eapcnet.eu

---

## When is the best time to initiate advance care planning in dementia?

There is much debate on when is the best time to offer ACP to people with dementia; many professionals feel that entering into discussions about ACP for end of life care in the early or diagnostic stage is both too soon and insensitive. However, in most cases, care and ACP needs to take place early, while the person has sufficient mental capacity to consider their preferences and make decisions or nominate and donate powers as supported by the statutes set out in the Mental Capacity Act (2005). Thus gaining a timely dementia diagnosis is important, (see Table 17.1).

## Personhood, autonomy, and dementia

To understand ACP in the context of dementia it is essential to understand what it is to be an autonomous person and being given the respect to make decisions. Kitwood stated that personhood is a status that is bestowed upon one human being by another (34) and an outcome of a relationship between two or more people that relies on the action of the bestowal of personhood, one to another. However, Nolan et al. (35) felt that Kitwood's view of person-centred care fails to capture the interdependencies and reciprocities that underpin caring relationships, especially across family members. In practice, family carers can often fear what the future holds for the person with dementia but also their own future health. In a recent poll, those over the age of 55 feared dementia (58%) more than any other condition, including cancer (47%) (8) often keenly felt by families of a person with dementia.

However, biomedical ethics does not specifically address the subject of personhood or nonpersonhood in dementia but appears to prefer to use terms such as competency and non competency (36). Adopting a solely **person**-centred approach to ACP in dementia care may cause

**Table 17.1** Milestones which can act as triggers to engage in ACP

| Transition points | Healthcare events |
|---|---|
| ◆ Making a will or dealing with the death of spouse / family member | ◆ Time of diagnosis of dementia |
| ◆ When undertaking a Lasting Power of Attorney for finance (consider LPA personal welfare) | ◆ Person presenting with complex symptoms and social care needs |
| ◆ Care plan/package review for community home care because changing need | ◆ Deterioration or decline in the persons condition from organ-specific or general frailty issues |
| ◆ Changes of care setting; transfer to acute care or residential care setting, etc. | ◆ Medical decisions related to or reflecting the consequence of dementia such as assisted nutrition / hydration, attempting cardio-pulmonary resuscitation |
| ◆ Changes in family/ carer situation to preventing meeting the needs of the person (practical issues, illness, stress, death, etc.) | ◆ Non-dementia related treatment or care issues |
| | ◆ Safeguarding concerns / DOLS orders |

Source: data from The Irish Hospice Foundation, 'Advance care planning and advance healthcare directives with a person with dementia, Guidance Document 2', 2016

conflict with the wishes, preferences, and perspectives of a family carer and vice versa. Therefore perhaps a focus should be more appropriately on **relationship**-centred care, including the whole family, where the interests of each are explored.

Autonomy is an important concept in decision making and is demonstrated by one who is able to decide on a course of action and is the central premise of the concept of informed consent (37). Locke (38) states that autonomy depends upon consciousness: that is to say, we are conscious of our past and *future* thoughts and actions in the same way as we are conscious of our present thoughts and actions. Dementia perhaps confounds this because, as dementia progresses, the ability to consider future thoughts and actions becomes compromised affecting decision-making abilities (7). It is important never to assume that if a person with dementia is unable to communicate in a conventional way, that they no longer have the capacity to understand and make decisions (as the first case study demonstrates).

## Case study (39)

The author of *Inside Alzheimer's*, Nancy Pearce, tells us the case of 'Robert', a very proud and independent man in the late stage of Alzheimer's disease who was living in a residential care setting. He was not taking enough nutrition to sustain himself. Most of the food offered was pocketed in his cheeks, or dribbled down his chin. A family meeting was called and even though Robert appeared unable to communicate or comprehend his situation, his daughter knowing his history of always wanting to be in charge suggested he be present for the discussions to include him and also in case there was any way he could signal his understanding.

The doctor explained Robert's clinical situation, but Robert seemed to stare blankly, without showing any sign of comprehension, His daughter asked him some questions directly, such as whether he would want to use intravenous antibiotics in case of infection, but he continued to show no response.

The doctor then went on to tell Robert's daughter about the option of gastric tube through which to feed him directly into his stomach and described the surgical procedure. 'Suddenly Robert began back and forth in his chair, his brow furrowed, his eyes wide open and his breathing twice the rate of what it had been. We had to ask ourselves, why now?' (p. 241)

The connection seemed to be related to the discussion of the feeding tube, so as the family meeting progressed they checked and rechecked Robert's response to the tube feeding issue as well as other discussing other treatments in his presence. 'The only times Robert consistently showed agitated reactions were those when we mentioned placement of a G-tube. By the day's end, we were convinced that he was quite clearly making his wishes known' (pp. 241–2). All those attending the family meeting could scarcely believe it possible, that given Robert's stage of dementia and seemingly inability to understand and communicate, that this was possible. Robert's daughter told him that they would not continue to talk about this and that they would not insert a feeding tube, he became more relaxed, his breathing slowing to his normal rate and gave a comforted sigh. The outcome of the family meeting and decisions reached was that they felt that Robert had made his wishes known, despite his impaired communication due to his dementia.

# Communication, dementia and advance care planning

Good communication is essential in ACP and this is especially important for people with cognitive, perceptual, and broader dementia problems. Guidance is given in this chapter to support communication. Sometimes subtle changes in the progressive disease and resultant behaviours can cause significant communication difficulties or misunderstandings. Good communication is essential not only in the process of decision making and potential testing of the mental capacity of the patient but in broader terms facilitating equally difficult discussions about their past and present wishes or preferences with the person and or their family. If a person lacks capacity and there is no Lasting Power of Attorney, the people closest to the patient have to be identified and must be consulted. Their views can only be disregarded for a very good reason, such as if they do not seem to be in the patient's best interest or are impossible. There are several 'best practice' points to consider when attempting ACP discussions with a person who has a diagnosis of dementia, (see Box 17.3).

AFIRM (see case study for definition) is an acronym which provides professional carers with a framework to guide informal conversations and use these as opportunities to pick up on any underlying apprehensions or queries the person with dementia (and/or their family member) may have.

## Case study

### Using the AFIRM framework (40)

Janet has just received a diagnosis of dementia and is concerned about what her future holds as she has no family experience of dementia. She is concerned that she will lose all control over her life. You might use the AFIRM framework to guide your conversation:

**A** Acknowledge Janet's distress:
 In acknowledging Janet's distress you might say: "The diagnosis of dementia has clearly distressed you."
**F** Find out what Janet knows:
 "What do you understand about the diagnosis?"
 "What is your biggest worry for the future?"
**I** Immediate concern addressed.
"That I will lose control of what happens to me as the disease progresses."
**R** Respond to further questions.
"So, let us explain what dementia is and what changes might you experience as your illness  progresses."
"We can help you to plan ahead to try and ensure that your wishes and preferences in certain possible
 circumstances are well recorded to ensure future care is commensurate with these."
**M** Meeting suggested.
"This is a good time to start to identify what is important to you and plan a meeting with the people who
 are important to you; family, GP, etc."
"Would you like me to arrange a meeting?"

> ## Box 17.3  Guidance on communication with people with dementia
>
> 1. It may take a person with dementia longer to process what you are saying to them and to think of their response—give the person sufficient time to respond
>
> 2. To ensure a person-centred approach try and find out their values and preferences as an opening to ACP development; what is important to them; their history, likes, strengths, beliefs, etc.
>
> 3. Face the person directly and make good eye contact; ensure you give them every opportunity to understand you are focused on them
>
> 4. They may, or may not wish their family carer/member to be present; ensure you ask
>
> 5. Use short, clear sentences that are free of clinical jargon; a useful resource to guide into what to ask and how can be found in *Difficult Conversations for Dementia* (see resource section)
>
> 6. Use language and words that are familiar to them
>
> 7. Ensure the space chosen to have the conversation(s) is quiet and calm. A person's own, familiar surroundings is best
>
> 8. Be aware and maximise upon your non-verbal communication: tone of voice, facial expressions, hand gestures, etc.
>
> 9. Use active listening and be fully attentive to what the person is saying and what their body language and expressions are telling you.
>
> 10. Use other ways to communicate if helpful; written word, pictures (e.g. www.talkingmats. com/), etc.
>
> 11. Focus on one question at a time. Mirror what they say (repeat back to them) for affirmation. For example; '. . . so you say having your family around you at the end of your life is the most important thing to you . . .?'
>
> 12. Use the AFIRM approach (41) to guide your conversations

## Families and decision making

Making decisions about end of life care and treatment on behalf of a family member with dementia is not straightforward and can at times be extremely difficult. It will often involve complex issues around whether to treat or whether to withhold treatment. There may be several treatment options to choose from, and the context of the decision will also be important (e.g. in a crisis as compared to states of chronic ill health). Overlaid on this are the perspectives, preferences, and wishes for the future care of the person for whom decisions are to be made. For clinicians it will often be difficult to know whether family decision making and treatment choices are consistent with the wishes of the family member with dementia, if at all ever expressed. However, professionals often assume family carers already know what any such decisions would have been had the person with dementia had not lost capacity. Thus, carers find themselves increasingly in a position whereby they are called upon to inform, or directly make decisions on behalf of the person with dementia. Successful decision making for a family affected by dementia involves:

◆ Information and support to understand of the prognosis of dementia

◆ Anticipating health and care issues as the disease progresses

◆ Knowledge of options available and support to access services

◆ How to care for themselves and their own needs

## Balancing the wishes and preferences of the person with dementia and those of the carer

ACP that promotes primarily the wishes and preferences of the person with dementia may, at times challenge the views and or needs of the carer. Delivering good dementia care and maintaining a positive relationship with the family or carers reduces (but does not remove) the chance of conflict of interest and helps prepare for bereavement at an early stage. Admiral Nurses, specialist dementia nurses are skilled at care management for families affected by dementia and support a balancing of needs (41).

Family carers often experience increasing demands in making decisions as the dementia progresses. Not surprisingly, carers often find decision making difficult and studies have reported on certain emotional and practical issues, including:

◆ Difficulties in deciding what to do about day to day care (42)
◆ Distress in making health related decisions
◆ Having insufficient information about any possible alternatives and their effects (43)
◆ Negative emotional effects, such as stress, guilt, self doubt (44)

But do carers 'get it right"'? Dening et al. (45) undertook a cross-sectional study to examine the accuracy of family carers to predict the wishes and preferences for end of life care and treatments of the person with dementia for whom they care. They found that a carer's ability to accurately predict the person with dementia's treatment preferences (in the absence of an ACP) was no better than chance (lower that 35% accuracy). Thus, questioning the professional reliance on family members in decision making. Livingston et al. (46) conclude that the most difficult decisions families have to make are those for end of life care made more difficult in the presence of family disharmony. In the absence of family cohesion the role of the surrogate decision maker becomes isolated and even more difficult.

## Summary

There will be large numbers of people with dementia as the population continues to age. Dementia is a progressive, irreversible, neurodegenerative condition that greatly reduces life with one in three of the population expected to die with or from dementia. People with dementia (and their families) are much in need of palliative care services, especially through ACP and support with decision making in preparation for end of life.

The process of ACP in dementia is far from straightforward; as dementia progresses, the ability to consider future thoughts and actions becomes compromised, thus affecting decision making abilities.

Family carers find themselves increasingly in a position whereby they are called on to inform, or directly make, decisions on behalf of the person with dementia. It is often assumed they know what the person with dementia's decisions might have been when capacity is lost even though wishes and preferences have not been articulated. We need to have greater confidence to initiate ACP conversations to directly involve the person with dementia themselves if we are to ensure their wishes and preferences are realised at a time where they have lost capacity to make these themselves in real time. Of equal importance is for professionals to support family carers to make decisions on behalf the person with dementia to enable them to effectively navigate the various transition points along the trajectory of dementia, such as seeking a diagnosis, access to support services, admission to a care home, end of life care options.

## References

1. **Berrio M** and **Levesque M**, (1996). 'Advance directives: Most patients don't have one, do yours?' *American Journal of Nursing* **8**: 25–8.
2. **World Health Organisation** (2012). *World Health Statistics 2012 Indicator compendium.* Available from: http://www.who.int/gho/publications/world_health_statistics/WHS2012_IndicatorCompendium.pdf. (Accessed 23 Dec 2016.)
3. **ONS (2016).** UK Perspectives 2016: *The changing UK population.* Available from: http://www.visual.ons.gov.uk/uk-perspectives-2016-the-changing-uk-population. (Accessed 23 Dec 2016.)
4. **ONS** (2013). *Population Estimates for UK, England and Wales, Scotland and Northern Ireland.* Available from: http://www.ons.gov.uk/ons/rel/pop-estimate/population-estimates-for-uk--england-and-wales--scotland-and-northern-ireland/2009/index.html. (Accessed 23 Dec 2016.)
5. **Stephan B** and **Brayne C**, (2008). 'Prevalence and projections of dementia'. In: Downs M, and Bowers S, (eds) *Excellence in Dementia Care: Research into practice.* Maidenhead: McGraw-Hill.
6. **Wilcock G, Bucks R'** and **Rockwood K**, (1999). *Diagnosis and Management of Dementia: A Manual for Memory Disorders Teams.* Oxford: Oxford University Press.
7. **Fratiglioni L** and **Qiu C**, (2013). 'Epidemiology of dementia'. In: Dening, T. and Thomas, A. (eds) 2nd edition, *Oxford Textbook of Old Age Psychiatry*, Oxford: Oxford University Press.
8. **NUFFIELD COUNCIL ON BIOETHICS** (2009). *Dementia: ethical issues*, London: Nuffield Council on Bioethics.
9. **Luengo-Fernandez R, Leal J,** and **Gray A** (2010). *Dementia 2010*, London: Alzheimer's Research Trust.
10. **Matthews FE, Arthur A, Barnes LE, Bond J, Jagger C, Robinson L,** and **Brayne C** (2013). 'A two-decade comparison of prevalence of dementia in individuals aged 65 years and older from three geographical areas of England: results of the Cognitive Function and Ageing Study I and II'. *Lancet* **382**(9902): 1405–12.
11. **Froggatt K, Mccormack B.** and **Reed J.** (2006). 'End-of-life issues in long-term care—implications for practice'. *International Journal of Older Peoples Nursing* **1**(1): 44. doi: 10.1111/j.1748-3743.2006.00011.x.
12. **Kulmala J, Nykanen I, Manty M,** and **Hartikainen S** (2014). 'Association between frailty and dementia: a population-based study'. *Gerontology* **60**(1): 16–21.
13. **Sampson EL,** and **Harrison Dening K** (2013). 'Palliative care and end of life care'. In: *Oxford Textbook of Old Age psychiatry*, 2nd edition, Dening T, and Thomas A (eds). Oxford: Oxford University Press.
14. **Mitchell SL, Kiely DK,** and **Hamel MB** (2004). 'Dying with advanced dementia in the nursing home'. *Archives of Internal Medicine* **164**(3): 321–6.
15. **Mitchell SL,** et al. (2009). 'The clinical course of dementia'. *New England Journal of Medicine* **361**(16): 1529–38.
16. **Morrison RS** and **Siu AL** (2000). 'Survival in end stage dementia following acute illness'. *Journal of the American Medical Association* **284**(1): 47–52.
17. **Sampson EL,** et al. (2009). 'Dementia in the acute hospital: prospective cohort study of prevalence and mortality'. *British Journal of Psychiatry* **195**(1): 61–6. doi: 10.1192/bjp.bp.108.055335.
18. **Xie J, Brayne C,** and **Matthews FE** (2008). 'Survival times in people with dementia: analysis from population based cohort study with 14 year follow-up'. *BMJ* **336**(7638): 258–62.
19. **Wilcock J, Froggatt K** and **Goodman C** (2008). 'End of life care'. In: DOWNS M and BOWERS, S (eds) *Excellence in Dementia Care: Research into Practice*, Maidenhead: Open University Press, pp. 359–78.
20. **Foley KM** and **Carver AC** (2001). 'Palliative care in neurology'. *Neurologic Clinics.* **19**(4): 789–99.
21. **Martyn CN** and **Pippard EC** (1998). 'Usefulness of mortality data in determining the geography and time trends of dementia'. *Journal of Epidemiology and Community Health* **42**: 134–7.
22. **Boyd CM** and **Fortin M** (2010). 'Future of Multimorbidity Research: How Should Understanding of Multimorbidity Inform Health System Design?' *Public Health Reviews* **32**: 451–74.
23. **Cigolle CT,** et al. (2007). 'Geriatric conditions and disability: the Health and Retirement Study'. *Annals of Internal Medicine* **147**(3): 156–64.

24. **Sampson EL, Gould V, Lee D**, and **Blanchard M** (2006). 'Differences in care received by patients with and without dementia who died during acute hospital admission: a retrospective case note study'. *Age and Ageing* **35**(2): 187–9.

25. **Addington-Hall JM** and **Mccarthy M** (1995). 'Regional study of the care for the dying: methods and sample characteristics'. *Palliative Medicine* **9**: 27–35.

26. **Addington-Hall JM** and **Mccarthy M** (1995). 'Dying from cancer: results of a national population-based investigation'. *Palliative Medicine.* **9**: 295–305.

27. **Cleary JF** and **Carbonne PP** (1997). 'Palliative medicine in the elderly'. *Cancer* **80**(7): 1335–47.

28. **National Collaborating Centre For Mental Health (NCCMH)** (2006). *The NICE/SCIE Guideline on Supporting People with Dementia and their Carers in Health and Social Care: National Clinical Practice Guideline Number 42*. London: The British Psychological Society, The Royal College of Psychiatrists and Gaskell.

29. **DH** (2008). *End-of-Life Care Strategy,* London: Department of Health.

30. **DH** (2009). *Living Well with Dementia: A National Dementia Strategy*, London: Department of Health.

31. **Harrison Dening K, Jones L**, and **Sampson EL** (2011). 'Advance care planning for people with dementia: a review'. *International Psychogeriatrics* **23**(10): 1535–51.

32. **Harrison Dening K, Jones L**, and **Sampson EL** (2012). 'Preferences for end-of-life care: A nominal group study of people with dementia and their family carers'. *Palliative Medicine* **27**(5): 409–17.

33. **The Irish Hospice Foundation** (2016). *Dementia Guidance Document 2: Advance care planning and advance healthcare directives with a person with dementia*. The Irish Hospice Foundation: Ireland.

34. **Van Der Steen JT**, et al. (2013). 'White paper defining optimal palliative care in older people with dementia: A Delphi study and recommendations from the European Association for Palliative Care'. *Palliative Medicine* **28**(3): 197–209.

35. **Kitwood T** (1997). *Dementia Reconsidered: The person comes first*. Buckingham: Open University Press.

36. **Nolan MR, Ryan T, Enderby P**, and **Reid D** (2002). 'Towards a more inclusive vision of dementia care practice'. *The International Journal of Social Research and Practice* **1**: 193–211.

37. **Beauchamp TL** and **Childress JF** (2013). *Principle of Medical Ethics*. Oxford: Oxford University Press.

38. **Post S** (2006). 'Respectare: Moral Respect for the Lives of the Deeply Forgetful'. In Hughes J, Louw S, and Sabat, SR, (eds) *Dementia: Mind, Meaning and the Person*. Oxford: Oxford University Press.

39. **Jolley N**, (1999). *Locke: His philosophical thought*. Oxford: Oxford University Press.

40. HSE. The National Dementia Training Programme. Available from: https://www.hse.ie/eng/about/Who/ONMSD/eductraining/dementiaeducation. (Accessed 23 Dec 2016.)

41. **Webb R** and **Harrison Dening K** (2016). 'In whose best interests? A case study of a family affected by dementia'. *British Journal of Community Nursing* **21**(6): 300–4.

42. **Vig EK**, et al. (2007). 'Surviving surrogate decision-making: what helps and hampers the experience of making medical decisions for others'. *Journal of General Internal Medicine* **22**(9): 1274–9.

43. **Hirschman KB, Kapo JM**, and **Karlawish JHT** (2006). 'Why doesn't a family member of a person with advanced dementia use a substituted judgment when making a decision for that person'. *American Journal of Geriatric Psychiatry* **14**(8): 659–67.

44. **Wendler D** and **Rid R** (2011). 'Systematic review: the effect on surrogates of making treatment decisions for others'. *Annals of Internal Medicine* **154**(5): 336–46.

45. **Harrison Dening K, King M, Jones L**, and **Sampson E** (2016). 'Advance Care Planning in Dementia: Can family carers predict the preferences of people with dementia?' *Plos One* **11**(8): e0161142. doi: 10.1371/journal.pone.0159056

46. **Livingston G**, et al. (2010). 'Making decisions for people with dementia who lack capacity: qualitative study of family carers in UK'. *BMJ* **341**: c4184. doi: 10.1136/bmj.c4184.

Section 3

# Experience of advance care planning internationally

Chapter 18

# Advance care planning in Australia

Karen Detering and Josephine Clayton

'I think people are more and more educated these days. Unlike in the olden days where people would make a huge deal about such things, people these days are more accepting of issues related to life and death.'
*Research participant*

---

**This chapter includes**

◆ An overview of the development and implementation of advance care planning (ACP) in Australia

◆ Discussion of the legislation, policy, funding, and implementation contexts

◆ Information on Advance Care Planning Australia (ACPA), Decision Assist and the Advance programmes

---

**Key Points**

◆ The Respecting Patient Choices programme (now known as ACPA) has played a key role in the development of ACP provision and evaluation in Australia

◆ ACP implementation has occurred in a range of settings including acute health services, aged care facilities, and community care, including general practice

◆ The Australian federal and state/territory governments recognise the importance of ACP, and have developed strategy, legislation and a range of resources and programmes to promote ACP, and to facilitate access and uptake

◆ This has included resources and education programmes for health professionals, community, and aged care workers, and consumers

---

**Key Message**

There remain significant challenges to the access and uptake of ACP in Australia, requiring new, cost effective, and sustainable models of implementation to be trialled and evaluated.

## The Australian population and health system

Australia, with a population of 24.5 million people, is an ethnically diverse society; 26% of the population having been born overseas and 60% of these originate from non-English speaking countries. Three per cent of the Australian population are Aboriginal and Torres Strait Islander people. Most of the population (85%) are urban dwelling; three per cent of the population live in remote or very remote areas of Australia. Like other developed countries, the Australian population is aging, with increased numbers of people reaching advanced age, and developing multi-morbidity conditions, frailty, and dementia (1).

All Australians have access to publically funded healthcare services, and almost half of the Australian population also has private health insurance, facilitating access to private hospitals and private ancillary services. Australia is a federation of six states and two territories (jurisdictions), which have their own constitutions, parliaments, governments, and laws. Under this federal system, responsibility for public funding and regulation of health is shared between governments. The federal government is responsible for national coordination, leadership, policy, and financing in health matters and focuses on the areas of public health, research, and national information management. The jurisdictions are largely responsible for the delivery of public sector hospital, palliative care, and emergency services. Aged care is financed and regulated by the federal Government and largely provided by the non-government sector (religious, charitable, and for-profit providers). The federal government mostly funds primary care (2).

## Advance care planning in Australia

### Legislation

In the 1980s, South Australia and the Northern Territory enacted Natural Death Acts, which allowed end of life medical preferences to be documented. In Victoria, the importance of respecting patient autonomy in the setting of end of life care was recognised in 1987 by the Victorian Parliament Dying with Dignity Inquiry, and resulted in legislation, the Medical Treatment Act. This enabled people to appoint a medical substitute decision maker and to refuse unwanted medical treatment. Since this time, similar legislation relating to legally appointed medical substitute decision makers and advance care directives (ACDs), have been developed in other jurisdictions.

Although the specifics of legislation vary between jurisdictions, all permit the formal appointment of a substitute decision maker(s), and most have legislation related to ACDs (3). See also: www.advancecareplanning.org.au.

Implementation of advance care planning (ACP) in Australia has also relied on the common-law respect for autonomy, ACDs, and substitute decision making. However, the legal standing of common-law directives has only been tested in New South Wales. In 2009, the New South Wales Supreme Court ruled that common-law directives are valid ways for people to indicate their objection to particular treatment(s) (3).

### A national framework for advance care directives

National, state, and territory health ministers recognised the need for a standardised national approach and format for ACDs. Subsequently, a working group of the Clinical, Technical and Ethical Principles Committee of Australian Health Ministers Advisory Council developed a national framework. The working group membership included people with backgrounds in health law, health ethics, health and aged care policy development, and clinical care.

The framework, published in 2011 (4) was intended to be aspirational, and as such describes the goals for which policy and practice should aim rather than just incorporating the current situation. Key components of the framework are summarised in Box 18.1. Whilst the framework has helped to facilitate change and assist with ACP implementation nationally, ongoing issues with harmonisation and best-practice ACDs exist.

---

## Box 18.1 A national framework for advance care directives: key elements

**Nationally** consistent terminology (inclusive of definitions for the following)

- Advance care planning
- Advance care plan
- Advance care directive
- Substitute decision maker
- Clinical care plans

### Code of ethical practice for advance care directives

- Set of 15 principles to guide practice

### Best practice standards for Advance Care Directives

Describe best practice for the development and use of ACDs regarding:

- Law and policy
- Forms
- Guidelines for the community
- Information for health and aged care sectors
- Decision-making guidance for SDM, health and aged care professionals
- ACP programmes using ACDs

### The framework also places ACDs within a broad context

- ACDs may be prescribed by legislation or operate under common law
- ACDs may record a range of preferences including values, life goals, specific treatments appoint a decision maker or a combination of these
- ACDs are relevant to adults at all stages of life, and may be activated at any time of future incapacity, not just at end of life

Source: data from 'A national framework for advance care directives', The Clinical, Technical and Ethical Principal Committee of the Australian Health Ministers' Advisory Council, Copyright © 2011 Australian Health Ministers' Advisory Council, (4) http://www.health.wa.gov.au

Although ACDs are widely available in Australia

◆ Uptake remains low (5)

◆ Jurisdictional variability makes it difficult to legally recognise ACDs from other jurisdictions

◆ Lack of harmonisation and national legislation poses challenges for delivering national ACP initiatives including education, tools for consumers, health, aged, and community workers, and incorporation of ACDs into 'My Health Record' the national patient controlled electronic health record

◆ There is lack of case law in Australia to provide direction on the legality of non-statutory ACDs

## Early coordinated advance care planning—the Australian Respecting Patient Choices programme

Towards the end of the last century, there were pockets of expertise and ACP-related work occurring in Australia. In 2001 following a review of national and international approaches to ACP, the successful US-based Respecting Choices programme was identified as being suitable for adoption in Australia. This programme reported increased rates of ACD documentation, and compliance with patients' wishes at the end of life (6).

In 2002 the Austin Hospital in Melbourne, Australia successfully trialled the Respecting Choices programme utilising a National Institute of Clinical Studies grant. The Australian Federal and Victorian State Governments subsequently funded the expansion of this programme, named the Respecting Patient Choices (RPC) programme, to other health services within Victoria, and in other Australian jurisdictions. The programme was also implemented into some aged care facilities, and more recently into primary care, and community care. See Box 18.2 for details of the RPC model.

---

### Box 18.2 Respecting patient choices model of advance care planning

**The ACP conversation includes the following elements:**

◆ Clarifying the person's understanding of their illness and treatment options

◆ Identifying (and appointing) their preferred substitute decision-maker

◆ Discussing their goals and values, in relation to their illness and preferences for future care

◆ Identifying their views regarding an acceptable outcome from treatment

◆ Considering particular treatments (if any) that they would *not* want

**Key elements of the RPC model:**

◆ Utilising trained non-medical staff to facilitate conversations, working in conjunction with treating doctors

◆ The person's family/decision makers are encouraged to be involved in the conversations

◆ Organisational systems are present, for storage and retrieval of documents

◆ Implementing systematic education of staff regarding ACP and their respective roles

One important aspect of the RPC programme, believed to be associated with its' success, was the extensive modification of the Respecting Choices programme to Australian conditions, taking into account the difference between the health systems in the US and Australia. A second key aspect of the RPC programme evolution has been the importance placed upon evaluation and research in order to improve the model and likely outcomes of the programme.

## Advance care planning implementation in hospitals

In 2010 a randomised controlled trial assessing the impact of coordinated ACP, on end of life care in elderly patients was published (7). In this study of 309 legally competent medical inpatients aged under 80 years, patients were randomly allocated to receive either coordinated ACP using the RPC model or usual care (control group). One hundred and fifty-four patients were randomly allocated to the intervention group; of which 125 patients (81%) participated in ACP conversation(s) lasting a median of 60 minutes, over one to three meetings. One hundred and eight patients (84%) taking part in ACP expressed preferences for end of life care, appointed a surrogate, or both.

The key findings of the study were:

◆ Of the 56 patients who died within six months, end of life preferences were more likely to be known and followed in the ACP intervention group (25/29, 86%) compared with controls (8/27, 30%, P<0.001)

◆ In the ACP group, family members of patients who died had significantly less stress (P<0.001), anxiety (P=0.02), and depression (P=0.002) than control patients

Since this study was conducted, the predominant provision of ACP at the Austin hospital has been by non-medical facilitators utilising the RPC model. These facilitators have accumulated experience supporting more than 1,000 patients per year to participate in ACP. Although elderly patients and those with poor prognoses are targeted (cancer, frailty, and chronic illness), the service is available to all patients. Similar to the 2010 study, one-third to one-half of patients complete ACDs, nominated substitute decision makers or both. Most conversations take less than 90 minutes over one or more meetings. The ACP facilitators also provide education and support to other staff thereby assisting them to undertake ACP, and consequently improving access for patients. Despite this approach, many Austin patients are unable to access ACP due to limited resources.

In the original study, only English-speaking competent patients were included. Subsequently, work has shown that ACP can be successfully delivered to inpatients from non-English speaking backgrounds (8), and non-competent hospital patients (9). In these circumstances, the person's family/substitute decision makers often have crucial roles in ACP discussions.

Some other Australian hospitals have adopted a similar approach to that of the Austin, and now employ dedicated ACP facilitators, whilst others incorporate ACP into current staff roles. As yet, limited data are available to assess outcomes from these differing models of ACP provision. Irrespective of the approaches taken however, there remain significant challenges to adequate provision of ACP in hospitals. These include the increasing age, complexity and illness severity of inpatients, reducing lengths of stay in acute care, and perceived and real lack of time and staff skills to undertake ACP.

## Implementation of advance care planning in aged care facilities

In 2004–2005 the RPC programme was piloted in 17 aged care facilities (approximately 1000 residents) in Melbourne. Important elements of this implementation comprised focus on engagement with senior management and on system changes, including development of ACP policies/procedures, ACP training for senior management, as well as other staff and involvement of general practitioners.

During this pilot, 51% of residents were offered ACP, 52% of these completed advance care plans; with most completed by families of residents lacking decision-making capacity. The most common preferences were for no life-sustaining measures, and good symptom management. Only 20% requested hospital transfer. During the six-month follow-up, 161 residents died; 58% had an advance care plan, and all had care consistent with their preferences. Of those who completed ACP, only 14% died in hospital compared to 46% of those who did not undertake ACP.

A further structured aged care ACP implementation occurred in 2010–11 involving 19 facilities (10). In additional to the elements outlined already, this project also included:

◆ Development of an aged care-specific ACD [11]

◆ Incorporation of education on palliative care

◆ Three one-day workshops separated in time giving participants time to practice skills and share experiences

◆ Task completion: including formulation of policies, engagement with general practitioners, and meetings with other participants to encourage peer support and networking

The aged care-specific ACD was adopted by 18 facilities and the quality of the documentation improved (11). Further assessment of this implementation occurred in 2012, and showed sustainability remains an issue. In particular, whilst many systematic changes continued, staff turnover, and need for subsequent education, was suboptimal, and staff identified lack of time and skills required for ACP.

## Implementation of advance care planning in the community

Despite the benefits of ACP, the availability and uptake within the Australian community healthcare is low (5). In Australia many elderly people living at home receive services through homecare package programmes. A national study exploring the attitudes, knowledge, and practice of ACP among home-care package services and managers found that whilst staff view ACP as valuable, worthwhile, and part of their role, there are fragmented organisational systems; low levels of support for case managers, and a lack of a normative approach to ACP (12). Subsequently an implementation study investigating two models of ACP occurred and showed that both facilitator (case managers facilitate ACP) and referral (client referred to a specialist ACP service) models of ACP achieved similar outcomes. Sixty-five per cent of 784 clients had ACP initiated, although only a small number completed ACDs (13).

Other community initiatives have recognised the important and central role of GPs in ACP. In collaboration with the Royal Australian College of General Practitioners, ACP resources specifically aimed at making ACP part of routine general practice care were developed, see: www.racgp.org.au. An education programme, called 'next steps', demonstrated success in supporting GPs to undertake ACP. This interactive multi-modality-training programme was specifically designed for junior doctors and GPs to build their confidence and ability to conduct ACP discussions with their patients (14). The training comprises pre-reading, a DVD (containing scenarios showing GPs discussing ACP with actor patients), an interactive e-simulation and a two-hour experiential workshop. The education follows a structured stepwise approach to ACP. More recently DVD scenarios have been incorporated into other training, such as decision assist training.

## Australian National Clinical Practice Guidelines: communicating prognosis and end of life issues

In 2007, Australian National Guidelines (15) were published regarding communication of end of life issues, including ACP with adults and their caregivers. These guidelines were funded by the Australian National Health and Medical Research Council in a Strategic Palliative Care Research Grant, informed by an extensive systematic review and input from an expert advisory group. The final recommendations were endorsed by multiple national professional and consumer organisations and widely disseminated by these organisations. The recommendations have been translated into various communication skills training resources for health professionals both in Australia and abroad, such as the National Palliative Care Curriculum for Undergraduates (PCC4U) funded by the Australian government and the UK Gold Standards Framework (www.goldstandardsframework.org.uk). There are general recommendations (PREPARED framework) applicable to all end of life discussions (Table 18.1), as well as specific recommendations for use during ACP discussions (Table 18.2).

## Contemporary advance care planning in Australia

Whilst the RPC model and other early initiatives have demonstrated success, key informant interviews across Australia in 2012 (5) showed low uptake and poor implementation of ACP. Suggestions for improvement included: increasing community awareness, encouraging health professional involvement, and system-wide implementation of a multifaceted approach to ACP with a focus on person-centred care. For some populations and settings, alternate approaches (e.g. utilising staff in usual care) to the RPC model may be more relevant, and achievable.

Over recent years the Australian Commonwealth Government has funded or led various initiatives to support ACP.

**Table 18.1** The PREPARED framework

| | |
|---|---|
| P | **Prepare for the discussion** |
| R | **Relate to the person** |
| E | **Elicit patient and caregiver preferences** |
| P | **Provide information** tailored to individual needs |
| A | **Acknowledge emotions & concerns** |
| R | (foster) **Realistic hope** |
| E | **Encourage question**s and further discussions |
| D | **Document** |

Source: data from Clayton J M, Hancock K M, Butow P N, et al. (2007) 'Clinical practice guidelines for communicating prognosis and end-of-life issues with adults in the advanced stages of a life-limiting illness, and their caregivers'. *The Medical Journal of Australia*, Volume 186, Supplement 12, p. 77

**Table 18.2** Strategies and example phrases for advance care planning discussions (15)

| Strategy | Example phrase or question |
|---|---|
| ◆ Describe ACP. Give a rationale for why these conversations can be helpful. | 'Have you thought about the type of medical care you would like to have if you ever become too sick to speak for yourself? This is the purpose of ACP to ensure that you are cared for the way you would want to be, even when communication may be impossible.' |
| | 'Have you ever talked about your wishes, values and beliefs about medical treatment and care in case you were ever injured or became too ill to speak for yourself?' |
| | 'It's often easier talk through tough decisions when there isn't a crisis.' |
| | 'Is this something that you would like to discuss further?' |
| ◆ Involve proxy decision-maker(s) in the discussions so they understand the patient's wishes. | 'Sometimes people with your type of illness lose the ability to make decisions or communicate their wishes as the illness progresses. Who would you like to make decisions for you if you were unable to do this yourself? *If the person can identify a substitute:* |
| | 'Have you spoken to this person about what would be important to you about your care if you were very ill?' |
| | 'Would you like to talk this through with them?' |
| | 'Would you like me to assist you with this?' |
| ◆ Use open ended questions to develop an understanding of the patient's values and to help them work out their goals and priorities. | 'What is most important to you now (or regarding your care in the future)?' 'What aspects of your life do you most value and enjoy?' |
| | 'When you look at the future:<br>◆ what do you hope for?<br>◆ What concerns you?' |
| | 'Do you have any thoughts about how you would like to be cared for in the future if you became more unwell?<br>◆ How would you want decisions regarding your care to be made?<br>◆ Is there a specific person that you would like us to speak to?' |
| | Is there anything you worry about happening?'<br>◆ What would you not want to happen to you in terms of your care? - Are there any situations where you would regard life-prolonging treatments to be overly burdensome?' |
| | 'Is there anything else you would like me to know about your values and priorities for care if you were very unwell?' |
| ◆ Consider using clinical scenarios to structure the discussion, particularly at early stage illness. | |
| ◆ Emphasise that ACP is an ongoing process, needing review periodically. | 'These are discussions we may need to revisit if there are changes in the course of the illness.' |
| ◆ Ensure that other health professionals involved with the patient's care are aware of the patient's wishes. | |

Source: data from Clayton J M, Hancock K M, Butow P N, et al. (2007) 'Clinical practice guidelines for communicating prognosis and end-of-life issues with adults in the advanced stages of a life-limiting illness, and their caregivers'. *The Medical Journal of Australia*, Volume 186, Supplement 12, p. 77

# Australian Federal Government funded or led advance care planning initiatives

- Development of the National Framework for Advance Care Directives
- Decision Assist Programme
- National palliative care programme projects
  - Advance Care Planning Australia (ACPA)
  - Advance project
  - ACP talk: religious and culturally sensitive ACP (www.acptalk.com.au)
  - 'Dying to Talk' discussion starter (www.dyingtotalk.org.au)
  - Other predominantly palliative care focus projects also include ACP
- ACP inclusion into accreditation for acute care, and aged care, via national agencies
- Incorporation of ACDs into the national electronic patient record, known as 'My Health' record. The Australian Digital Health Authority has responsibility for this

## Advance care planning Australia

In 2013, the RPC programme (see previous section) was renamed to ACPA. This decision followed confusion surrounding the nature of the programme, the emerging new models of ACP and the need to support health professionals, aged and community workers, lawyers, and consumers to access information, relevant to their specific needs and location within Australia. ACPA has a website, (www.advancecareplanning.org.au) and provides a national 'hub' facilitating access to resources, advisory services, and organises the national ACP conference. ACPA hosts e-learning modules, underpinned by key messages developed by ACPA. (Box 18.3) ACPA is also involved in curriculum development. All resources, including e-learning, are freely available.

ACPA supports engagement and collaboration amongst the variety of government and non-government stakeholders from a range of backgrounds. Other current ACPA projects include the

---

### Box 18.3 Key messages: Advance Care Planning Australia

#### Advance care planning:

- Is essential to person-centred care
- Promotes care that is consistent with a person's goals, values, beliefs, and preferences
- Prepares people and their substitute decision makers for making healthcare decisions
- Improves outcomes for people, their family and carers, health, aged and community care workers, and the health system
- Is part of routine care, and the person's healthcare journey
- Is an ongoing process
- May be initiated or completed by the person himself or herself, or by health, aged and community care workers
- Is most effective when it has a system-based approach

development of ACP resources for people from non-English speaking backgrounds and the training care workers caring for people with dementia in how to have ACP conversations.

ACPA receives national palliative care project grant funding.

## Decision Assist Program

The Decision Assist Program (www.decisionassist.org.au) is funded by the Australian government, and was established to enhance national provision of palliative care and ACP services to recipients of aged care services. A consortium of national agencies and universities with extensive experience in palliative care, ACP and aged care administer this programme. The primary objectives of Decision Assist are to:

♦ Provide specialist palliative care and ACP advice (website and telephone) to aged care providers and GPs caring for recipients of aged care services

♦ Improve linkages between aged care services and palliative care services

♦ Improve palliative care skills and ACP expertise of aged care service staff and GPs caring for recipients of aged care services

♦ Improve the quality of care for aged care recipients, prevent unnecessary hospital admissions, and shorten hospital stays

In October 2016, the initial three-year evaluation was finalised, and showed that the programme had implemented a comprehensive range of national initiatives; and had demonstrated significant reach in the general practice and aged care sectors nationally. Health professionals or aged care staff participating in education and linkages projects demonstrated a knowledge increase, some change in clinical practice, and a high rate of satisfaction with initiatives. Decision Assist activities have been promoted to large numbers of stakeholders, professional organisations, and leading agencies. The website has resulted in a large number of visits. Although uptake of phone advisory services was low, most callers were from target audiences and calls addressed symptoms management/medication and ACP information queries. The programme provides resources on ACP and palliative care suitable for different spiritual and faith-based perspectives, people from diverse backgrounds, people who identify as LGBTI (lesbian/gay/bisexual/transgender/intersex), and people who are homeless or at risk of homelessness. Other key findings of this project included identified benefits in key stakeholders working together rather than the traditional silo approach, although role and responsibility definition at the outset is important for optimal functioning.

## The Advance Project: initiating palliative care and advance care planning training for general practice nurses

The Advance Project (www.caresearch.com.au/advance) involves training and resources to enable nurses to work with GPs to initiate palliative care and ACP with elderly (over 75 years) or chronically ill patients as part of routine health assessments. The programme includes a toolkit of six screening and assessment tools; including an ACP screening tool; and a guide indicating how to implement these in a systematic way. The toolkit was informed by a literature review, input from a national and international expert advisory group and feedback from stakeholders including general practice nurses, GPs and Carers Australia. The project receives national palliative care grant funding.

Online modules demonstrate how to use the tools in clinical practice; aiming to increase nurses' skills and confidence in initiating conversations with older and/or chronically ill patients about

ACP and palliative care. Workshops are being delivered nationally to complement online training. Programme evaluation informs ongoing implementation.

The structured ACP tool has spaces within it to record the patient's responses. The completed tool can be included in the patient's practice records. The tool initially developed for acute care (16), has been adapted for use in general practice (13) and found to be feasible and acceptable tool for ACP initiation. The aims of the ACP screening tool are to:

◆ Introduce the topic of ACP

◆ Determine a patient's preferred substitute decision maker

◆ Ensure the general practice is aware of any ACP already completed by the patient

◆ Assess a patient's readiness to further discuss ACP

Further follow up to discuss ACP can then be arranged with either the general practice nurse or the GP if the patient wishes to do so. The training offered by other national programmes such as ACPA and Decision Assist complements these advance tools and training resources.

## Jurisdictional-based initiatives

In addition to the Australia-wide initiatives, many Australian states and territories have also developed specific strategies and initiatives to improve the uptake of ACP. Some states/territories have specific ACP strategies (for example Victorian and NSW) whilst others include ACP under areas such as palliative care or end of life care (Queensland). Coordinated approaches have common features such as emphasis on 'normalising' ACP, establishing systems and resources to support the public, healthcare professionals, aged and community care workers, and lawyers. Resources for the individual jurisdictions are available via individual websites. The national Advance Care Panning Australia website has links for each jurisdiction and resources to enable relevant information and documents to be accessible.

A strategy for Victorian health services 2014–18, has information and resources aimed at facilitating healthcare services and staff to undertake ACP. The strategy includes four priority action areas with practical implementation guidance and support for the evaluation framework. These priority areas relate to robust systems, evidenced-based and quality approaches, workforce capacity, and enabling the the person to have the conversation (17).

Advance Planning for Quality Care at End of life—Action Plan 2013–18, aimed to implement ACP in the public health system over five years. It seeks to normalise ACP and improve end of life care by integrating patients' wishes into the management of chronic life-limiting illness. Resources are available to support professionals and consumers (18).

## Conclusion

In summary the RPC model, utilising ACP facilitators to conduct discussions has played an important role in the development of ACP implementation and evaluation within Australia. However, there remain significant challenges to adequate provision of and access to ACP within Australia and newer models, such as utilising existing staff to undertake ACP conversations, are being developed and evaluated. Currently there is limited data comparing these different approaches, and limited information as to how best to use these differing models. The Australian Federal Government and the jurisdictions recognise the importance of ACP; fund initiatives are actively working on ways to enhance ACP.

## References

1. **Australalin Bureau of Statistics**. Available from: http://www.abs.gov.au/population.

2. **Health in Australia: a quick guide**. Available from: http://www.aph.gov.au/About_Parliament/Parliamentary_Departments/Parliamentary_Library/pubs/rp/rp1314/QG/HealthAust

3. **Carter RZ, Detering KM, Silvester W**, et al. (Nov 2015). 'Advance care planning in Australia: what does the law say?' *Australian health review:* a publication of the Australian Hospital Association.

4. **The Clinical, Technical and Ethical Principal Committee of the Australian Health Ministers' Advisory Council**. *A national framework for advance care directives.* Available from: http://www.health.wa.gov.au/advancecareplanning/docs/AdvanceCareDirectives2011.pdf.

5. **Rhee JJ, Zwar NA**, and **Kemp LA** (Feb 2012). 'Uptake and implementation of Advance Care Planning in Australia: findings of key informant interviews'. *Australian Health Review* **36**(1): 98–104.

6. **Hammes BJ** and **Rooney BL** (Feb 1998). 'Death and end-of-life planning in one midwestern community'. *Archives of Internal Medicine* **158**(4): 383–90.

7. **Detering KM, Hancock AD, Reade MC**, et al. (2010). 'The impact of advance care planning on end of life care in elderly patients: randomised controlled trial'. *BMJ* **340**: c1345. PubMed PMID: 20332506. Pubmed Central PMCID: 2844949. Epub 2010/03/25. eng.

8. **Detering K, Sutton E, Fraser S**, et al. (2015). 'Feasibility and acceptability of advance care planning in elderly Italian and Greek speaking patients as compared to English-speaking patients: an Australian cross-sectional study'. *BMJ open* **5**(8): e008800.

9. **Detering K, Fraser S, Whiteside K**, et al. (2015) 'Not competent but not silent—a pilot study of ACP with dementia patients. *BMJ Support Palliat Care* **5**: A22–A23. doi: 101136/bmjspcare-2015-00097870.

10. **Silvester W, Fullam RS, Parslow RA**, et al. (Sep 2013). Quality of advance care planning policy and practice in residential aged care facilities in Australia'. *BMJ Support Palliat Care* **3**(3): 349–57.

11. **Silvester W, Parslow RA, Lewis VJ**, et al. (Jun 2013). 'Development and evaluation of an aged care specific Advance Care Plan'. *BMJ Support Palliat Care* **3**(2): 188–95.

12. **Sellars M, Detering KM, Silvester W** (2015). 'Current advance care planning practice in the Australian community: an online survey of home care package case managers and service managers'. *BMC palliative care* **14**: 15.

13. **Detering KM, Carter RZ, Sellars MW**, et al. (2017). Prospective comparative effectiveness cohort study comparing 2 models of advance care planning provision for Australian community aged care. *BMJ Supportive and Palliative Care.* doi: 10.1136/bmjspcare-2017-001372

14. **Detering K, Silvester W, Corke C**, et al. (Sep 2014). Teaching general practitioners and doctors-in-training to discuss advance care planning: evaluation of a brief multimodality education programme. *BMJ Support Palliat Care* **4**(3): 313–21.

15. **Clayton JM, Hancock KM, Butow PN**, et al. (Jun 2007). 'Clinical practice guidelines for communicating prognosis and end-of-life issues with adults in the advanced stages of a life-limiting illness, and their caregivers'. *Med J Aust* 18;186(12 Suppl): S77, S9, S83–108.

16. **Cheang F, Finnegan T, Stewart C**, et al. (Oct 2014). 'Single-centre cross-sectional analysis of advance care planning among elderly inpatients'. *Intern Med J* **44**(10): 967–74.

17. **Victoria**: 'Advance care planning: have the conversation; A strategy for Victorian health services 2014–2018,' (www.health.vic.gov.au/acp/strategy).

18. **New South Wales: Statewide plan**: 'Advance Planning for Quality Care at End-of-life—Action Plan 2013-2018' (www.**health.nsw**.gov.au).

Chapter 19

# Advance care planning in Canada

Doris Barwich, John You, Jessica Simon,
Louise Hanvey, and Cari Borenko Hoffmann

'It sounds to me like there's, um . . . a very large
amount of training that needs to go on with health care
professionals. But there's also a huge amount of education
that needs to be given to the general public.'
*(Public participant, ACP CRIO qualitative study)*

---

**This chapter includes**

♦ A broad overview of the development of ACP in Canada, including the development of
a national ACP framework

♦ A summary of the key activities, including Canadian ACP research, the public engagement strategy: Speak Up: Start the conversation about end of life care, educational initiatives and accountability

♦ A discussion regarding opportunities and barriers to ACP in Canada

---

**Key Points**

♦ National framework for ACP (education, engagement, structure, continuous quality
improvement) has helped organise an approach to implementing ACP in Canada

♦ Informal and formal network of champions—including healthcare providers, lawyers,
non-governmental organisation (NGO) leaders, and decision makers—has helped communicate opportunities and seed key changes

♦ Research and audit data has helped prioritise ACP initiatives with decision makers and
stakeholders

♦ ACP invites new thinking and behaviours from public, patients, healthcare providers, lawyers, and government. Such change takes investment, time, energy, and change
management

---

**Key Message**

Implementation of ACP in Canada has followed a multifaceted approach, with significant
national leadership, key stakeholder participation, and consumer engagement strategies,
with important outcomes demonstrated.

## 'Advance care planning in Canada'—a national initiative

Canada, with a population of approximately 35 million people, is a geographically immense country. There are ten provinces and three territories in Canada, each with their own provincial/territorial governments. Canadians are a diverse population representing many cultures and ethnic groups. A national poll in Canada revealed that there was a lot of work required regarding engaging Canadians in and raising their awareness about advance care planning (ACP). While 80% of Canadians believed that it was important to talk about wishes for future healthcare, less than half (45%) had had a conversation with anyone, and only 5% had ever talked to their doctor about their wishes for future care (1).

In 2007, an Inaugural Canadian Symposium on Advance Care Planning was held with the support of Calgary Health Region and Fraser Health, along with the Canadian Hospice Palliative Care Association and the Health Quality Council of Alberta—featuring speakers from across Canada, the United States and Australia. After the Symposium, Health Canada, along with these four agencies, sponsored a National ACP Workshop, which resulted in an Implementation Guide to Advance Care Planning in Canada: A Case Study of Two Health Authorities.

In follow-up, in 2008, the Canadian Hospice Palliative Care Association, a national non-governmental organisation that advocates for improved access to palliative care in Canada, brought together leaders from across the country who decided to work together to promote ACP in Canada. The result was the initiative, 'Advance Care Planning (ACP) in Canada'. This initiative is facilitated by the Canadian Hospice Palliative Care Association, which acts as the Secretariat. To support the initiative, the Canadian Hospice Palliative Care Association has secured funding from a variety of sources, including the private sector, government agencies, research agencies and other health charities. 'ACP in Canada' operates under the guidance of a National ACP Task Group. This Task Group is comprised of representation from the major national professional health and legal associations including the Canadian Medical Association, the College of Family Physicians of Canada, the Canadian Society of Palliative Care Physicians, the Canadian Nurses Association, and the Canadian Bar Association, among others. The Task Group also includes consumers such as experts in ACP from major non-governmental organisations (NGOs) representing major disease groups in Canada, e.g. The Canadian Cancer Society; bioethicists; and researchers. 'ACP in Canada' officially partners with Canadian Researchers at End of Life Network (CARENET). This provides the opportunity to develop evidence-based tools and approaches and to collaborate in knowledge dissemination and knowledge translation activities. (See Box 19.1) For instance,

## Box 19.1 Canadian advance care planning research: partnering with stakeholders to respond to patient and family priorities

ACP research in Canada is notable for its direct engagement of patients and families, and its partnerships with healthcare providers and decision makers. Originally funded through a New Emerging Teams grant from the Canadian Institutes of Health Research, the Canadian Researchers at End of Life Network (CARENET) is a national, multi-disciplinary group of healthcare professionals who aim to improve the quality of end of life communication and decision-making. When directly asked by CARENET researchers, hundreds of seriously ill, hospitalised patients across Canada, and their families, identified end of life communication and decision making as the top priority for improving the quality of end of life care (2,3). This work led to the creation of a conceptual framework of end of life communication and decision-making (Figure 19.1) to guide quality improvement efforts in this area (4). This framework was developed by a multi-disciplinary panel of 28 experts, who were healthcare professionals or researchers working in palliative or end of life care drawn from five Canadian provinces.

Guided by this framework, and in partnership with policy and decision makers (notably in the provinces of British Columbia and Alberta), CARENET led a multi-site audit of ACP. Key audit findings were:

◆ The majority of hospitalised patients with serious illness could express preferences for end of life care

◆ Clinicians often did not engage patients in ACP or goals of care conversations

◆ There is frequent (70%) disagreement between patients' expressed preferences for end of life care and prescribed orders in the medical record (5)

A complementary multi-centre survey of clinicians also identified inadequate preparation of patients and families as important barriers to end of life communication and decision-making (6).

This work has given rise to new initiatives that are refining and evaluating multi-faceted tools to support patients, families and clinicians in ACP and goals of care activities in primary care, hospital, and long-term care settings.

Active partnerships between researchers and knowledge users are ongoing and are striving to increase the uptake and impact of ACP. Researcher-stakeholder partnerships continue to thrive at multiple levels, including with national groups (e.g. the National ACP Task Group), with provincial decision-makers (e.g. through the ACP Collaborative Research & Innovation Opportunities Program in Alberta and the BC Centre for Palliative Care), with government agencies, with clinical programmes (e.g. Northern Alberta Renal Program) (7) and the legal profession. The Canadian Frailty Network (CFN), established in 2012, is a recently launched federally-funded Network of Centres of Excellence that is dedicated to the improvement of ACP for frail older adults and is expected to sustain and catalyse ACP initiatives in Canada.

through this partnership, 'ACP in Canada' has been able to mobilise research findings generated by CARENET and others by partnering with researchers to disseminate new evidence to its diverse and nationwide network of stakeholders using e-mail blasts, its website, newsletters, traditional media (radio, television, and newspapers), and co-hosting webinars with investigators.

## National advance care planning framework

In 2012, the National ACP Task Group further developed a National Framework for Advance Care Planning in Canada, through a nation-wide consultative process. The consultation involved the federal government; the provincial and territorial governments; national/provincial/territorial non-governmental and professional organisations; and provincial/territorial and local health agencies. This Framework provides a model for ACP that is used across the country to guide related activity, programme development, and practice. The Framework features the patient and family at its centre and is based on four basic building blocks: engagement; education; system infrastructure; and continuous quality improvement. (See Figure 19.2.) Engagement involves engaging all relevant participants and sectors—the general public; the healthcare system; healthcare professionals; and the legal sector/professionals. Education refers to the education of the general public and of healthcare professionals. System infrastructure involves the development and implementation of ACP policies and the development of tools to support conversations and to document the process and results of ACP. Continuous quality

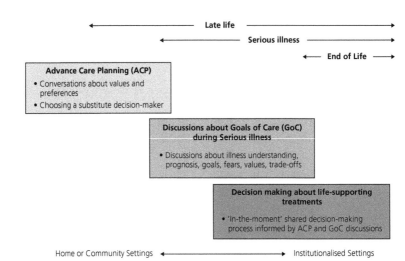

**Figure 19.1** Conceptual framework of end of life communication and decision making

**Advance care planning (ACP)** refers to an upstream communication process—which should occur when patients have decision-making capacity and are relatively well—among patients, family members, future substitute decision maker(s), and healthcare providers to identify patients' values and preferences about future care.

**Goals of care (GoC) discussions** become relevant as patients experience serious illness in later life. These are illness-specific, patient-centred conversations framed around illness understanding and prognosis which seek to elicit patients' values, goals, fears, concerns, and acceptable trade-offs that relate to their care.

**'In-the-moment decision making'** is a shared decision-making process, informed by ACP and GoC discussions, to make specific medical decisions about care, including the use or non-use of life-sustaining treatments including cardiopulmonary resuscitation, mechanical ventilation, intensive care unit admission, dialysis, tube feeding, and intravenous hydration.

Adapted from *Journal of Pain Symptom Management,* Volume 49, Issue 6, Sinuff T, Dodek P, You JJ, et al. 'Improving End of Life Communication and Decision Making: The Development of a Conceptual Framework and Quality Indicators', pp. 1070–80, Copyright © 2015 American Academy of Hospice and Palliative Medicine, Published by Elsevier Inc., with permission from Elsevier. http://www.sciencedirect.com/science/article/pii/S0885392415000445

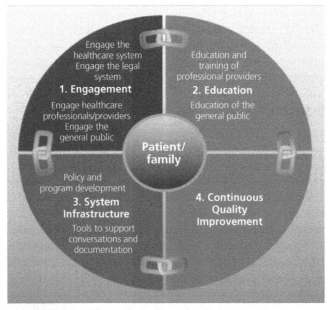

**Figure 19.2** A National Framework for Advance Care Planning

Adapted from 'Implementation Guide to Advance Care Planning in Canada: A Case Study of two Health Authorities', March 2008, http://www.hc-sc.gc.ca/hcs-sss/alt_ formats/pdf/pubs/palliat/2008-acp-guide-pps/acp-guide-pps-eng.pdf, with permission from Health Canada

improvement ensures that ACP policies and practices are based on evidence and are continually informed by relative outcomes (8).

## Engagement in advance care planning

'ACP in Canada' works with community organisations, professional organisations (national and local), and NGOs to engage ACP Champions and facilitate their work to promote ACP with their constituents. This is accomplished through the development of a Community of Practice, a group of professionals that works together to share learnings and solve problems.

'ACP in Canada' strives to raise Canadians' awareness about the importance of ACP, normalise ACP conversations across the life span, and to give the general public the tools they need to achieve these conversations. In addition, 'ACP in Canada' works to assist professionals; healthcare, legal and financial and funeral planning—with the tools they need to facilitate ACP with their patients and clients. The activities of 'ACP in Canada' are directed to engage a number of target audiences including community organisations; the general public; patients with acute and/or chronic illness and families/caregivers; professionals—healthcare, legal, financial, and funeral planning; policy makers and ACP professionals. This is achieved primarily through the 'Speak Up Campaign' which is directed at both the general public and professionals. (See Box 19.1.)

With its partners and stakeholders, 'ACP in Canada' invites new thinking and behaviours from the public, patients, healthcare providers, lawyers, and governments. Such change takes investment, time, energy, and change management.

## Facilitators to advance care planning in Canada

There are a number of facilitators, which have helped the progress and uptake of ACP in Canada. Canada has a publicly funded healthcare system, which means that the majority of Canadians have access to healthcare. The fact that all of the major national professional associations and NGOs are engaged in 'ACP in Canada' and have endorsed the implementation of ACP has had a significant impact. For example, Choosing Wisely Canada has included early ACP in their recommendations along with resources from 'ACP in Canada' (9,10). Recently in Canada, there have been high-profile legal cases related to end of life decision making. As well, medical aid in dying has recently been legalised. This has led to an increased public discourse regarding planning for end of life care, which has provided an opportunity to draw attention to ACP. A number of educational initiatives have taken place to educate healthcare professionals regarding the importance of ACP and how to engage with their patients. (See Box 19.3.)

## Challenges

There are a number of challenges that make it difficult to implement ACP programmes in Canada. One key barrier to the implementation of a national approach to ACP in Canada is that the legislation that governs healthcare consent and ACP is enacted at the provincial/territorial level with significant differences between the provincial/territorial laws regarding terminology and how ACP and consent are legally constituted. For example, in some provinces written advance directives, or personal directives are legal documents, in others they are not. In order to help reduce confusion, 'ACP in Canada' has focussed on three key messages: ACP is about reflecting on values and wishes for future health and personal care,

## Box 19.2 Engagement: Speak Up: Start the conversation about end of life care

In order to engage with the general public and professionals 'ACP in Canada' launched a national campaign—**Speak Up: Start the Conversation About End of Life Care**. One of the primary mechanisms of engagement is the **national website**—www.advancecareplanning. ca/www.planificationprealable.ca. This website hosts all of the tools and resources of 'ACP in Canada' and the Speak Up Campaign for the general public and professionals. These tools are all freely downloadable from the site or can be purchased from the Canadian Hospice Palliative Care Association. 'Speak Up' is directed to a number of target audiences including community organisations; the general public; patients with acute and/or chronic illness and families/caregivers; professionals including healthcare, legal, financial/funeral planning; policy makers, and ACP professionals.

In addition, the National ACP Task Group established 16 April as **National Advance Care Planning Day in Canada** which has been ongoing since 2011. Each year the Speak Up Campaign has a Campaign Kit to enable community organisations, professional groups and institutions to facilitate their constituents' participation in ACP. The Campaign tools are available in template format so that community organisations can add their own branding. These include template news releases, template articles, infographics and posters, videos, PSAs and concrete examples of activities for celebrating National ACP Day. (The Speak Up Campaign Toolkit is found at www.advancecareplanning.ca / www.planificationprealable.ca.)

'ACP in Canada' has developed a **suite of tools**—for the general public and professionals— to enable them to engage in ACP. The flagship tool is the Advance Care Planning Workbook (originally adapted from the Fraser Health My Voice Workbook). This workbook is an interactive tool which enables the general public to engage in the five steps of ACP—thinking about their values, beliefs, and wishes for care; learning about their health and medical interventions; deciding on their substitute decision maker; talking with their substitute decision maker, family/friends, and healthcare team; and recording their wishes. There is a national workbook, along with co-branded workbooks specific to provinces. There are also tools for healthcare providers—to help them get started in ACP conversations with their patients. For example, a 'Just Ask' discussion guide that help facilitate conversations. There are also a number of tools, which can be used to promote ACP at the community and agency level. All tools are freely downloadable in French and English on the website or they can be ordered through the Canadian Hospice Palliative Care Association. ACP in Canada has developed a number of videos which are used to start conversations, as educational tools in workshops and waiting rooms and as public service announcements.

*Communications* is central to engagement—and 'ACP in Canada' utilises a number of communications strategies. The website is a key mode of communication and is used along with social media—with a YouTube channel, Facebook page, and Twitter feed. In addition, ACP in Canada has relationships with journalists and media outlets across the country to communicate their messages.

deciding on a substitute decision maker and having conversations with that substitute decision maker and others about values and wishes. Professionals and the public are then directed to resources specifically describing the legal parameters in their province/territory.

In Canada, while both the federal and provincial/territorial governments have a role in health and healthcare, the actual provision of healthcare falls within the jurisdiction of the provinces and

## Box 19.3 Education

ACP educators in Canada are a small but connected group of people who have been sharing resources and information informally for several years. With the support of 'ACP in Canada', in 2012, the Canadian ACP Educators Community of Practice was formed. This once small group has grown into 79 participants from nine provinces/territories who meet regularly to promote sharing of information, experiences and educational resources.

The province of British Columbia (BC) has been a leader in developing education for health-care providers from all sectors to ensure access to standardised education relating to ACP, goals of care, and serious illness conversations. Several initiatives have been led at the provincial level by different sectors and, at times, by specific disciplines. There are a number of provincial organisations, including Doctors of BC, BC Cancer Agency, BC Renal Agency, and now the BC Centre for Palliative Care who have led various provincial initiatives relating to ACP. These approaches have all been instrumental in moving ACP forward for the citizens of BC.

For example, in September 2011 the BC General Practice Services Committee and the provincial Practice Support Program, supported by ACP and palliative care experts, developed an End of Life Module targeting primary care physicians. The Module was created to address a gap in education for family physicians regarding the new provincial ACP legislation (2011) and other issues relating to end of life care. The goal was to provide consistent education and practice support regarding identifying patients, initiating and documenting the outcomes of ACP, serious illness and goals of care conversations, and developing patient and family centred care plans.

Three half-day learning sessions were separated by action periods supported by local coaches to help interdisciplinary primary care teams throughout BC make changes to improve care for patients with life-limiting and chronic illnesses. These teams included General Practitioners (GPs), medical office assistants and home health staff. Over 1000 physicians completed this module. Following the completion of this education, 96–100% GPs stated they were confident in identifying and engaging with patients and families regarding ACP, goals of care, and serious illness conversations (11).

Most education however is delivered at local or regional levels. British Columbia has five regional health authorities, serving 4.6 million people. All five regional health authorities have developed ACP on-line learning modules which are accessible to all staff as well as ACP classroom learning for physicians, nursing, and allied health clinicians.

The implementation of standardised medical orders (commonly known as Medical Orders for Scope of Treatment or MOST) in all sectors within the health authorities prompted additional educational sessions in ACP, goals of care, and serious illness conversations. This initiative has been most successful at normalising these conversations for those with serious illness and supporting access to the documentation of the outcomes of these conversations across care settings.

territories. The federal government is responsible for setting and administering national principles for the healthcare system under the *Canada Health Act*. The federal government provides financial support to health in the form of cash transfers to the provinces and territories. However, the provinces and territories administer and deliver most of Canada's healthcare services. The provinces and territories are required to provide reasonable access to medically necessary hospital and doctors' services (2). ACP is not specifically delineated in the *Canada Health Act* or the national principles set out by the federal government. Therefore, the 13 provinces and territories are autonomous with regard to the focus they place on ACP and how they implement policies and programmes. There has been relatively little provincial and federal funding provided for ACP. Only a few provinces have provincial policies regarding ACP.

## Shifting culture takes time

Common to other countries, Canada's attempts to normalise ACP as a process suitable for all adults represents a significant shift from current behaviours, including the acceptance of talking about serious illness, death, and end of life care. This involves change within multiple cultures, including the medical culture (where eliciting patient values in relation to the care offered is still relatively new), the legal system culture, distinct provincial cultures and across the diverse ethnic and socio-cultural perspectives of Canadians, including indigenous peoples and those who have immigrated from other countries.

Tools in this culture shift include the iterative nature of audits, polls, and research evaluation, the intentional qualitative exploration of multiple perspectives, tailoring messages, tools, and

---

### Box 19.4 Structure and continuous quality improvement: Alberta Health Services, provincial policy and procedure for advance care planning and goals of care designations

Alberta Health Service (AHS) is Canada's first province-wide, fully-integrated health system, delivering health services to four million people in Alberta. In April 2014 AHS introduced a province-wide policy (13) and procedure (14) for guiding ACP and implementing the 'Goals of Care Designation' (GCD) framework. GCDs are medical orders for 'shorthand' communication of the general intention of care, the types of interventions, transfers, and locations that might be used or withheld. There are a total of seven GCDs divided between resuscitative, medical, and comfort care-focused categories. In addition AHS introduced a procedure for communication and documentation that supports the transfer of information across time and between health sectors. This policy and procedure were built on those implemented six years previously in one local region within the province and designed to be consistent with relevant legislation in the province (15).

The current structural element is a 'green sleeve'; a green plastic folder that is owned by the patient and is used to store and transport ACP GCD documents. At home this is kept on or near the patient's fridge as a readily identifiable location for emergency medical services. It contains a GCD medical order form completed by a physician or nurse practitioner and an 'ACP GCD tracking record' used to record the conversations that are part of ACP or determining the GCD order. In addition it stores a copy of the patient's 'Personal Directive' (and other relevant legal forms once enacted). Other structural elements include an e-module for teaching healthcare providers about GCD, a public and healthcare provider website of resources (www.conversationsmatter.ca), as well as printed resources.

Continuous quality improvement has been a central part of the policy implementation. For example, AHS has conducted serial chart audits to assess use of GCD and the tracking record, which have been use to prioritise improvement activities. In 2016, a research (16)/ AHS partnership developed nine performance indicators (of structures, processes, and outcomes in Institute of Medicine healthcare quality domains) that will be adopted to monitor and further improve ACP and GCD practice.

interventions to be appropriate to those perspectives and the intentional 'silo-bridging' nature of the collaborations. Recognising the complexity of the systems and the change also helps set realistic targets and timelines for efforts to engage the public and professionals in ACP.

## Accountability and opportunities

To date ACP efforts in Canada have been driven mostly by healthcare systems and within them frequently by palliative care or seniors' services. Indeed 'ACP in Canada', is hosted by Canadian Hospice and Palliative Care Association and has drawn on the communication strengths of that specialty. It is important now to reframe ACP as a public health issue and health promotion activity with ACP programmes within pan-system portfolios (akin to infection prevention). Being aware of the funding priorities of granting agencies, new innovations, and driving trends is essential to creating new opportunities for ACP. For example, in Canada, we can make connections and draw attention of the relevance of ACP to precision or personalised medicine and to health services research (focused on cost, value, and quality) and to patient-oriented research, (such as the Canadian Institutes of Health Research's Strategy for Patient Oriented Research), which are all current priorities in the Canadian context. (See Box 19.4.)

## References

1. **Canadian Hospice Palliative Care Association, (CHPCA)** (2013). 'What Canadians Say: The Way Forward Survey Report, for The Way Forward initiative', Harris/Decima. Available from: http://www.hpcintegration.ca/resources/what-canadians-say.aspx#sthash.R4qgG5B4.dpuf (Accessed November 25, 2016.)
2. **Heyland DK, Dodek P, Rocker G**, et al. (2006). 'What matters most in end-of-life care: perceptions of seriously ill patients and their family members'. *CMAJ* **174**(5): 627–33.
3. **Heyland DK, Cook DJ, Rocker GM**, et al. (2010). 'Defining priorities for improving end-of-life care in Canada'. *CMAJ* **182**(16): E747–E752.
4. **Sinuff T, Dodek P, You JJ**, et al. (2015). 'Improving end-of-life communication and decision making: the development of a conceptual framework and quality indicators'. *J Pain Symptom Manage* **49**(6): 1070–80.
5. **Heyland DK, Barwich D, Pichora D**, et al. (2013). 'Failure to engage seriously ill hospitalized patients and their families in advance care planning: results of a multicenter prospective study'. *JAMA Intern Med* **173**(9): 778–87.
6. **You JJ, Downar J, Fowler RA**, et al. (2015). 'Barriers to goals of care discussions with seriously ill hospitalized patients and their families: a multicenter survey of clinicians'. *JAMA Intern Med* **175**(4): 549–56.
7. **Davison SN** and **Torgunrud C** (2007). 'The creation of an advance care planning process for patients with ESRD'. *Am J Kidney Dis* **49**(1): 27–36. *Review* PubMed PMID: 17185143.
8. Advance Care Planning in Canada National Task Group. (2012). *Advance Care Planning in Canada: National Framework*. Ottawa: Canadian Hospice Palliative Care Association. Available from: http://www.advancecareplanning.ca/wp-content/uploads/2016/08/ACP-Framework-2012-ENG.pdf (Accessed November 25, 2016.)
9. **Choosing Wisely Canada** (2014). *Palliative Care: Five Things Patients and Physicians Should Question*. Available from: http://www.choosingwiselycanada.org/recommendations/palliative-care/ (Accessed 1 December 2016.)
10. **Choosing Wisely Canada** (2014). *Palliative Care: Support At Any Time During a Serious Illness*. Available from: http://www.choosingwiselycanada.org/materials/palliative-care-support-at-any-time-during-a-serious-illness/. (Accessed December 1, 2016.)

11. **Hollander MJ** (2013). *Evaluation of the Full Service Family Practice Incentive Program and the Practice Support Program.* Synthesis Report for Work Completed to June 2013. British Columbia Ministry of Health Services and the General Practice Services Committee. Available from: http://www.gpscbc.ca/sites/default/files/Synthesis-Report-2_2013-06-13.pdf

12. **Health Canada**. 2011. *Canada's Health Care System.* Available from: http://www.hc-sc.gc.ca/hcs-sss/pubs/system-regime/2011-hcs-sss/index-eng.php#a4. (Accessed 25 November 2016.)

13. 'Advanced Care Planning and Goals of Care Designation'. (2014). Available from: https://extranet.ahsnet.ca/teams/policydocuments/1/clp-advance-care-planning-hcs-38-policy.pdf (Accessed 20 Nov 2016.)

14. 'Advance care planning and goals of care designation'. Available from: https://extranet.ahsnet.ca/teams/policydocuments/1/clp-advance-care-planning-hcs-38-01-procedure.pdf (Accessed 20 Nov 2016.)

15. **Province of Albert** (2008). *Adult Guardianship and Trusteeship Act.* Available from: http://www.qp.alberta.ca/documents/Acts/A04P2.pdf (Accessed 20 Nov 2016.)

16. **University of Calgary** (2016). *The Alberta Advance Care Planning CRIO Research Program (ACP CRIO).* Available from: www.acpcrio.org (Accessed 20 Nov 2016.)

# Chapter 20

# Advance directives and advance care planning: the US experience

Maria J. Silveira and Phillip Rodgers

In preparing for battle, I have always found that plans are useless, but planning is indispensable.
*Attributed to Dwight D. Eisenhower in Richard Nixon, Six Crises, 1962*

---

**This chapter includes**

- The history of advance directives (ADs) and advance care planning (ACP) in the United States
- Review of the evidence base for ADs and ACP in the US
- Description of successful ACP programmes in the US
- Discussion of technology in ACP and AD

---

**Key Points**

- Advance directives have a long history in the US, with more recent data showing positive outcomes.
- There are three types of AD used in the US: the living will (LW), Durable Power of attorney for Healthcare (DPAHC), and combined LW and DPAHC. All states have a DPAHC, and most use LW or combined directives.
- ACP mostly occurs within multifaceted programmes, and has a growing evidence base for its effectiveness.
- In 2016, Medicare successfully established payment for ACP services. Following Medicare's example, some private insurers and Medicaid plans have also instituted reimbursement for ACP services.

---

**Key Message**

There is increasing evidence that Americans welcome ACP discussions and complete ADs, and that doing so helps to ensure they receive medical care consistent with their preferences.

## The flip side to modern medicine

Improvements in public health and biomedical technology during the latter half of the twentieth century substantially extended life expectancy in the US from 47 in 1900 to 79 by 2014 (1). This accomplishment, paired with the aging of America's largest generation (known fondly as the 'Baby Boomers'), is largely responsible for an exponential increase in expenditures related to healthcare over the last 20 years. The US spends a greater proportion of its GDP on healthcare than any other country in the world (18%) (2).

A significant proportion of healthcare expenditures in the US relates to care provided near the end of life. Medicare (government provided insurance for adults who are either older than 65 or disabled) spends more on care in the last six months of life than it spends during the rest of the life span (3). It is fair to assume that most of this cost relates to invasive, life sustaining interventions given through the end of life. Despite most wishing otherwise, a significant proportion of older adults die in the hospital (4). While that proportion has been decreasing over the last two decades (largely due to the increased use of hospice care before death), the average number of hospital days during the last six months of life has remained high (4). During the same period, there have been increases in lengths of stay in the intensive care unit (ICU) (4).

Research has shown that many interventions intended to prolong life only extend it marginally, while significantly reducing its quality (5). As a result, there is increasing recognition that decisions to start therapies like feeding tubes, dialysis, and artificial ventilation must be thoughtfully discussed with patients and their families, ideally long before the treatments are needed. Advance care planning (ACP) is the name that has been given to this process. In the last twenty years, ACP in the US has grown from a nebulous concept known only to palliative care specialists, to a well-defined, reimbursable service that is becoming a routine part of healthcare, especially for older adults. Advance directives (ADs), while a much older concept than ACP, have fallen from the spotlight to become one piece of ACP, rather than the primary purpose of these discussions.

## Advance care planning

ACP is a process whereby a patient's medical condition and prognosis are reviewed and options for treatment and non-treatment are discussed (6). In an ideal ACP discussion, clinicians, the patient, and his or her loved ones think through particular approaches to follow as the patient's health declines (7). ACP discussions can also address the patient's preferences for when to hospitalise, place of death, as well as a surrogate decision maker. ACP is meant to occur through a series of conversations over time, not as a singular discussion. It is iterative and ideally occurs within the context of an existing and continuing medical relationship. There are three objectives for ACP (see Box 20.1).

---

### Box 20.1 Key goals of advance care planning conversations

1. Patients learn something about their current medical condition and prognosis.
2. Patients come to understand what treatment options they have.
3. Patients evaluate this information using their personal calculus of benefits and burdens and formulate broad goals of care.

Source: data from Gillick MR, 'A broader role for advance medical planning', *Annals of Internal Medicine*, Volume 123, Issue 8, pp. 621–4, Copyright © 1995 The American College of Physicians, doi: 10.7326/0003-4819-123-8-199510150-00009

# Advance directives

Advance directives are means of documenting and disseminating patient preferences for medical care and choice of a surrogate decision maker. Any written documentation of a patient's preference is considered an AD, but only those meeting the requirements codified in the legal code of each US state are deemed legally valid. This legal backing becomes important when patients lose decisional capacity and there is disagreement (within a family or between the family and the patient's providers) about what to do. Only 15 states recognise oral advance directives (i.e. not in writing) (8).

Advance directives can only be authored by a person with decisional capacity (i.e. not by a surrogate or proxy decision maker), and they only come into effect when that person has lost decisional capacity. In the US, decisional capacity is determined by the bedside physician based on the patient's ability to understand his or her circumstances, appreciate the options (with risks and benefits), express a choice, and explain its rationale (9). In cases where there is any ambiguity, confirmation from another provider (usually a psychiatrist or ethicist) without direct responsibility for the patient is recommended. Advance directives can be revoked by a decisional patient at any time, in writing or otherwise.

There are three types of AD used in the US:

1. **Living will (LW).** The living will is any written documentation of a patient's preferences for future medical care in the event she/he needs it and has lost the capacity to speak for himself or herself. The typical living will in the US addresses cardiopulmonary resuscitation (CPR) and intubation/ventilation; some will address artificial nutrition, dialysis, the decision to hospitalise, antibiotics, and/or pain control. Many types of living wills have been proposed over the years, from one that documented values instead of precise preferences (knowns as the 'values history' (10)), to another that went through a myriad of scenarios that patients might face (known as the 'instructional directive' (11)); to date, there is no evidence that one type of living will is any better than the rudimentary living will recommended by most US States.

   Most US States have suggested language for the living will codified in their statutes, however, any documentation that meets certain requirements for content and/or witnessing can have the official backing of the state; thus, while patients are strongly encouraged to use statutory advance directives, no state mandates their use.

2. **Durable Power of Attorney for Healthcare (DPAHC).** The DPAHC gives a preferred surrogated decision-maker authority to make healthcare decisions on behalf of its author. Just like the LW, the DPAHC does not come into effect until a patient loses decisional capacity. Additionally, it can be revoked with a patient's say-so.

   All 50 states have sanctioned DPAHCs. Most states limit who can serve as a surrogate and usually exclude direct care providers or proprietors of healthcare facilities (in-which the patient resides) from serving in this capacity. In all states, DPAHCs must be witnessed or notarised and the limitations on who can serve as witness can vary by state. Some states require that the appointed surrogate accept the role by co-signing the document.

   When patients do not have a DPAHC, a 'default' surrogate is typically appointed for the patient; 44 states and the District of Columbia have laws in place that guide this process (12).

3. **Combined AD.** Twenty-five US states have a 'combined AD', one that merges the LW and DPAHC into a single document (8). This practice is patterned after model legislation (the Uniform Healthcare Decisions Act (13)) first proposed by the American Bar Association (ABA) in 1993 to standardise AD content, process, and language across the 50 states (see Additional Resources). Additionally, a number of highly respected groups have developed

> ## Box 20.2 Five Wishes, content
>
> 1. The person I want to make care decisions for me when I can't.
> 2. The kind of medical treatment I want or don't want.
> 3. How comfortable I want to be (related to pain, depression, mouthcare, bathing, music, readings, hospice).
> 4. How I want people to treat me (to be accompanied, prayers, pictures, die at home etc.).
> 5. What I want my loved one to know (love, forgiveness, fears, funeral arrangements etc.).
>
> Source: data from Five Wishes, Aging with Dignity, 2013, http://www.agingwithdignity.org/5wishes.html

more 'user-friendly' combined ADs that meet the requirements for most if not all US states; this includes Five Wishes, a very popular programme developed by the non-profit Aging with Dignity with the guidance of the ABA (14) (see Box 20.2).

## Do not resuscitate orders

In the US, advance directives are meant to guide physicians' clinical decision making and do not carry the authority of physicians' orders. Because many first-contact clinicians such as emergency medical technicians, bedside nurses, or nursing home aides, can follow only physicians' orders, patients are at risk of resuscitation even when they have a LW stating otherwise. Thus, when patients choose not to undergo CPR, physicians of record are responsible for writing an order directing medical staff NOT to resuscitate the patient. This 'do not resuscitate' (DNR) order must be entered into the medical record each time a patient is admitted or transferred to any healthcare facility. It is highly recommended that community-dwelling patients have such orders at home as well in case they arrest at home. Without a so-called 'out of hospital DNR' emergency medical service personnel are obligated to do everything possible to resuscitate the patient, regardless of what their living will says (12).

### POLST

Physicians' Orders for Life Sustaining Treatment (POLST) were created in Oregon in the 1990s as a combined advance directive that pairs patients' wishes with a DNR order (15,16). The POLST form was designed to narrow the gap between patients' wishes and the implementation of the plan of care. In states that have adopted POLST, there are agreements in place whereby all segments of the healthcare system agree to respect the orders written on a POLST, regardless of where it originated, so long as it is consistent with the patient's wishes (see Additional Resources).

## A history of advance directives and advance care planning in the US

As far back as 1914, US case law established the requirement that health professionals obtain a patient's consent for invasive medical procedures based on their right to self-determination. The term 'living will' first appeared in the US in 1969, with the introduction of a document designed to allow a patient to consent or refuse life-sustaining measures in 'advance', in case she/he ever lost decisional capacity (17,18).

Consumer rights and hospice advocates began to demand that states adopt living will legislation in the mid 1970s, largely in response to the case of Karen Ann Quinlan. Ms. Quinlan was a 21-year-old who was left in a persistent vegetative state after a cardiac arrest in 1974. Because her wishes were not known, she was resuscitated and put on life support. She would have been kept on life support indefinitely had her parents not been granted the right to withdraw care by the New Jersey Supreme Court in 1976. The Court held, based on the principle of autonomy, that the onset of incapacity did not mean Ms. Quinlan lost her right to refuse medical treatment (19). The Court recognised her parents as her legitimate proxies and allowed them to make decisions on her behalf based on their knowledge of what they thought Ms. Quinlain would have wanted (19).

As the Quinlan case proceeded through the courts, California passed the Natural Death Act in 1976, officially sanctioning the first statutory living will in the US. Soon after, Arkansas followed suit. Today every state in the US, except Michigan has codified living wills (8).

Durable Powers of Attorney for Health Care (DPAHC) were created in order to assert a patient's right to choose his surrogate, especially when the next of kin would not be the patient's first choice. In 1983, Pennsylvania became the first state to enact legislation establishing the legal basis for the DPAHC. Today, all 50 states and the District of Columbia have statutes sanctioning DPAHCs (8,18,20).

Not long after the Quinlan case, a similar case caught the country's attention. Nancy Cruzan was a young woman who had been left in a persistent vegetative state after an automobile accident in 1983. Like Quinlan, Ms. Cruzan had never authored a living will. Initially, Ms. Cruzan's parents hoped for neurologic recovery and consented to life support in the form of tube feeding. After many years of disappointment at her lack of neurologic recovery, however, her parents changed their minds and asked her doctors to withdraw her feeding tube. Fearing legal repercussions, her doctors refused to do so without a court order. Initially, local courts affirmed the parents' right to withdraw life support, citing Quinlan. In an appeal of this ruling, however, the Missouri State Supreme Court reversed the decision on the grounds that Ms. Cruzan's parents lacked 'clear and convincing evidence' that their choice reflected the patient's known prior wishes. Ultimately, the case made it to the US Supreme Court where, in 1990, they affirmed the parents' right to discontinue life-sustaining treatment for Ms. Cruzan, but also emphasised that states have the constitutional authority to set their own standards for surrogate decision making (19).

To date, the level of evidence required to substantiate a non-decisional patient's prior wishes about life support (when there is no living will) varies depending upon the state. Some states, like New York require 'clear and convincing evidence' of the patient's prior wishes; this can be in the form of attestations from friends and family. Other states, like Ohio, do not allow life support to be withdrawn from a patient unless she/he has specifically granted their surrogate that authority in writing, in advance. The majority of states, however, allow clinicians to use their discretion to ensure that surrogates who withdraw life support do so in good faith and the patient's best interest.

Partly motivated by the Cruzan case, but mostly concerned about the exponential growth in healthcare expenditures, the US Congress passed the Patient Self Determination Act (PSDA) in 1991 encouraging completion of ADs (21). The PSDA requires that healthcare facilities that receive Medicare or Medicaid (health insurance for the poor) funding ask all incoming patients whether they have an advance directive and, if not, to provide them the educational materials and forms necessary to craft one. The law represents the first national attempt to promote AD completion in the US.

Realising there were many limitations to ADs, the Institute of Medicine (22) recommended something more expansive and meaningful in 1997, coining the term 'advance care planning' (ACP). ACP would focus attention away from the completion of forms, to the communication between patients, families, and clinicians. Additionally, ACP would go beyond the topics of CPR and life support to include other kinds of treatment, decisions to hospitalise, use of hospice, and psychosocial services.

While ACP is consistent with the ideals of medicine and nursing, as well as what American patients and families want (23), the reality of ACP meant longer, more frequent conversations with patients and families. To this day, clinicians complain that their busy practices do not allow for ACP to take place. In 2008, to incentivise clinicians to engage in ACP, Congress attempted to add ACP to the list of services included in the initial physical exam patients receive when they enroll in Medicare; however, this idea was dropped after public accusations of healthcare rationing ('death panels') were voiced by conservative activists.

In the years that followed, diverse stakeholders continued to advocate for reimbursement for ACP by Medicare. In 2016, with broad-based support from the physician and consumer advocacy groups, Medicare successfully established payment for ACP services through regulatory reform as opposed to legal reform. Now physicians and certain eligible practitioners (e.g. advanced practice nurses and physician assistants) can be paid for the time spent in ACP with patients and their families at rates comparable to those paid for more complex services. Following Medicare's example, some private insurers and Medicaid plans have also instituted reimbursement for ACP services.

## Evidence base for advance directives and advance care planning in the US

Early on, many clinicians, especially those in critical care, complained that ADs were ineffective at driving the care patients received (24). Few patients completed them (18). When patients did complete them, most physicians were unaware of their existence (25). When completed, ADs often were not available at the bedside when needed (25,26). When AD were completed and available, the preferences voiced in the ADs rarely helped inform the decision at hand (27) and were largely disregarded by physicians at the bedside (26). In addition, there was evidence suggesting that the underlying conversations that needed to happen prior to completion of AD were not occurring (28).

In recent years, more favourable data has emerged. Although the research has not been consistent, there is good evidence that:

1. **Many Americans complete ADs when given the chance.** A 2006 survey by the Pew Research Center found that 29% of the general American population reported having a living will. These numbers are much higher among certain populations. Community-dwelling older Americans, for example, complete them 70% of the time (29). Patients with chronic illness do so in high proportions as well. Americans who are young, African American, Hispanic, poor, or less educated, however, complete them at far lower rates (30,31) and there is increasing recognition that ADs are not for people of all cultural backgrounds (31,32).

2. **ADs decrease the rates of hospitalisation and the chances of dying in a US hospital (33).**

3. **ADs decrease the use of life-sustaining treatment (33).**

4. **ADs increase the use of hospice and palliative care (33,34).**

5. **The preferences voiced in AD are relatively stable over time, especially if they concern life-sustaining treatment (35).**

6. **ADs increase preference concordant care (36).**

7. **No harm comes to patients who complete ADs (34,37).**

The impacts of POLST are better understood due to systematic efforts to track their impact among populations adopting them. Research from Oregon (38) has shown that 31% of decedents have a POLST and that those decedents whose POLST requests aggressive care are more likely to die in the hospital than those whose POLST requests comfort care (38). Evidence also suggests that where they are implemented, POLSTs ensure that patients preferences are followed (39).

Research suggests that many Americans welcome ACP discussions (40). However, ACP discussions rarely occur outside of the context of a multifaceted programme. A study by Zhang et al. (41) showed that only 37% of patients with advanced cancer had an ACP conversation before death. When ACP discussions occur, patients receive less intensive care (5) and more hospice care (5), and are more satisfied with their care (42,43).

Simple educational or promotional efforts to increase AD completion or ACP discussions have been universally ineffective. Providing patients with a pamphlet, clinicians with education, or triggers in the medical record are not enough to ensure patients' wishes are routinely assessed, documented, and followed. Better results are seen with systematic interventions that integrate standardised processes for ACP and documentation of preferences with ongoing care (44). The best understood programme in the US is 'Respecting Choices'.

Respecting Choices is a commercial product that involves a coordinated approach to ACP whereby trained non-medical facilitators, in collaboration with treating physicians, assist patients and their families to reflect on the patients' goals, values, and beliefs, and discuss and document their future choices about care. The programme has been in effect in LaCrosse, Wisconsin since 1991. Data from LaCrosse suggests Respecting Choices has increased the rates of AD completion, AD documentation, and compliance with patients' wishes at the end of life (45).

There are other ACP programmes that are less well known, but equally effective (33,44). Successful ACP programmes typically include:

◆ Skilled facilitators to initiate discussions and develop individualised plans

◆ Standardised documentation and AD forms

◆ Proactive, but appropriately timed ACP discussions

◆ Systems and processes that ensure planning and documentation occur

◆ Ongoing evaluation and quality improvement

## Technology and advance directives and advance care planning

In 2016, the US government required that all health institutions adopt electronic medical records (EMRs) and this has resulted in a blossoming of technology to facilitate documentation of AD. Several EMRs have the functionality to store and disseminate ADs (e.g. EPIC). Many EMRs can link across institutions making AD available across providers and settings of care. A few US regions have been able to develop regional health information exchanges with success allowing this information to travel even further.

Nine states have created 'advance directive registries' to provide a central place where residents of each state can store their AD; however, state registries have numerous limitations. Many registries require patients 'snail mail' paper versions of their AD and pay a $10 to $20 fee to register it with the state. Most registries do not allow patients to edit their AD online, and many require that either patients give permission to specific providers and surrogates, or that providers and surrogates apply for permission before accessing individual ADs. State registries do not cross state lines, limiting the dissemination of ADs to the local community only. Lastly, registries are a challenge to sustain; one, Washington State, closed after losing its funding from the state. Private online AD registries (profit and non-for-profit) do exist, but face similar challenges relating to uptake, sustainability, and the balance between privacy and usability.

Technology has been tested to facilitate ACP as well, although many find the use of technology in this capacity distasteful. One programme using a website to engage patients and caregivers in ACP was shown to increase the completion of ADS by 10% (46).

## References

1. **Kochanek K, Murphy S, Xu J,** and **Tejada-Vera B** (2016). Deaths: Final data for 2014. Hyattsville, MD.: National Center for Health Statistics.

2. **Services** (2015). CfMaM. National Health Expenditure Fact Sheet Washington DC: CMS. Available from: https://www.cms.gov/Research-Statistics-Data-and-Systems/Statistics-Trends-and-Reports/NationalHealthExpendData/NHE-Fact-Sheet.html.

3. **Hogan C, Lunney J, Gabel J,** and **Lynn J** (2001). 'Medicare beneficiaries' costs of care in the last year of life'. *Health affairs* **20**(4): 188–95.

4. **Goodman DC, Esty AR, Fisher ES, Chang CH** (2011). 'Trends and variation in end-of-life care for Medicare beneficiaries with severe chronic illness'. Dartmouth Institute for Health Policy and Clinical Practice. Center for Health Policy Research, New Hampshire.

5. **Wright AA, Zhang B, Ray A, Mack JW, Trice E, Balboni T,** et al. (2008). 'Associations between end-of-life discussions, patient mental health, medical care near death, and caregiver bereavement adjustment'. *JAMA* **300**(14): 1665–73.

6. **Sudore RL** and **Fried TR** (2010). 'Redefining the "planning" in advance care planning: preparing for end-of-life decision making'. *Ann Intern Med* **153**(4): 256–61.

7. **Kass-Bartelmes BL, Hughes R,** and **Rutherford MK** (2003). 'Advance care planning: prefernces for care at the end of life'. In: *J Pain Palliat Care Pharm* **18**(1): 8–109.

8. **Sabatino C** (2010). 'The evolution of health care advance planning law and policy'. *Milbank Quarterly* **88**(2): 211–39.

9. **Appelbaum PS** and **Grisso T** (1988). 'Assessing patients' capacities to consent to treatment'. *N Engl J Med* **319**(25): 1635–8.

10. **Doukas DJ** and **McCullough LB** (1991). 'The values history. The evaluation of the patient's values and advance directives' [see comments]. *J Fam Pract* **32**(2): 145–53.

11. **Emanuel LL** and **Emanuel EJ** (1989). 'The Medical Directive. A new comprehensive advance care document' [see comments]. *Jama* **261**(22): 3288–93.

12. **Sabatino CP** (2010). 'The evolution of health care advance planning law and policy'. *Milbank Q* **88**(2): 211–39.

13. **Uniform Law Commission** (1993). Uniform Healthcare Decisions Act; 1993.

14. **Dignity.** Aw. Available from: https://www.agingwithdignity.org/five-wishes/about-five-wishes.

15. **Tolle SW, Tilden VP, Nelson CA,** and **Dunn PM** (1998). 'A prospective study of the efficacy of the physician order form for life-sustaining treatment' [see comments]. *J Am Geriatr Soc* **46**(9): 1097–102.

16. **Cantor MD** (2000).' Improving advance care planning: lessons from POLST. Physician Orders for Life-Sustaining Treatment'. *J Am Geriatr Soc* **48**(10): 1343–4.

17. **Andersen RM, Yu H, Wyn R, Davidson PL, Brown ER, Teleki S** (2002). 'Access to medical care for low-income persons: how do communities make a difference?' *Medical care research and review: MCRR* **59**(4): 384–411.

18. **Brown BA** (2003). 'The history of advance directives. A literature review'. *J Gerontol Nur.* **29**(9): 4–14.

19. **Gostin LO** (1997). 'Deciding life and death in the courtroom. From Quinlan to Cruzan, Glucksberg, and Vacco—a brief history and analysis of constitutional protection of the "right to die"'. *Jama* **278**(18): 1523–8.

20. **Meisel A** (1992). The legal consensus about foregoing life-sustaining treatment: its status and its prospects. *Kennedy Institute of Ethics Journal* **2**(4): 309–45.

21. Omnibus Budget Reconciliation Act of 1990.

22. **Institute of Medicine** (1997). 'Approaching Death: Improving Care at the End of Life'. Field MJ CC, ed. Washington, DC: National Academy Press.

23. **Steinhauser KE, Christakis NA, Clipp EC** et al. (2000). 'Factors considered important at the end of life by patients, family, physicians, and other care providers'. *JAMA* **284**(19): 2476–82.

24. **Tonelli MR** (1996). 'Pulling the plug on living wills. A critical analysis of advance directives'. *Chest* **110**(3): 816–22.

25. **Teno JM, Licks S, Lynn J, Wenger N, Connors AF, Jr., Phillips RS**, et al. (1997). 'Do advance directives provide instructions that direct care? SUPPORT Investigators. Study to Understand Prognoses and Preferences for Outcomes and Risks of Treatment' [see comments]. *J Am Geriatr Soc* **45**(4): 508–12.

26. **Kass-Bartelmes BL** and **Rutherford HR** (2003). 'Advance care planning: preferences for care at the end of life'. Rockville, MD. *AHRQ* Contract No.: 03-0018.

27. **Teno JM, Stevens M, Spernak S**, and **Lynn J** (1998). 'Role of written advance directives in decision making: insights from qualitative and quantitative data'. *J Gen Intern Med* **13**(7): 439–46.

28. **Virmani J, Schneiderman LJ**, and **Kaplan RM** (1994). 'Relationship of advance directives to physician-patient communication'. *Arch Intern Med* **154**(8): 909–13.

29. **Silveira MJ, Wiitala W**, and **Piette J** (2014). 'Advance directive completion by elderly Americans: a decade of change'. *J Am Geriatr Soc* **62**(4): 706–10.

30. **Kwak J, Haley WE** (2005). 'Current research findings on end-of-life decision making among racially or ethnically diverse groups'. *Gerontologist* **45**(5): 634–41.

31. **Bullock K** (2011). 'The influence of culture on end-of-life decision making. Journal of social work in end-of-life & palliative care'. **7**(1): 83–98.

32. **Blackhall LJ, Frank G, Murphy ST, Michel V, Palmer JM**, and **Azen SP** (1999). 'Ethnicity and attitudes towards life sustaining technology'. *Social Science & Medicine* **48**(12): 1779–89.

33. **Brinkman-Stoppelenburg A, Rietjens JA**, and **van der Heide A** (2014). 'The effects of advance care planning on end-of-life care: a systematic review'. *Palliative medicine* **28**(8): 1000–25.

34. **Teno JM, Gruneir A, Schwartz Z, Nanda A**, and **Wetle T** (2007). 'Association between advance directives and quality of end-of-life care: a national study'. *J Am Geriatr Soc* **55**(2): 189–94.

35. **Auriemma CL, Nguyen CA, Bronheim R, Kent S, Nadiger S, Pardo D**, et al. (2014). 'Stability of End-of-Life Preferences: A Systematic Review of the Evidence'. *JAMA internal medicine* **174**(7): 1085–92.

36. **Silveira MJ, Kim SY**, and **Langa KM** (2010). 'Advance directives and outcomes of surrogate decision making before death'. *N Engl J Med* **362**(13) :1211–8.

37. **Fischer SM, Min SJ, Sauaia A**, and **Kutner JS** (2012). ' "They're going to unplug grandma": advance directive discussions and documentation do not decrease survival in patients and at baseline lower risk of death'. *Journal of hospital medicine*: an official publication of the Society of Hospital Medicine. **7**(1): 3–7.

38. **Schmidt TA, Zive D, Fromme EK, Cook JN**, and **Tolle SW** (2014). Physician orders for life-sustaining treatment (POLST): lessons learned from analysis of the Oregon POLST Registry. *Resuscitation* **85**(4): 480–5.

39. **Hickman SE, Nelson CA, Perrin NA, Moss AH, Hammes BJ**, and **Tolle SW** (2010). 'A comparison of methods to communicate treatment preferences in nursing facilities: traditional practices versus the physician orders for life-sustaining treatment program'. *J Am Geriatr Soc* **58**(7): 1241–8.

40. **Smucker WD, Ditto PH, Moore KA, Druley JA, Danks JH**, and **Townsend A** (1993). 'Elderly outpatients respond favorably to a physician-initiated advance directive discussion'. *The Journal of the American Board of Family Practice/American Board of Family Practice* **6**(5): 473–82.

41. **Zhang B, Wright AA, Huskamp HA, Nilsson ME, Maciejewski ML, Earle CC**, et al. (2009). 'Health care costs in the last week of life: associations with end-of-life conversations'. *Arch Intern Med* **169**(5): 480–8.

42. Tierney WM, Dexter PR, Gramelspacher GP, Perkins AJ, Zhou XH, and Wolinsky FD (2001). The effect of discussions about advance directives on patients' satisfaction with primary care. *Journal of General Internal Medicine* **16**(1): 32–40.

43. Kiely DK, Shaffer ML, and Mitchell SL (2012). 'Scales for the evaluation of end-of-life care in advanced dementia: sensitivity to change'. *Alzheimer Dis Assoc Disord* **26**(4): 358–63.

44. Lorenz KA, Lynn J, Dy SM, Shugarman LR, Wilkinson A, Mularski RA, et al. (2008). 'Evidence for improving palliative care at the end of life: a systematic review'. *Ann Intern Med* **148**(2): 147–59.

45. Hammes BJ and Rooney BL (1998). 'Death and end-of-life planning in one midwestern community'. *Arch Intern Med* **158**(4): 383–90.

46. Sudore RL, Knight SJ, McMahan RD, Feuz M, Farrell D, Miao Y, et al. (2014). 'A novel website to prepare diverse older adults for decision making and advance care planning: a pilot study'. *J Pain Symptom Manage* **47**(4): 674–86.

47. Gillick MR (1995). 'A broader role for advance medical planning'. *Ann Intern Med* **123**(8): 621–4.

# Chapter 21

# Advance care planning in New Zealand: our Voice—tō tātou reo

Leigh Manson and Shona Muir

'I feel more relaxed knowing that I won't be leaving my family guessing'
*NZ consumer*

---

**This chapter includes**

- A brief background of the development of advance care planning (ACP) in New Zealand; the ACP Cooperative (the Cooperative) and the ACP deployment model
- The deployment of ACP includes organisational and community engagement, health workforce and consumer education, system infrastructure and continuous quality improvement all underpinned by a conducive policy environment
- Information on the New Zealand ACP training programme

---

**Key Points**

- ACP in New Zealand has grown as a people's movement
- This people's movement is a whole of systems approach led by the national ACP Cooperative (the Cooperative)
- The approach has provided a permissive platform for the national evolution of ACP which has allowed ACP to quickly gain momentum
- It has facilitated collaboration of multiple interest groups with consumers at the centre and has provided an environment for innovation
- The movement has focused on engaging health sector leadership and the community, educating clinicians and the public, whilst keeping the patient and their family/whānau values at the centre of the process

---

**Key Message**

ACP in New Zealand is a systems approach to increasing consumer health literacy and engagement. While it is specifically crafted to help with end of life, the Cooperative is acutely aware that ACP forms the foundation of people powered health, the cornerstone of the transformation of the health sector.

## Introduction

This chapter will discuss the evolution of advance care planning (ACP) in New Zealand (NZ). Included in the discussion is a brief background of NZ demographics, detail on the ACP Cooperative (the Cooperative), and the ACP deployment model. The chapter will focus on the work undertaken in the engagement and education quadrants of the deployment model.

## Background on New Zealand

NZ is a collection of islands in the south western Pacific Ocean. The country is long and narrow with a landmass of 268,000 square kilometres and 18,000 kilometres of coastline (1). New Zealanders have a reputation for ingenuity, innovation, sporting accomplishments, and exploration.

NZ's population is 4.73 million (2), half of whom live in four main urban areas (3). In the 2013 census, 74% of NZ residents identified ethnically as European and 15% as Māori. Other major ethnic groups include Asian (12%) and Pacific peoples (seven per cent) (4).

The NZ government, through the Ministry of Health (MoH) leads and funds the healthcare system. Central funding of the health sector by the government is approximately $2.2 billion (NZD) per year. These funds are used to provide inpatient and out-patient hospital services, subsidies on prescription items and a range of support services for people in the community (5). There are 20 District Health Boards (DHBs) tasked with delivering care at local level.

In 2014, life expectancy of a New Zealander was 83.0 years for females, and 78.9 years for males (6). Compared with other industrialised nations NZ currently has a young population, however, the percentage of people 65 years and over is growing. By 2051 this group is projected to be around 1.14 million people, or 25% of the overall NZ population (6). The very elderly, those aged over 85 years, will increase to a quarter of a million people within the same timeframe (7). The major causes of death in NZ currently are ischaemic heart disease and cancer (8).

## The national advance care planning Cooperative

The Cooperative is a grass-roots movement of passionate people who advocate for and drive ACP activity in their spheres of influence. The group had its genesis in June 2010 when a small number of NZ healthcare staff attended the inaugural International Society of Advance Care Planning and End Of Life Care (ACPEL) conference in Melbourne, Australia. Prior to this, there were pockets of interest in ACP with a few organisations piloting ACP activities and exploring different models from Australia and the United Kingdom (UK), but there was no consistent or national approach.

Inspired by ACPEL, NZ attendees formed the Cooperative to drive a consistent approach to the development of ACP across NZ. The Cooperative's goal was that 'All people in New Zealand will have access to comprehensive, structured and effective Advance Care Planning' (9). Since then the Cooperative membership has grown from 60 to just over 1,500 members. Members include healthcare staff and those from the fields of ethics, disability representation, cultural teams, and consumers.

The Round Table governs the Cooperative and task teams work on specific components of the National ACP Programme as needed.

## The Cooperative advance care planning deployment model

The Cooperative Round Table reviewed the ACP deployment approaches used in Australia, the United States of America, Canada, and the UK. The Cooperative was looking for a whole of system approach with the individual at the centre of the healthcare initiative. The Canadian *'Advance*

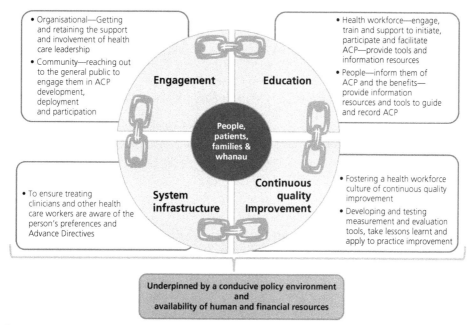

**Figure 21.1** New Zealand Advance Care Planning Deployment Model
Reproduced courtesy of the National ACP Programme

*Care Planning model: Four basic building blocks'* (10) met this 'whole of system' approach and was subsequently adapted by the Cooperative for NZ (see Figure 21.1).

The deployment model enabled the Cooperative to focus on the key ACP areas of patient-centric care provision, engagement, education, system infrastructure, continuous improvement and policy/funding. At the heart of the model, and of the ACP programme, were people, i.e. individuals, families, and whānau (11). Keeping people at the centre was the reason a co-design approach was used in the creation of the NZ ACP programme and all its resources. This model has ensured that the needs, values, and outcomes the person wanted for them self and their families/whānau were at the centre of the process.

## Organisational engagement

Securing and retaining the support and involvement of the leadership of the District Health Boards (DHBs) and others was a key challenge for the Cooperative, particularly as there was no consistent approach to ACP across the various organisations. The challenge was obtaining 'buy in' to the concept of a single national ACP service and set of resources for NZ. Consistency is a particular challenge within the NZ healthcare system where DHBs often act independently from one another. This can result in increased opportunity costs, confusion, and duplication. From an individual's perspective, one national plan and consistent information across the country is preferable.

For the first four years, the Cooperative membership met quarterly via videoconferencing during which individuals and organisations showcased developments in their area. Whilst these three-hour sessions were informative, the videoconferencing became increasingly challenging logistically as the number of participants increased. Latterly, best practice sharing and ACP promotion was done through distribution of a quarterly newsletter. In November 2016, the inaugural Advance Care Planning National Forum bolstered sharing developments and promoting ACP.

Hosting the forum was a joint venture between the Cooperative and the Health Quality and Safety Commission.

The Cooperative promoted its vision and established relationships with each of NZ's 20 DHBs, leading non-government organisations, such as, Hospice and the Cancer Society, education organisations, registration bodies, and others. Cross-sectoral work with the Ministry of Social Development and bodies such as Age Concern is also being undertaken. The Cooperative is recognised as the national lead for ACP in New Zealand.

The Cooperative has effectively engaged with most of the healthcare organisations in NZ and successfully supports local and regional leaders to fund and promote the Cooperative approach. The ACP training and consumer information resources developed by the Cooperative are consistently used by all healthcare organisations.

## Community engagement

In 2010 New Zealanders did not routinely think about, talk about, and plan for future healthcare and treatment. Because of this, individuals and their family/whānau were not empowered to make treatment decisions that supported the outcomes they wanted for themselves. In recognition of the need to socialise the idea of ACP with the public, and to provide information and a service that met their needs, the Cooperative worked with consumers from the outset. The ACP programme and all the information resources, for example: guides, pamphlets, websites, awareness campaigns, and a short film were created with consumers using the co-design methodology.

Co-design is, 'a way of improving healthcare services with patients. Many service improvement projects have patient involvement but co-design focuses on understanding and improving patients' experiences of services as well as the services themselves' (12). Through co-design consumers have determined what an ACP service should look like, what resources are required, branding, and how individuals should be enabled to engage with ACP resources. In addition, consumer participation in the Advance Care Planning National Forum successfully increased the profile of consumer experiences. This highlighted the urgency to increase ACP activity for attendees from the health sector.

ACP is personal to each and every one of us. Tapping into this, the Cooperative launched Conversations that Count (CtC) Day a national annual ACP awareness raising campaign. This is held on the 16 April to coincide with the ACP awareness days in the US and Canada. The day aims to get people thinking and talking about what matters to them, and how they might want to plan their future and end of life care. A national steering group comprised of key ACP staff and consumers lead the campaign. Each year, the campaign theme and approach is decided through co-design and with input from specialist communication and design teams. To support and enable local ACP activity on the day, printed resources and communication briefs are distributed across NZ.

Within healthcare settings, 'morning tea' with ACP was used to encourage clinical teams to take time out over a cup of tea and talk about ACP and how they might increase conversations with their patients.

Since 2015, CtC Day activity has included promotion of ACP by Tammy Wells, a NZ television celebrity. Twitter and Facebook have also been used to actively promote ACP during the campaigns.

## Community education

A desire by consumers to advocate for ACP within their own communities was identified during the co-design workshops with consumers and through feedback from the national awareness campaigns. The Cooperative developed a programme with the community called CtC Training to up-skill train volunteers to deliver community education sessions, initiate conversations and raise awareness of ACP.

## Health-workforce education

At the inaugural meeting of the Cooperative in 2010 the need for a clinical training programme for ACP was identified as a key component of successful deployment. A training task team was formed to investigate this further. The Cooperative learnt that the greatest barrier to staff increasing ACP activity was a lack of skill and confidence to start ACP conversations. This was supported by research which showed that the health workforce did not have the necessary skills required to support patients and their families/whānau to think about what is important to them, talk about how that might impact on the choices they might make, and how to plan for their future health and treatment (13).

The task team developed a Competency Framework (see Figure 21.2). Training for the skills and knowledge required by each level of competency was not readily available in NZ. While some could be developed by the Cooperative, the advanced communication component required for Level 2 and the training of Level 3 facilitators could not. After discussions with Australia, Canada, and the UK it was decided that the CONNECTED (14) Group within the NHS was the best option. CONNECTED agreed to adapt their evidence-based and proven advanced communication course for the NZ ACP Programme. This was done in partnership with the Cooperative training programme leads.

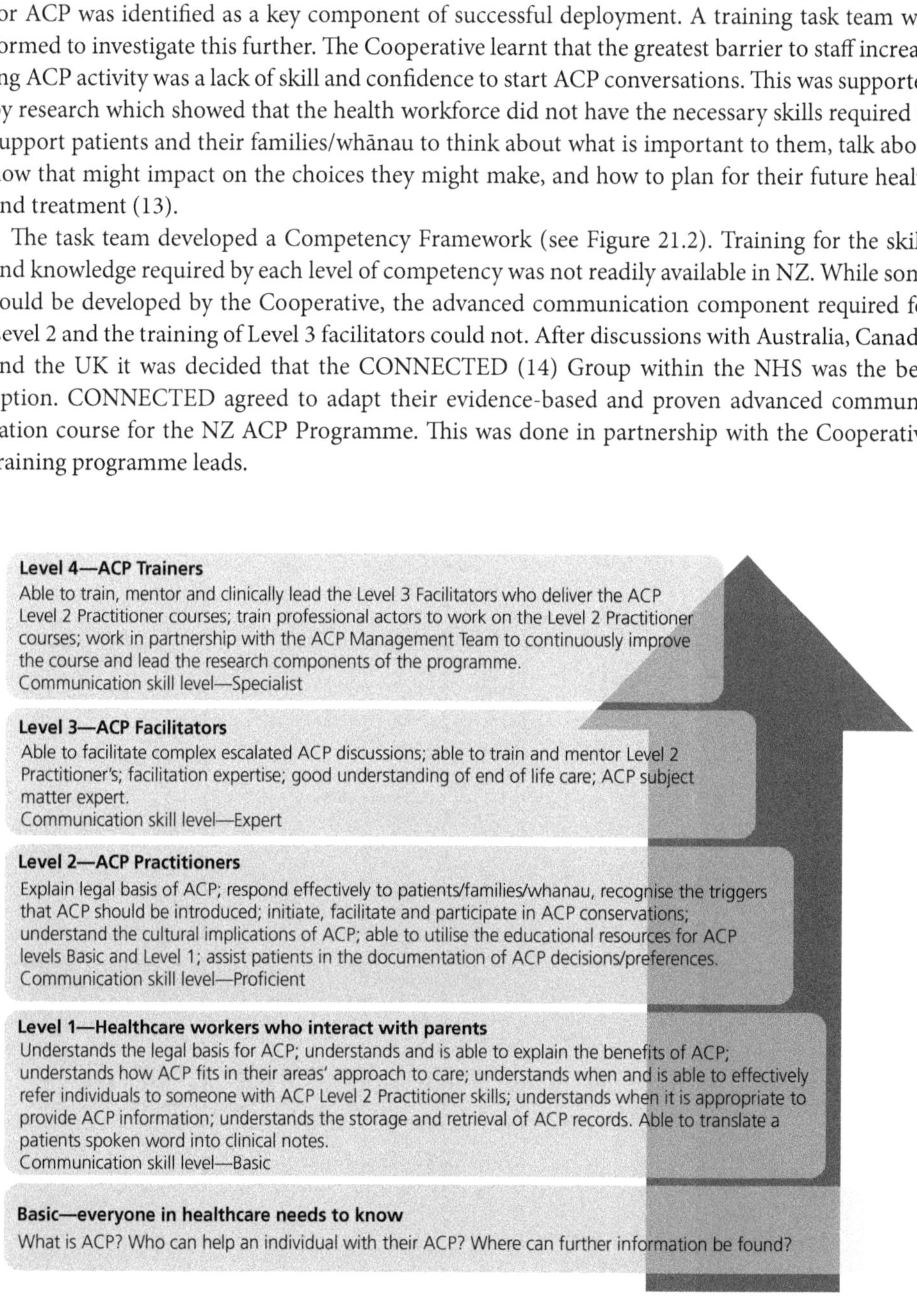

**Level 4—ACP Trainers**
Able to train, mentor and clinically lead the Level 3 Facilitators who deliver the ACP Level 2 Practitioner courses; train professional actors to work on the Level 2 Practitioner courses; work in partnership with the ACP Management Team to continuously improve the course and lead the research components of the programme.
Communication skill level—Specialist

**Level 3—ACP Facilitators**
Able to facilitate complex escalated ACP discussions; able to train and mentor Level 2 Practitioner's; facilitation expertise; good understanding of end of life care; ACP subject matter expert.
Communication skill level—Expert

**Level 2—ACP Practitioners**
Explain legal basis of ACP; respond effectively to patients/families/whanau, recognise the triggers that ACP should be introduced; initiate, facilitate and participate in ACP conservations; understand the cultural implications of ACP; able to utilise the educational resources for ACP levels Basic and Level 1; assist patients in the documentation of ACP decisions/preferences.
Communication skill level—Proficient

**Level 1—Healthcare workers who interact with parents**
Understands the legal basis for ACP; understands and is able to explain the benefits of ACP; understands how ACP fits in their areas' approach to care; understands when and is able to effectively refer individuals to someone with ACP Level 2 Practitioner skills; understands when it is appropriate to provide ACP information; understands the storage and retrieval of ACP records. Able to translate a patients spoken word into clinical notes.
Communication skill level—Basic

**Basic—everyone in healthcare needs to know**
What is ACP? Who can help an individual with their ACP? Where can further information be found?

**Figure 21.2** Overview of the ACP Competency Framework
Reproduced courtesy of the National ACP Programme

## The ACP training programme

The NZ ACP Training Programme follows a modular framework (Figure 21.3). There are 13 modules moving through basic to Level 4.

## Basic training ('What is ACP?')

Basic training is provided through the ACP website (www.advancecareplanning.org.nz) and includes a short film which explains what ACP is, discusses the benefits of ACP for patients and

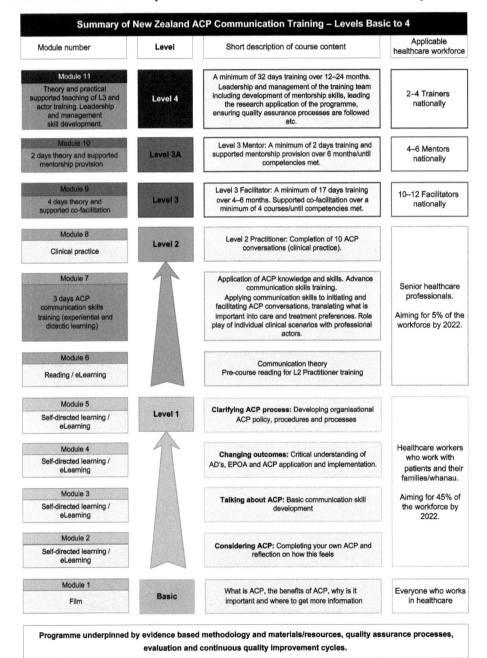

**Figure 21.3** The New Zealand ACP Training Programme

Reproduced courtesy of the National ACP Programme

healthcare staff, and explains where to find further information. This is an open-access resource for both the general public and healthcare staff. This resource was developed after co-design input from the healthcare sector and the general public. Basic training is not evaluated.

## Level 1 e-learning training ('How can I start a conversation with a patient or my loved one?')

ACP Level 1 (L1) training is provided through four e-learning modules on the ACP website:

1. **Considering ACP**—healthcare staff write their own ACP so they understand the process and are better placed to support patients to complete an ACP.
2. **Talking about ACP**—basic communication skill information.
3. **Changing outcomes**—the legal and ethical framework around clinical decision making.
4. **Clarifying ACP process**—creating systems and processes to facilitate recording and retrieving ACP conversations and plans.

The L1 e-learning training modules started in August 2013. The online modules are compulsory pre-work for both the Level 1A workshop and the Level 2 practitioner training. Level 1A participants evaluate the e-learning modules in the written feedback they provide at the end of Level 1A training.

## Level 1A one day workshop ('How do I convert an individual's spoken word into clinical notes?')

The one-day workshop consolidates the online modules and supports healthcare staff to hear and translate a patient or individual's spoken word into clinical notes. One of the workshop aims is to ensure ACP conversations are noted in clinical documents in a way that they can be developed further during subsequent staff and patient interactions see Figure 21.4).

The workshop is evaluated through participant self-assessments. These evaluations consistently show a statistically significant increase in confidence to document ACP conversations post-course.

Since May 2016, 309 healthcare practitioners have attend this training (62% nurses, 7.4% doctors, 17% allied health, and 13.5% other) with 92% of participants noting they would **definitely recommend** the course to other healthcare staff (14).

## Level 2 advance care planning practitioner training ('How can I improve my communication and better facilitate in-depth advance care planning conversations?')

Level 2 (L2) training is evidence-based training (15,16,17) delivered to a maximum of ten delegates per course and involves experienced facilitated communication practice with professional actors. Actors are specifically taught to work in the role-play component of the training. The 2013 Cochrane Review (18) supports this approach to teaching communication skills. Figure 21.5 provides an overview of the Level 2 training.

Key competencies for Level 2 practitioners include:

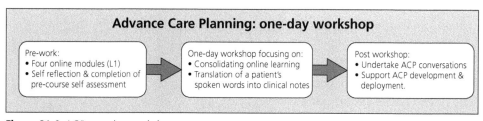

**Figure 21.4** ACP one-day workshop

Reproduced courtesy of the National ACP Programme

◆ Acknowledging your own feelings and experiences and how that might impact on ACP facilitation

◆ Explaining ACP and its benefits

◆ Responding appropriately to patient cues

◆ Initiating discussion with patients identified as potentially benefiting from ACP

◆ Contextualising a person's culture into discussions

◆ Demonstrating empathy and active listening skills

◆ Acknowledging emotions

◆ Assisting people to frame what is important to them and helping them to translate that into treatment preferences

Since February 2012, 1,140 healthcare practitioners have attend Level 2 training (63% nurses, 18% doctors, 12% allied health, and 7% other) (19).

Analysis of the participant self-assessment pre-and post-course confidence scores show statistically significant increases in confidence to:

◆ Explain what ACP is, structure conversations, and explain the benefits of ACP

◆ Explain the NZ legal and ethical framework

◆ Develop patient cues and work with patient's agenda

◆ Discuss future care options

◆ Discuss with patients that they might be dying

Positive feedback was received in both the course evaluation forms and post-course communication, for example:

◆ 'This is one of the best learning experiences of my professional career. . . Since doing the course I am applying the things I learnt, and this has made a very positive difference to my practice. I would recommend this course to all health professionals. It has changed the way I communicate with staff, patients and even at home with family and friends.'—Healthcare professional

◆ 'We all felt safe and encouraged. Pushed us out of comfort zone skillfully.'—General Practitioner

◆ 'Post course: I have reflected on the course content more than I normally would, over the last few weeks; and as part of the commitment is to engage in ACP conversations this has kept this learning alive. I have enjoyed sharing my experiences of the course with colleagues and family.'—Primary health care nursing practice development leader

Since January 2012, 93% of individuals who have attended the Level 2 training noted they would **definitely recommend** the course to other healthcare staff.

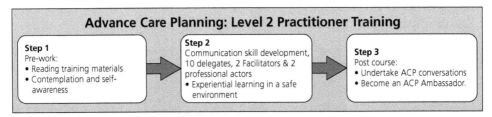

**Figure 21.5** ACP Level 2 Practitioner course detail

Reproduced courtesy of the National ACP Programme

## Level 3 facilitators: a train-the-trainer model for training Level 2 practitioners

Level 3 facilitators are trained by Level 4 trainers to deliver Level 2 practitioner courses. The training takes place over four to six months and includes theoretical classroom based teaching, mentored Level 2 course delivery, and continuing personal development plan review and assessment.

The ten Level 3 facilitators working on the programme include: renal, palliative care and gerontology consultants, a nurse practitioner, clinical nurse specialists, senior nurses, and a university lecturer. Level 3 facilitators have delivered 23 Level 1A workshops and 120 Level 2 courses.

Feedback has been positive with participants noting that the training meets their needs and prepares them for the role they undertake on the programme.

## Level 4 trainers: clinical leads for the training programme

Level 4 training is only open to Level 3 facilitators. Level 4 trainers also deliver Level 2 courses and are the clinical experts for the programme who work alongside the management team to ensure course content and training approaches remain current and effective.

The remaining components of the deployment model are summarised below:

- **Continuous Quality Improvement.** All the Cooperative work is underpinned by continuous quality improvement. All aspects of the programme are evidence or best practice based with robust data collection, analysis, review, innovation, and iteration practices. The improvement approach is based on a hybrid model of lean six sigma and co-design which enables the Cooperative to easily adapt to the evolving nature of end of life care and ACP.

- **Systems and Infrastructure.** A national ACP information system is required to support the use and retrieval of ACP Plans and documented conversations. The deployment model focus on systems ensures that accessibility to electronically held ACP conversations and plans is considered as various healthcare organisations' IT systems evolve. Nationally several information technology projects are underway to develop systems to share clinical records across secondary care services, primary care, community pharmacies, and aged residential care homes. Despite an increase in the availability of documented conversations and plans online, a national solution remains a number of years away.

- **Under pinned by policy.** The development and use of ACP policies and processes for organisations and services is encouraged and supported as best practice. Over the past six years NZ health policy has grown from little awareness of ACP to acknowledging, clarifying, and most recently incorporating ACP into policy. This includes ACP and related policy initiation and development at organisational, regional, and national level.

# National growth and support for advance care planning

Everyone approached and engaged with in the six years of the NZ programme has embraced ACP, and the core principles that underpin it. This includes NGOs, the cancer networks, the public trust, law societies, the disability community, aged residential care facilities, St Johns (ambulance service), New Zealand Medical Association, Royal New Zealand College of General Practitioners, New Zealand Nurses Organisation, and the Health and Disability Commissioner. Across New Zealand, there has been almost universal adoption of the Cooperative's approach, the training programme, website, and printed resources.

In 2011, the Ministry of Health published *Advance Care Planning: A guide for the New Zealand health care workforce* (20) and in 2014 New Zealand Ethical Advisory Commission published Advice on the ethical challenges healthcare professionals face in ACP (21).

Increasing recognition of the benefit and value of ACP across the NZ health sector has resulted in ACP being included as a specific action of the *New Zealand Health Strategy* 2016 (22), a key component of a respectful end of life in the *Healthy Ageing Strategy* (23), and an action in many district health board strategies (24,25,26,27,28,29).

## Conclusion

ACP is a systems approach to increasing consumer health literacy and engagement. While it is specifically crafted to help with the end of life, the Cooperative is acutely aware that ACP forms the foundation of people-powered health, the cornerstone of the transformation of the health sector.

ACP in NZ has grown as a people's movement, resourced by passionate individuals across the country supported by their organisations. Until very recently, it was led largely by staff at the Auckland District Health Board with some regional (Northern Regional Alliance) and national (Health Workforce New Zealand) funding. This model has provided a permissive platform for the national evolution of ACP and has allowed ACP to quickly gain momentum. It has facilitated collaboration of multiple interest groups with consumers at the centre and has provided an environment for innovation. From September 2016, ACP has been included in the remit of the National Health Quality Safety Commission with national funding from all the district health boards.

The Cooperative's hope is that the people who make up NZ healthcare workforce systematically seek to understand what matters to individuals i.e. what outcomes they want for themselves and their families/whānau, and work with them to provide the care and treatment that supports that. The continued evolution of ACP into how we do things for all people, not only those approaching the end of their lives, is an opportunity not to be missed.

## References

1. **King, M** (2003). *The Penguin history of New Zealand*. Auckland: Penguin Group.
2. **Statistics New Zealand** [internet] (2016). *New Zealand: Population Clock*. Available from: http://www.stats.govt.nz/tools_and_services/population_clock.aspx. (Accessed 1 Dec 2016.)
3. **The New Zealand Government** [internet] (2015). *The Encyclopaedia of New Zealand*. Available from: http://www.teara.govt.nz/en/society/page-2. (Accessed 1 Dec 2016.)
4. **New Zealand Government** [internet] (2015). *Statistics New Zealand*. (.) Available from http://www.stats.govt.nz/Census/2013-census/profile-and-summary-reports/infographic-culture-identity.aspx. (Accessed 1 Dec 2016.)
5. **IndexMundi** [internet] (2016). *New Zealand life expectancy at birth*. Available from: http://www.indexmundi.com/new_zealand/life_expectancy_at_birth.html. (Accessed 1 Dec 2016.)
6. **Statistics New Zealand** [internet] (2016). *Population Aging in New Zealand*. Available from: http://www.stats.govt.nz/browse_for_stats/people_and_communities/older_people/pop-ageing-in-nz.aspx. (Accessed 1 Dec 2016.)
7. **Statistics New Zealand** [internet] (2016). *Population Aging in New Zealand*. Available from: http://www.stats.govt.nz/browse_for_stats/people_and_communities/older_people/pop-ageing-in-nz.aspx. (Accessed 1 Dec 2016.)
8. **Ministry of Health** [internet] (2015). *Major causes of death (all ages)*. Available from: http://www.health.govt.nz/nz-health-statistics/health-statistics-and-data-sets/maori-health-data-and-stats/tatau-kahukura-maori-health-chart-book/nga-mana-hauora-tutohu-health-status-indicators/major-causes-death-all-ages. (Accessed 1 Dec 2016.)

9. **The Ministry of Health** [internet] (2011). *Advance Care Planning: A guide for the New Zealand Workforce.* Auckland: Ministry of Health; 2011. Available from: https://www.health.govt.nz/system/files/documents/publications/advance-care-planning-aug11.pdf. (Accessed 1 Dec 2016.)

10. **Health Canada** [internet] (2008). *Implementation Guide to Advance Care Planning in Canada: A Case Study of Two Health Authorities.* Available from: http://www.hc-sc.gc.ca/hcs-sss/alt_formats/pdf/pubs/palliat/2008-acp-guide-pps/acp-guide-pps-eng.pdf (Accessed 1 Dec 2016.)

11. *Māori for family—however the concept is much wider and extends to a family grouping spanning generations, other familial bonds or close friends.*

12. **Boyd H, McKeron S,** and **Old A** (2010). *Health Service Co-design: Working with patients to improve healthcare services.* Auckland: Waitemata District Health Board, p. 4.

13. **John J. Harford Foundation** (2016). [internet]. *We need to talk: How conversations starters' can improve advance care planning.* Available from: http://m.marketwired.com/press-release/we-need-to-talk-how-conversation-starters-can-improve-advance-care-planning-2180204.htm (Accessed 1 Dec 2016.)

14. **NHS England.** *Communication training team who have an international reputation for excellence in evidence based communication training.*

15. **ACP Training Programme: Level 1A Evaluation Database.** (Accessed 13 Feb 2016.)

16. **Maguire P, Booth K, Elliott C,** and **Jones B** (1996). 'Helping health professionals involved in cancer care acquire key interviewing skills—The impact of workshops'. *European Journal of Cancer.* **32A**: 1486–9.

17. **Fallowfield L, Jenkins V, Farewell V, Saul J, Duffy A, Eves R** (2002). 'Efficacy of a Cancer Research UK communication skills training model for oncologists: a randomised controlled trial'. *Lancet* **359**(9307): 650–6.

18. **Wilkinson S, Perry R, Blanchard K,** and **Linsell L** (2008). 'Effectiveness of a three-day communication skills course in changing nurses' communication skills with cancer/palliative care patients: a randomised controlled trial'. *Palliative Medicine* **4**: 365–75. doi: 10.1177/0269216308090770.

19. **Moore PM, Rivera MS, Grez Artigues M, Lawrie TA** (2013). 'Communication skills training for healthcare professionals working with people who have cancer'. *Cochrane Database of Systematic Reviews* **3**: CD003751. doi: 10.1002/14651858.CD003751.pub3.

20. **ACP Training Programme: Level 2 Evaluation Database.** (Accessed 13 Dec 2016.)

21. **The Ministry of Health** [internet] (2011). *Advance Care Planning: A guide for the New Zealand Workforce.* Auckland: Ministry of Health; 2011. Available from: https://www.health.govt.nz/system/files/documents/publications/advance-care-planning-aug11.pdf (Accessed 1 Dec 2016.)

22. **Health Quality and Safety Commission** [internet] (2015). *About the commission.* Available from: https://www.hqsc.govt.nz/about-the-commission/. (Accessed 1 Dec 2016.)

23. **Minister of Health** [**internet**] (2016). *New Zealand Health Strategy: Future direction.* Wellington: Ministry of Health; 2016. Available from: http://www.health.govt.nz/publication/new-zealand-health-strategy-2016 (Accessed 1 Dec 2016.)

24. **Ministry of Health** [**internet**] (2016). *Health of Older People Strategy: Consultation draft.* Available from: http://www.health.govt.nz/our-work/life-stages/health-older-people/health-older-people-strategy-update (Accessed 1 Dec 2016.)

25. **Bay of Plenty DHB** [**internet**] (2015). *Annual Plan 2015/16 Incorporating the statement of intent and statement of performance expectations.* Available from: http://www.bopdhb.govt.nz/media/58478/bopdhb_2015-16_annual_plan.pdf (Accessed 13 Dec 2016.)

26. **Auckland District Health Board** [**internet**] **Strategy** (2020). Available from: http://www.adhb.health.nz/assets/Documents/About-Us/Planning-documents/Master-ADHB-Strategy-25-August-2016.pdf (Accessed 5 Dec 2016.)

27. **Waitemata District Health Board** [internet] (2015/16). *Annual Plan Incorporating the statement of intent and statement of performance expectations.* Available from: http://www.waitematadhb.govt.nz/dhb- planning/organisation-wide-planning/annual-plan/ (Accessed 13 Dec 2016.)

28. **South Canterbury DHB** [internet] (2016/17). Annual Plan 2016–17 Which incorporates Statement of intent 2016–20 statement of performance expectations 2016–17. Available from: http://www.scdhb. health.nz/__data/assets/pdf_file/0018/95022/Annual-Plan-2016-17.pdf (Accessed 1 Dec 2016.)

29. **Hutt Valley DHB** [internet] Annual Plan (2016–17). Incorporating Statement of intent and statement of performance expectations 2016/17–2019/20. Available from: http://www.huttvalleydhb.org.nz/ about-us/reports-and-publications/annual-plan/2016-17-hutt-valley-dhb-annual-plan.pdf (Accessed 13 Dec 2016.)

Chapter 22

# Advance care planning in Germany: on track for nationwide implementation

Georg Marckmann, Kornelia Götze, and Jürgen in der Schmitten

---

**This chapter includes**

- Background to advance care planning (ACP) and advance directives in Germany
- The ACP programme *'beizeiten begleiten®'* and the RESPEKT study
- Information on national legislation in Germany
- The work of the German ACP task force
- Barriers to and reflections on the implementation of ACP in Germany

---

**Key Points**

- ACP is a rather new development in Germany
- Despite legal regulation of advance directives in 2009, there was limited uptake
- The German ACP programme *beizeiten begleiten®*, based on Respecting Choices(R), has demonstrated success, firstly at a regional level, and more recently at national level

---

**Key Message**

With new legislation in place, Germany has a regulatory basis for the nationwide implementation of ACP. However, major obstacles are yet to be overcome. Over the next few years it will become clearer as to whether the nationwide ACP implementation in German nursing homes and institutions caring for people with disability will live up to the high-quality standards of comprehensive regional ACP programmes like Respecting Choices and *beizeiten begleiten®*. Also, ACP must soon become a regular healthcare service also for wider target populations.

# Introduction

While respect for patient autonomy is a constitutive element of the legal frame for medical practice, Advance Care Planning (ACP) is a rather new development in the German healthcare system. A first attempt to develop and introduce a regional ACP programme (in the region of Münster) was to some extent successful locally (1). Beyond local implementation, however, it received little national or scientific attention. From 2008–11, the Federal Ministry for Research and Education funded the first prospective inter-regionally controlled trial of the regional implementation of *beizeiten begleiten*°, a German ACP programme adapted from the US programme Respecting Choices.

In September 2015 the fifth International Society on Advance Care Planning and End of Life Care (ACPEL) conference in Munich was held. This provided both a platform for the exchange of research results and implementation experiences from around the world and stimulated the ACP development in Germany.

In December 2015 legislation was enacted which provides funding from the sickness funds to German nursing homes and care institutions if they offer ACP to their residents. This was part of a broader initiative of the Federal Ministry of Health to improve the care for seriously ill patients approaching the end of life. Currently, the details of the implementation are negotiated between the sickness funds and the nursing home organisations. With this legislation, Germany has become one of the few countries in the world which has a financing framework for the national implementation of ACP. However, this is currently limited to nursing homes and care institutions for people with disabilities.

This chapter explains the historical and legal background of advance decision-making in Germany, reports the experiences of the regional ACP programme *beizeiten begleiten*, and describes the current process of implementing ACP in German nursing and care homes. We conclude with reflections on the upcoming challenges for implementing ACP in Germany.

# Background

## Germany's health insurance

Germany has one of the oldest statutory health insurance systems in the world covering almost 90% of the population. The remaining 10% opt for private health insurance which is open for individuals above a certain income threshold or self-employed persons (only some 0.2% who fall through the statutory network have no healthcare coverage, e.g. certain self-employed people or illegal immigrants). The legal frame of the system, including statutory provisions for the coverage of healthcare services, is laid down in the fifth Social Code Book (Sozialgesetzbuch V, SGB V). The details of the statutory health insurance plan are negotiated between the national representatives of physicians, dentists, hospitals and sickness funds in the Federal Joint Committee (Gemeinsamer Bundesausschuss, G-BA). The G-BA specifies which services are covered by the statutory health insurance system. Any ACP initiatives have to be implemented within this general regulatory and organisational framework.

## Advance directives in Germany

Written documents in which individuals specify how they want to be treated when they have lost decision-making capacity were first mentioned in Germany as a 'patient letter', later 'patient will' and then 'patient advance directive' in the late 1970s. Nevertheless, advance directives (ADs) did not receive much attention during the following two decades, and the prevalence of ADs in Germany remained at a low level of 2.5% in 1998 (2). After the turn of the century, however, there was increasing discussion in medical and legal communities about appropriate standards of substitute decision-making. A first high court ruling stated that patients' prior wishes have to be respected in decisions about life-sustaining treatment when the patient has lost decision-making capacity (XII ZB 2/03, 17.03.2003).

The prevalence of ADs, however, remained low. In 2007, a cross-sectional survey in all 11 nursing homes of a German city, which included 1,089 residents, showed only 11% of the residents had a personal AD and a further 1,4% an AD by proxy (3). Most ADs were of questionable validity and did not cover relevant clinical scenarios like acute care decisions. 23 of the analysed 119 ADs implied a DNR status for the currently given chronic condition (i.e. incapability of decision making due to severe dementia), but in 14 (61%) of these cases, the responsible nursing staff declared that in case of cardiac arrest the residents would be resuscitated.

After controversial discussions in parliament and society over many years and a number of failed attempts to introduce legislation, ADs finally received legal standing in 2009 (4). Accordingly, medical treatment preferences in written ADs must be respected for incapacitated patients (just like actual informed decisions) if they apply to the medical situation at hand, irrespective of the stage or prognosis of the disease. In absence of a written AD, the decisions have to follow prior oral wishes or substituted judgements about what the patient would have chosen if he or she had decision-making capacity. Furthermore, regardless of whether there is an AD or not, the law strengthens the position of the legal proxy who is strictly obliged to act in line with the will of the patient and has to discuss both the medical situation and the advance directive (or the presumed wishes) with the treating physician in a process of shared decision-making. Although not explicitly laid down in law, it is now widely accepted that also in the absence of a proxy, physicians and other healthcare staff are to follow the written AD to the best of their understanding.

However, as in other countries, the legal regulation of ADs did not impact on the prevalence and quality of ADs in Germany. Still, only ten to 20% of the population have completed an AD (5,6). Counselling for advance directives (be it facilitation in the sense of ACP, or any advice or information) is not legally required and not offered regularly; where it is provided, it varies considerably in content and quality (7). As a consequence, the requirements for effectively respecting patients' wishes when they have lost decision-making capacity are currently not fulfilled in Germany. Specifically, less than one fifth of the elderly population has completed ADs, and these ADs often do not cover clinically relevant situations, are of questionable validity, are not available when needed, and are not honoured reliably by medical staff (3,8).

## The advance care planning programme *beizeiten begleiten*® and the RESPEKT study

In the 1990s, a conceptual alternative to traditional ADs emerged in the US (9,10): ACP programmes which provide both a qualified facilitation process preceding every single AD (on the micro-level) and the systematic implementation of standards and routines how to handle and honour effectively the resulting ADs (on the meso-, i.e. institutional, and macro-, i.e. regional level). With funding of the German Federal Ministry of Education and Research, GM, JidS and others developed a regional ACP programme based on the US ACP-programme Respecting Choices (11). The programme *beizeiten begleiten*® was implemented as a prospective, interregionally controlled study assessing the effect of the ACP intervention (see Table 22.1) on the prevalence and quality of ADs in nursing homes (12). Data from 136 residents in the three intervention nursing homes were compared with the data from 439 residents in ten control nursing homes.

**Table 22.1** The Seven Elements of the German regional ACP programme *beizeiten begleiten®* (6), closely derived from the 'Five Promises' of the US programme Respecting Choices

| 1 | Active promotion | All persons in the target population are offered professional assistance in ACP and completing an AD |
|---|---|---|
| 2 | Qualified support (facilitation) | Specifically trained medical and non-medical personnel supports the development and documentation of treatment preferences for hypothetical future medical decisions |
| 3 | Professional documentation | Preferences are documented in standard forms providing clear instructions also for emergency care |
| 4 | Archiving, access and transfer | The regional institutions establish standards and routines to guarantee that the ADs are available when needed |
| 5 | Regular updating | ACP is an ongoing communicative process involving regular updates, especially after changes in health status |
| 6 | Reliably consideration in clinical practice | All regional healthcare personnel are trained to reliably honour the documented wishes in patient care |
| 7 | Continuous quality insurance | Mechanisms are established to continuously monitor and improve process and outcome quality of the ACP system |

The core of the intervention consisted of offering professional ACP facilitation to the residents and their proxies to support ACP and the completion of a written AD after at least two conversations. The non-physician facilitators received a 20-hour training course, the cooperating primary care physicians four hours of training (plus two two-hour meetings later on), complemented by educational sessions for the nursing home and hospital staff, medical and paramedic emergency staff, and professional guardians. Given the low quality of widespread AD forms in Germany, the following standardised forms were developed:

1. Personal ADs for residents with decision-making capacity

2. ADs completed by the legal surrogate decision-makers (ADs by proxy (13,14)) for the legal representatives of residents with permanent loss of decision-making capacity

3. A physician order for life-sustaining treatment in emergency situations (POLST-E) (15), adapted from the US POLST form

Evaluation showed a significant increase in ADs in the intervention nursing homes compared to control nursing homes during the 16.5 month observation period from February 2009 to June 2010 (see Table 22.2). Due to the high number of residents with permanent loss of decision-making capacity and no prior ACP, considerably more ADs by proxy than personal ADs were completed during the observation period (30 vs. 19). The difference was considerable and statistically significant, even though the control region performed better than another set of nursing homes we had studied earlier (3). Importantly, not only the number but also the quality of the ADs increased: in the intervention group more ADs included the designation of a proxy (94.7% vs. 50.0%), were signed by a third party (95.9% vs. 77.8%), particularly by a physician (93.9% vs. 16.7%), included an emergency plan (POLST-E, 98% vs. 44.4%), and clearly defined the resuscitation status (95.9% vs. 38.9%) (6).

RESPEKT was the first study to demonstrate the feasibility and procedural efficacy of introducing a regional ACP programme in Germany. Internationally, it was the first prospective inter-regionally controlled study of the implementation of an ACP programme. In contrast to other

**Table 22.2** Incidence of new ADs during the intervention period and prevalence of ADs at the end of the intervention period (6)

| *New* advance directives since t0 (incidence) | IR (n=136) | CR (n=439) | P |
|---|---|---|---|
| Personal ADs | 19 (14.0%) | 8 (1.8%) | <0.001 |
| ADs by proxy | 30 (22.1%) | 10 (2.3%) | <0.001 |
| All ADs | 49 (36.0%) | 18 (4.1%) | <0.001 |
| **All directives at t1 (prevalence)** | | | |
| Personal ADs | 40 (29.4%) | 83 (18.9%) | 0.092 |
| ADs by proxy | 33 (24.3%) | 33 (7.5%) | <0.001 |
| All ADs | 71 (52.2%) | 109 (24.8%) | <0.001 |

Source: data from in der Schmitten J et al. (2014) 'Implementing an Advance Care Planning Program in German Nursing Homes', *Deutsches Ärzteblatt International*, Volume 111, Issue 4, pp. 50–7, doi: 10.3238/arztebl.2014.0050

implementations in Canada (16) and Australia (17), but in line with the Respecting Choices programme in La Crosse (11), our study chose the regional rather than the institutional or individual level as the focus of the intervention, because the systemic changes required for improved respect of patients' prior preferences cannot be achieved at an institutional level alone. However, in this study it was not possible to investigate whether the regional ACP programme had a significant impact on clinically relevant endpoints like unwanted days in hospital. Further studies are therefore required in order to evaluate the outcome quality of comprehensive ACP programmes in Germany.

## National legislation to implement advance care planning in German nursing homes and care institutions

In 2014, after completion of the RESPEKT study and publication of the results (6), GM and JidS approached the Federal Ministry of Health and presented ACP as a viable concept to realise shared decision-making and a valid informed consent process for patients' choices on future medical treatment, thus strengthening the autonomy of patients, especially when they have become fragile and vulnerable as in old age, chronic multimorbidity, and care dependency.

At that time, the Ministry had a legislative proposal in preparation which aimed to strengthen hospice and palliative care (Hospiz- und Palliativgesetz [HPG]). The Ministry endorsed the concept of ACP (18) and concluded that implementation of ACP in Germany would be a worthwhile investment and a justified use of limited public healthcare resources (19). As a first step, the Ministry decided to include a new paragraph 132g into the Social Code Book V (as an element of the then coming law, the HPG) which would warrant funding for facilitated ACP conversations to residents of nursing homes and institutions caring for people with disabilities. The Ministry was aware that this initiative would narrowly focus ACP on a population which, on the one hand has probably the highest need for ACP, but, on the other hand, is already (often chronically) incapable of decision making. In the best case scenario, ACP in these settings will become a nucleus for wider implementation of ACP in the ambulatory care sector.

In September 2015, GM and JidS hosted the fifth International Society for Advance Care Planning and End of Life Care (ACPEL) Conference in Munich (www.acpel2015.org). In addition to facilitating the exchange of recent international advances in research and implementation in the field of ACP, the conference contributed also to the ACP implementation process in Germany. Firstly and importantly, participants from all over Germany interested in implementing ACP in their institution or region got valuable input and inspiration from successful international ACP programmes. Secondly, a workshop on the implementation of the new §132g involved key representatives of the Federal Ministry of Health, the National Association of Statutory Health Insurance Funds, and representatives of the nursing and care home organisations. Thus, these leaders were able to encounter and better appreciate the still unfamiliar concept of ACP and learn from national and international experiences.

In December 2015, the German parliament passed the Hospice and Palliative Care Law which included the new 'ACP paragraph' 132g. Accordingly, care institutions can receive funding from the sickness funds for qualified healthcare staff, so they can offer individualised professional guidance and information to their residents. These facilitated conversations enable residents to make informed and well-reflected decisions about future medical situations, including the use of emergency, palliative, and psychosocial care in health crises in line with their individual wishes. Further provisions of the law include:

◆ The nursing homes can qualify their own staff for ACP, or cooperate with other regional care providers (e.g. hospice and palliative care)

◆ A GP or palliative care physician should be involved in the planning process and will also be reimbursed

◆ Cooperation of regional healthcare institutions and professionals shall ensure that the resulting plans are available and honoured when needed. However, the legislation does not budget for a regional ACP coordinator responsible for the regional implementation of the ACP system, despite the fact that such regional and institutional coordination is a mandatory complement to the facilitation of individual ACP conversations (20)

Currently, the details of the ACP implementation are negotiated between the sickness funds and the national representatives of nursing homes and institutions for the care of the disabled. The results of these negotiations are currently overdue and will eventually (probably by autumn 2017) take the form of a Ministry decree regulating what minimal standards have to be met, especially in terms of facilitator qualification, in order for the new service to trigger reimbursement by the statutory health insurance.

## The German advance care planning task force

The way how ACP was implemented into the German healthcare system by means of the new § 132g SGB V is probably a unique incident in German social legislation. Usually, new concepts to be introduced to nursing homes derive in a bottom-up process from the nursing sciences, are then broadly discussed, tested, further developed in the nursing homes, and subsequently endorsed by their carriers, for example the large welfare organisations like Caritas, or private enterprises, before they are eventually (and often reluctantly) picked up by the legislator so they can be reimbursed by the statutory health insurance.

ACP, in contrast, remained a concept known only to a very small group of scientists and palliative care experts until 2015, the year of the ACPEL conference in Munich. When ACP nevertheless became part of the new law (HPG) in its first draft version in November 2014 and even when it was passed in December 2015, this was a top-down introduction, and very few people (if any) in the welfare organisations or nursing sciences (or the society as a whole) were aware of what this concept exactly implied. Thus, while the law assigned the task to negotiate the necessary concrete qualification standards and regulations triggering the reimbursement of ACP facilitations to the national representation of the sickness funds on the one hand and the national representatives of the large nursing home carriers on the other hand, many of these representatives were until then not aware of the existence of a concept called ACP, let alone that they would appreciate its details.

Thus, in order to support the negotiations between sickness funds and nursing home carriers with scientific, evidence-based advice and thereby contribute to an effective, patient-centred and sustainable national ACP implementation, an ACP expert task force established itself under the umbrella of the German Society for Palliative Medicine in April 2016, financially supported by the German Federal Ministry of Health. The task force brought together most German ACP experts and practitioners, including representatives of relevant academic and professional societies, covering the fields of nursing, social work, law, ethics, hospice and palliative care, and medical disciplines including primary care, palliative care, neurology, oncology, and intensive care medicine. A representative from Switzerland participates in the task force to exchange experiences and harmonise ACP implementation across both countries.

The ACP task force has been providing the negotiating partners with scientifically consented:

(a) Recommendations for the implementation of ACP in general, specifically in nursing homes and care institutions for persons with disabilities

(b) Specific, detailed curricula for the qualification of the new professional ACP roles in healthcare, especially the facilitators, based on the current state of the art of national and international scientific evidence and implementation experiences

The task force recommendations emphasise the need for:

(1) Well-trained and regularly re-certified facilitators as the backbone of a high-quality ACP process resulting in clinically relevant, valid ADs

(2) An effective institutional and regional project coordination, providing support and resources for the necessary change management and network building, given the significant cultural change coming along with the implementation of ACP

(3) Sufficient palliative care resources available for care home residents who have used ACP to opt for limited life-sustaining measures or a palliative treatment goal in case of critical disease

It may be noteworthy that the ACP task force's expert recommendations have so far not been unanimously welcomed by all partners involved in the negotiating process for the implementation of ACP in nursing and care homes according to the new § 132g SGB V. In particular, it seems that the large carriers of nursing homes, i.e. the charity organisations and others, have reservations to accept the suggested high standard of facilitator qualification (currently adding up to altogether 118 hours of training). This may have several reasons:

◆ The nursing home carriers have a natural interest to direct the additional reimbursement for ACP (through the new § 132g SGB V) to their nursing staff, given the ubiquitary problem of understaffing. However, qualification of nursing home nurses is much lower in Germany than, for example, in Anglo-American countries, and in pilot projects, most nurses who attended the facilitator workshops for various reasons ended up not working as facilitators. Therefore, the task force recommendations address mainly academic staff employed in nursing homes, for example social education workers. If facilitation were to become a task for the nursing staff in care institutions, the high qualification standard envisaged by the task force could likely not be met.

◆ There is a tendency among some representatives of the palliative care and hospice scene to claim that the counselling reimbursed through the new § 132g SGB V should mainly cover palliative care themes, so they suggest a different understanding of ACP, resulting in a different facilitator qualification that focuses rather on discussing future palliative care issues than on fostering autonomous choices for medical decisions. This significant shift of focus, compared with the task force's perspective on ACP, is endorsed by some of the carrier organisations as it strengthens the eligibility of nurses as facilitators.

◆ It seems that ACP becomes a projection area for a deeper status conflict between physicians and nurses in Germany. The historic focus of ACP on shaping future medical decisions is perceived by some to represent an undue predominance of medical issues, whereas important nursing (and spiritual, psychosocial, cultural etc.) issues are felt to be neglected. The task force's counter argument that an urgent need for medical ACP has been documented for decades, whereas nursing care (and palliative nursing care in particular) is a matter of custom-tailored provision at the time when it is needed rather than one of advance planning, is not accepted. Thus, the pre-existing status conflict between health professions may be reflected in a conflict on who defines ACP. This conflict creates a rather unspecific irritation that may well strengthen the two preceding points

## The German-Speaking Interprofessional Union for Advance Care Planning (DiV-BVP e.V.)

On Feb 20th 2017, a German-Speaking equivalent to the International ACPEL Society was founded. Key issues of this German-Speaking ACP Union will be the continuous development of

◆ ACP concepts (including regional implementation), adapted to local medico-cultural and legal needs,

◆ education and training for the new professional roles in ACP, ensuring uniform (re)certification procedures,

◆ uniform AD forms which reflect and validly document the ACP conversation process and provide clear guidance in the clinical application,

◆ institutional and regional coordination of ACP implementation, and

◆ providing and sharing resources for individuals, institutions and regions interested in adopting and promoting ACP.

## Barriers to and critical reflections on the implementation of advance care planning in Germany

Not all societal groups and individuals embrace the idea of introducing ACP. Critical arguments and objections include:

◆ Some physicians and clerical circles claim that ADs should be confined to situations where dying is irreversible and death imminent. They argue that patient autonomy deserves to be honoured to a certain extent, but must not render medical indication and 'the trustful relationship' between doctor and patient meaningless (21). The concept of relational autonomy (i.e. autonomy that only becomes effective in relations) underlying ACP offers potential to accommodate these groups and help to support them to engage with ADs, since it counteracts the widespread misunderstanding that signing an AD form without counselling is an expression of autonomy.

◆ Some palliative care experts recognise ACP as part of what they feel they are already doing, or consider ACP as little more than part of good palliative care, becoming relevant only or mainly when patients face an incurable disease. This view tends to shift the meaning of ACP to encompass a wide range of socio-cultural, spiritual, nursing, and psycho-social needs and concerns, while neglecting the advance planning of medical treatment decisions where the prognosis is open and the choice truly autonomous.

◆ There is a legitimate worry that ACP may easily be interest driven and therefore manipulated by the stakeholders concerned, be it heirs, institutions, or the society as a whole (22,23). Comparable to the US death panel debate (24) some insinuate that the protagonists of ACP are mainly driven by personal interests or by the fact that they felt necessity to save limited resources (25).

◆ Critics who share the above worries often argue that implementing ACP in institutions will unfold a dynamic of its own, and residents will eventually feel a social pressure to participate in an ACP process even if they do not want to (22).

## Current status of advance care planning implementation in Germany (late 2017)

While the negotiations between sickness funds and care institution organisations are ongoing, since 2015 several regions in Germany have started to implement the ACP programme *beizeiten begleiten*®, often initiated by already existing regional care networks, e.g. palliative care and hospice networks. There are a few German ACP initiatives other than *beizeiten begleiten*®, and it remains to be seen whether a single, uniform standard for ACP will evolve for Germany as it is advocated by the national task force. Further initiatives in ACP research and implementation are developing in special fields like psychiatry and paediatrics.

ACP facilitator training according to *beizeiten begleiten*® and to the newly founded German-speaking ACP Union (DiV-BVP), has undergone several updates in the past years. In its current version (as from autumn 2017), it adds up to 120 hrs (= teaching units of 45 min):

◆ 24 hrs private study (e-learning module currently in development)
  - altogether 92 workshop hrs (in three workshop blocks of 2.5 days each, separated by four to six weeks respectively), including 24 units of small group role play training with trained actors as simulated patients;
  - altogether at least 20 documented training facilitations with real patients (six between workshop blocks A and B, six between blocks B and C, and eight after block C),

◆ two plenary sessions of two hrs each during the training period after block C.

Certification will from 2018 depend on passing an ACP OSCE (objective structured clinical exam) with patients simulated by trained actors.

## Perspectives

With new legislation in place, Germany has a regulatory basis for the nationwide implementation of ACP. However, major obstacles have yet to be overcome. First of all, creating a sufficient work force of highly qualified facilitators constitutes a critical bottleneck. Furthermore, the effectiveness of the ACP system will significantly depend on the regional implementation of appropriate routines and standards for the reliable transfer and respect of the resulting ADs, certainly a major challenge in the fragmented German healthcare system—especially as the new legislation does not include a regional ACP coordinator. Over the next few years, it will become clearer as to whether the nationwide ACP implementation in German nursing homes and institutions caring for people with disability will live up to the high-quality standards of comprehensive regional ACP programmes like Respecting Choices and *beizeiten begleiten*®. In addition, ACP must become a standard available healthcare service also for other (wider) target groups, like for example all persons receiving ambulatory care. Further empirical studies are needed to provide sound scientific evidence of the complex impact of comprehensive ACP programmes on patient-relevant outcomes and thereby bolster the implementation efforts in Germany.

## References

1. **Schulze UN** (2004). *Selbstbestimmt in der letzten Lebensphase—zwischen Autonomie und Fürsorge. Impulse aus dem Modellprojekt LIMITS Münster.* Münster: Lit Verlag Münster.

2. **Schröder C, Schmutzer G,** and **Brähler E** (2002). 'Repräsentativbefragung der deutschen Bevölkerung zu Aufklärungswunsch und Patientenverfügung bei unheilbarer Krankheit'. *Psychother Psychosom Med Psychol* **52**(5): 236–43.

3. **Sommer S, Marckmann G, Pentzek M, Wegscheider K,** and **Abholz HH, in der Schmitten J** (2012). 'Advance directives in nursing homes: prevalence, validity, significance, and nursing staff adherence'. *Dtsch Arztebl Int* **109**(37): 577–83.

4. **Wiesing U, Jox RJ, Hessler HJ,** and **Borasio GD** (2010). 'A new law on advance directives in Germany'. *J Med Ethics* **36**(12): 779–83.

5. **Hartog CS, Peschel I, Schwarzkopf D, Curtis JR, Westermann I, Kabisch B,** et al. (2014). 'Are written advance directives helpful to guide end-of-life therapy in the intensive care unit? A retrospective matched-cohort study'. *J Crit Care* **29**(1): 128–33.

6. **in der Schmitten J, Lex K, Mellert C, Rotharmel S, Wegscheider K,** and **Marckmann G** (2014). 'Implementing an advance care planning program in German nursing homes: results of an inter-regionally controlled intervention trial'. *Dtsch Arztebl Int* **111**(4): 50–7.

7. **Petri S** and **Marckmann G** (2016). [Advance directive consultations—A study of selected consultation services in the Munich region]. *Dtsch Med Wochenschr* **141**(9): e80–6.

8. **Evans N, Bausewein C, Menaca A, Andrew EV, Higginson IJ, Harding R,** et al. (2012). 'A critical review of advance directives in Germany: attitudes, use and healthcare professionals' compliance'. *Patient Educ Couns* **87**(3): 277–88.

9. **Teno JM, Nelson HL,** and **Lynn J** (1994). 'Advance care planning. Priorities for ethical and empirical research'. *Hastings Cent Rep* **24**(6): S32–6.

10. **Hammes BJ** and **Rooney BL** (1998). 'Death and end-of-life planning in one midwestern community'. *Arch Intern Med* **158**(4): 383–90.

11. **Hammes BJ, Rooney BL,** and **Gundrum JD** (2010). 'A comparative, retrospective, observational study of the prevalence, availability, and specificity of advance care plans in a county that implemented an advance care planning microsystem'. *J Am Geriatr Soc* **58**(7): 1249–55.

12. **in der Schmitten J, Rotharmel S, Mellert C, Rixen S, Hammes BJ, Briggs L,** et al. (2011). 'A complex regional intervention to implement advance care planning in one town's nursing homes: Protocol of a controlled inter-regional study. *BMC Health Serv Res* **11**(1): 14.

13. **Volicer L, Cantor MD, Derse AR, Edwards DM, Prudhomme AM, Gregory DC,** et al. (2002). 'Advance care planning by proxy for residents of long-term care facilities who lack decision-making capacity'. *J Am Geriatr Soc* **50**(4): 761–7.

14. **In der Schmitten J, Jox R, Rixen S,** and **Marckmann G.** (2015). 'Vorausplanung für nicht-einwilligungsfähige Personen—"Vertreterverfügungen" ' In: Coors M, Jox R, In der Schmitten J, eds. *Advance Care Planning—von der Patientenverfügung zur gesundheitlichen Vorausplanung.* Stuttgart: Kohlhammer-Verlag.

15. **In der Schmitten J, Rothärmel S, Rixen S, Mortsiefer A,** and **Marckmann G** (2011). 'Patientenverfügungen im Rettungsdienst (Teil 2). Neue Perspektiven durch Advance Care Planning und die "Hausärztliche Anordnung für den Notfall" '. *Notfall Rettungsmed* **14**(6): 465–74.

16. **Molloy DW, Guyatt GH, Russo R, Goeree R, O'Brien BJ, Bedard M**, et al. (2000) Systematic implementation of an advance directive program in nursing homes: a randomized controlled trial. *JAMA: the journal of the American Medical Association* **283**(11): 1437–44.

17. **Detering KM, Hancock AD, Reade MC, Silvester W** (2010). The impact of advance care planning on end of life care in elderly patients: randomised controlled trial. *BMJ* **340**: c1345.

18. **Widmannn-Mauz A** (2015). 'Geleitwort'. In: Coors M, Jox R, in der Schmitten J, eds *Advance Care Planning: Von der Patientenverfügung zur gesundheitlichen Vorausplanung*. Stuttgart: Kohlhammer.

19. **Klingler C, in der Schmitten J, Marckmann G** (2016). 'Does facilitated Advance Care Planning reduce the costs of care near the end of life? Systematic review and ethical considerations'. *Palliat Med* **30**(5): 423–33.

20. **Gilissen J, Pivodic L, Smets T, Gastmans C, Vander Stichele R, Deliens L**, et al. (2017). 'Preconditions for successful advance care planning in nursing homes: A systematic review'. *Int J Nurs Stud* **66**: 47–59.

21. **Dörner K** (2008). '"Der gute Arzt" im Spannungsfeld zwischen Patientenwille und medizinischer Indikation'. In: Charbonnier R, Dörner K, Steffen S, eds *Medizinische Indikation und Patientenwille*. Stuttgart: Schattauer Verlag. Pp. 1–6.

22. **Neitzke G**. 'Gesellschaftliche und ethische Herausforderungen des Advance Care Plannings' (2015). In: Coors M, Jox R, in der Schmitten J, eds. *Advance Care Planning: Von der Patientenverfügung zur gesundheitlichen Vorausplanung*. Stuttgart: Kohlhammer. Pp. 152–63.

23. **Neitzke G, Charbonnier R, Diemer W, May AT**, and **Wernstedt T** (2006). 'Göttinger Thesen zur gesetzlichen Regelung des Umgangs mit Patientenverfügung und Vorsorgevollmacht'. *Ethik Med* **18**: 192–4.

24. **MacGillis A** (Sep 2009). 'The Unwitting Birthplace of the "Death Panel" Myth'. *Washington Post*.

25. **Feyerabend E, Görlitzer K-P** (2015). 'Freiwillige Zwangsberatung pro Therapieverzicht? Eine kritische Analyse plus Aktionsvorschlag von BioSkop. BioSkop'.

Chapter 23

# Advance care planning in an Asian country

Irwin C A Wai Hoong Chung

'Many people think that ACP discussions are about death and dying. In actual fact, it's really about how well you want to live.'
*Heart failure patient*

---

**This chapter includes**

- The history and development of advance care planning (ACP) in Singapore
- Details of the 'Living Matters' ACP programme in Singapore, including facilitator training, and certification
- The current situation in Singapore regarding ACP
- A discussion regarding the challenges of implementation of ACP in Singapore, and how these are being addressed

---

**Key Points**

- For ACP to be meaningful and effective, the system of care must recognise and be prepared to be organised around a patient-centric approach that gives patients the ability to and supports them in exercising autonomy in decision making
- Apart from developing systems within healthcare to support the ACP process, the community at large also needs to be sensitised and empowered to embrace ACP as part and parcel of participating in the care process
- ACP needs to be culturally sensitive and appreciate that nuances and local belief systems around death and dying are crucial for effective messaging, obtaining buy-in and achieving activation of the general public

---

**Key Message**

Important lessons from the implementation of ACP in Singapore are likely to facilitate other Asian jurisdictions in formally adopting ACP as part of good care delivery. There are many similarities in cultural setting and social dynamics that will be critical to a successful adaptation of awareness building and public education efforts for ACP in Asia.

## Advance care planning in Singapore

Advance care planning (ACP) as a healthcare concept and principle of patient autonomy and choice and the way that it is practiced in Western civilisation is still rather new to Asia at large, even in cosmopolitan Singapore, home to 5.5 million residents largely of Asian ethnicities. Although its openness to trade and communication ensures that ideas flow freely in science, technology, business, and popular culture, its peoples still hold dear core values, preferences, and practices that are rooted in Asian precepts of respect, filial piety, and deference to authority or social and familial role.

## The case for ACP

Singapore has a rapidly ageing population, contributed in part by a low birth rate and a phenomenal increase in average life expectancy on par with most of Europe and Japan. The latter is attributable to vast improvements in public health and nutrition since the end of World War II. By 2030, Singapore's age-dependency ratio will be a worrisome 1:4, in large part due to post-war baby boomers surviving till advanced old age. With an ageing population comes increasing demand for health and social care, and healthcare expenditure as a percentage of gross domestic product (GDP) as well as total government expenditure (12.1% in 2014) has seen a continuous uptrend over the last decade (1).

It is in this context that ACP as a concept of practice is attractive on three counts:

1. Planning in advance deters hasty and often poorly-informed decision making on healthcare interventions, which are more likely to be aggressive and expensive

2. Involving the patient intimately in healthcare decision making not only respects patient autonomy, but is also appropriate to an increasingly educated, resourced, and vocal population

3. Having essential conversations on end of life decisions supports communication within the family and with the healthcare team, making for better care outcomes and patient satisfaction

With these in mind, the Ministry of Health commissioned the Agency for Integrated Care, a standalone entity tasked to develop and coordinate health and social care initiatives for the elderly, to develop ACP capacity and capability within and across Singapore's public healthcare system from 2011 to 2015. This effort was eventually extended into 2016 and totalled S$18.1 million, comprising of:

a. S$0.4 million to increase awareness of ACP and its importance among healthcare providers

b. S$12.4 million to recruit and train ACP facilitators

c. S$5.4 million to build and strengthen systems to support ACP implementation, including a centralised Information Technology system

## Living Matters®

ACP in Singapore is branded Living Matters®, and borrows heavily in form and process from Respecting Choices® which originated from the Gundersen Health System, Wisconsin, United States of America. It has undergone several iterations with adaptations made largely to language and nuances to better suit the understanding of Singapore residents as well as conform to healthcare contexts and options available. ACP is now available upon request across all public acute care hospitals, with the exception of the Institute of Mental Health, several community hospitals, all nursing homes and a variety of eldercare organisations. There are now 1,500 trained and certified

ACP conversation facilitators (from clinical and support professions) spread across the public acute care hospitals and another 500 in community-based health and social care services.

## Facilitator training and certification

Training and certification of facilitators are centrally coordinated by the ACP National Office residing in the Agency for Integrated Care, but largely delivered by the respective hospital and institutional ACP offices. Most facilitators in the hospitals are nurses, social workers, and counsellors by profession, with a smaller number of doctors from across various grades and disciplines. Service delivery is protected by institutional malpractice indemnity regardless of professional discipline. The hospital ACP offices coordinate all in-house ACP programmes and services, determine the training and supervision roadmap for facilitators, and also conduct outreach and education to their patients, staff members, and the wider community. This modus operandi has served well in enabling the spread of ACP awareness and practice across 60 distinct disciplines in the public acute care hospitals within four years.

## The national advance care planning information technology system

The process of ACP documentation is facilitated by an IT system that captures key decisions made on options of care and catalogues conversation transcripts as well as supporting documents in a single record. From April 2017, this record will also be made available at the point of care through the National Electronic Health Record (NEHR), which holds together the patient's key health information captured from the public healthcare system. This will ensure that the patient's ACP is available anytime at any point of care in any practice setting that has access to the NEHR.

## Other concurrent efforts

In 2013, three other initiatives spun off from the original programme:

1. ACP for the paediatric population
2. ACP for Community Care Providers
3. ACP Advocacy

In 2015, the ACP National Office started exploring ACP for mental health sufferers beginning first with dementia. And in 2017, the focus will be on ACP being delivered at primary care.

We will also focus on the development of ACP advocacy to help sensitise health and social care providers, their patients, clients, and the public at large to the merits of ACP in order for uptake to improve.

## Enhancing Living Matters®

In the first two years of ACP implementation (2011–12) much effort was put into establishing operating systems, designing conversation templates, the branding of Living Matters®, and training personnel in the conduct of ACP. Despite these pioneering efforts, reception and uptake of ACP was generally low and limited to sub-populations of patients within the hospitals. By the first half of 2014, only a few hundred plans had been formally lodged nationally. ACP progress was often hampered by lack of readiness for conversation on the part of either patients or their next of kin. There was an urgent need to increase public education as well as build a more personable approach to outreach and education.

The Ministry approved plans in 2014 to:

1. Outreach to the community through public messaging and education
2. Enable community care providers to conduct ACP for their clients
3. Develop institutional capability to integrate ACP as part of healthcare delivery

As part of community outreach, the concept of ACP advocacy was born. Advocates were trained to understand and appreciate the concept of ACP, be convinced of its importance and merits, and in turn to 'sell' the key ACP messages of autonomy in decision making and pre-emptive planning opportunistically within their social context. To support this outreach, new materials such as an ACP workbook that guides one to think through the concept of living well, describe personal beliefs and values, and can be used as a conversation starter before the documentation of an official ACP were developed and also made available online (https://www.livingmatters.sg/start-the-conversation/overview/).

To date, more than 1,000 community advocates from a spectrum of care providers, interest groups, and civic and religious bodies have been trained. More than 30 community-based organisations now offer ACP as part of their programmes or incorporate it into their outreach agenda. It is hoped that as this effort continues, more segments of society will come to know and appreciate ACP as a means to ensuring that care outcomes, particularly at the end of life, are commensurate with their beliefs, principles, means, and expectations. Within the hospitals, certified facilitators who are not active in practice are also encouraged to be familiar with the advocacy approach and leaven both staff and patients in their understanding and appreciation of ACP opportunistically, so that patients who are referred on for ACP conversation and documentation are more sensitised to the topic and better prepared psychologically for the process.

## The state of advance care planning in Singapore today

By late 2016, more than 6,000 plans have been officially lodged in the national ACP IT system, not including advance care plans documented on hard copy (from the earlier years of the effort) that will in time be captured electronically. We are also confident that a good number of informal conversations have already taken place, through awareness building and advocacy efforts, and will sooner or later translate into formal lodging, as evidenced by the online workbook receiving several thousand unique accesses since its launch in 2015. More than 20,000 hard copies of the workbook have also been disseminated, demonstrating the appetite for ACP among the public at large.

## Challenges to advance care planning in Singapore

Singapore is largely Confucian at heart, with its large Chinese population and main minority communities—the Malays and Indians—holding very similar life views and beliefs on issues surrounding death and dying, the role of the family under such circumstances, the appointment of a decision maker(s) and even how much the patient should know about his or her own condition. In the earliest days of the national effort, official communication around ACP as a concept was highly muted, due to concern that the public may misconstrue it as a covert government-led effort to reduce public healthcare burden. Such was the uproar over the Advance Medical Directive Act (2), passed in 1996, which garnered fierce debate and also stoked fear of euthanasia being legalised.

However, in recent years, public sentiment has been positive on the topic of death and dying, helped in part by the release of the Lien Foundation's Quality of Death Index Report, with Singapore placed at a healthy twelfth position among 80 jurisdictions and ranking fourth in the Asia-Pacific region after Australia, New Zealand, and Taiwan. People have also been surprisingly open towards the topic of ACP, as evidenced by a proliferation of testimonies, public letters, road shows, and even educational dramas advocating ACP.

That said, the topic of death and dying remains a highly emotive subject and is definitely not a dinner table favourite, and it remains a difficult conversation to have in a generally reserved Asian family environment.

## Taking advance care planning into the public sphere

Our public messaging effort, based on an understanding of what would resonate with the Asian psyche, is couched round three culturally sensitive or neutral precepts:

### Advance care planning is about planning to live

We emphasise that ACP plans for life *before* death, that it is about consciously deciding to live well in accordance to one's beliefs and values, and going about planning for it in advance. The key strategy in reinforcing this message is to dissociate ACP from death per se; we say that ACP is not like a will, which takes effect only when one is dead, but a plan for living life.

### Some conversation is better than no conversation

ACP advocacy encourages use of the ACP workbook as a reflection aid and conversation primer with the next-of-kin. The online version of the ACP workbook is designed in such a way as to make it easy to complete and share, with its contents mirroring closely the thinking process and conversation flow of a formal ACP. The reflections and preferences indicated within the workbook can be used as conversation primers should the time come for formal facilitated planning, but meanwhile, it serves to sensitise the person's decision making proxy (known as the nominated healthcare spokesperson) to the values and preferences of the person concerned to guide future deliberations on healthcare decisions.

### Having a conversation reduces the future decision making burden

One thing the Asian family is very conscious of is the concept of duty to care and the resulting care burden. In a fast-paced urban economy with its high cost of living and small family sizes, where many adults are at work most of the day, concurrent care for children, the elderly, and the infirm can be challenging. It is not surprising that oftentimes the elderly sick cannot be discharged from hospital due to insufficient feasible care options available, and many eventually end up being consigned to long-term institutional care. Having a conversation about options available, what is acceptable or unacceptable as care decisions and outcomes, helps to reduce the burden of decision making by the next of kin under pressurised circumstances.

## Real options MUST be available

There are still the practical aspects of actually delivering care that align with patient preferences. Until recently, the community-based care sector in Singapore comprising various eldercare centre-based services, home-based care services, as well as other forms of support like medical escort services, has been nascent and poorly coordinated. However, there has been a conscious shift in care model paradigm over the last decade to better support the care for the elderly and infirm, which has encouraged the mushrooming of health and social services outside of hospitals and institutional homes. The public is also now more aware of them due to concerted awareness building. This opens the opportunity for ACP conversations to be richer, with options for out-of-hospital care more acceptable and attainable.

Another challenge is found in insufficient medical support and access to stronger pain control medication such as opiates in the nursing homes. Whilst staff could be trained as facilitators and advocates for ACP, they very often found that they could not support the resident well at life's end with existing resources and skills. Under such circumstances, there was a high chance that the resident would perish in a hospital environment, regardless of preference for place of death.

## Quality of advance care planning in Singapore

Since formally adopting the Respecting Choices® in 2011 for the national effort, much has been added on to make Living Matters® resonate better with both providers and the public. The most notable of lessons are:

1. **Patient autonomy—How important is it?**

   The understanding of patient autonomy in an Asian context is different from that of Western civilisation at large, even though both appreciate this element of person-centred care. In Asia, it is not uncommon for a patient to 'forgo' autonomy in deference to a more significant person in the family; this could be, in more extreme circumstances, a patriarch or matriarch of the family, or the spouse, adult children, or a legal guardian. In many cases, autonomy could be devolved into a 'collective responsibility', wherein the extended family would confer and arrive at a consensus before a decision is made, most often seen in families where the patient has a large number of adult children. Regardless, many also simply 'toe the line' of professional judgement. Therefore in the ACP conversation here, the need for understanding and consensus building within the family is paramount, particularly with the person(s) selected as nominated healthcare spokesperson(s). Thus autonomy is exercised more by a 'we' rather than an 'I'.

2. **Decision bias—The need to review advance care planning regularly**

   In a recent unpublished surveillance on place of care and options of care data from our national ACP IT system database, we found that an overwhelming proportion of ACPs lodged by hospital-based facilitators tended to gravitate towards 'trial of treatment in hospital'. In contrast, a significantly larger proportion of ACPs completed in the community tended towards more conservative and non-hospital treatment, with home bring the preferred place of death. We cannot discount the possibility that staff perspectives and the 'clinically-safe' environment of a hospital play a role in leading patients to prefer whatever is perceptively more familiar to them at that point in time.

   It is therefore important that the ACP remains a dynamic document and fodder for ongoing conversations, with reviews conducted every time there is a change in the patient's circumstance and/or state of health. We have thus clearly steered the ACP away from legal promulgation as a directive and kept its conduct under the common law governance of good practice to reduce barriers of access and opportunities for review.

3. **Advance care planning needs to be integrated with care delivery**

   The whole care team, and not just the ACP facilitator, needs to be involved in the conversation by understanding and appreciating the need for the conversation to take place (awareness), encouraging the patient to make an ACP (advocacy), offering options of care and their foreseeable outcomes for consideration (professional input), respecting and supporting the care decision made (service delivery). Only in such a collaborative and corroborating environment can ACP's fulfilment be more assured.

## The future of advance care planning in Singapore and Asia

ACP continues to evolve even as I write as part of a larger system of integrated care, which by definition is necessarily person-centred, co-ordinated, and traverses care settings and institutional boundaries. In the coming years, consolidation of efforts and streamlining of ACP processes within each of the regional health systems in Singapore will be a priority as part of a push towards more accountable and equitable population health management. In tandem with that will be continuing quality improvement initiatives aimed at making ACP relevant and accessible in specific care settings and patient sub-populations, such as under-privileged communities, people in institutional care, people confined to home, those suffering from mental illness and dementia, end-stage organ failure, and the paediatric population.

As the national effort for ACP in Singapore continues, we are heartened that our work is being increasingly noticed, having received expressions of interest from the UK, Canada, New Zealand, Australia, the US, Taiwan, Japan, Hong Kong, and Malaysia. We hope that, in time to come, more Asian jurisdictions will formally adopt ACP as part of good care delivery. There are many similarities in cultural setting and social dynamics that will be critical to a successful adaptation of awareness building and public education efforts for ACP in Asia.

We are also grateful to Respecting Choices® for having shared with us their system of ACP implementation, training, and accreditation, as well as ongoing quality improvement. We also acknowledge the contribution of Professor Keri Thomas and her team from the Gold Standards Framework® to our understanding and appreciation of sound community-based end of life care that pivots on the application of good ACP. I thank Professor Keri Thomas and the editorial team for the opportunity to share this snippet of experience and opinion with you.

## Acknowledgements

The epigraph at the start of this chapter was reproduced with permission of Living Matters, Singapore, www.livingmatters.sg.

## References

1. **Department of Statistics**, (2016). Singapore. Accessed from: (http://www.singstat.gov.sg/home).
2. Advance Medical Directive Act. Chapter 4A (1996, revised 1997).

# Section 4

# Practicalities and areas of common ground

# Chapter 24

# Communication skills and advance care planning

## Sarah Russell

'See the person; not just the paperwork, prognosis or process'
*Russell S (2016) (1)*

---

**This chapter includes**

- Definitions of communication
- Discussion of the benefits and barriers to communication, and blocking behaviour
- Examples of facilitative skills
- Communication skills models to assist with advance care planning (APC) conversations
- Illustrative case scenario

---

**Key Points**

- Person-centred ACP is interactive conversations about what matters to people as they contemplate their future death
- This chapter covers some of the issues, evidence, and models for ACP conversations

---

**Key Message**

All clinicians have a part to play in ACP conversations and discussions are key in helping people to live well and prepare and plan for dying.

---

## Introduction

Advance care planning (ACP) imagines and contemplate ones' future death. This may be in the next few weeks, months, or years. It is about helping people to live well (where ever that may be) until they die within the context of their life and relationships with that or those who matter to them. Talking about dying is not always a familiar or comfortable experience. Considering how we carry out conversations and what those discussions may include enables them to be more person centered and rewarding for patients, their families, and clinicians.

---

### Box 24.1 Definitions of communication

'The process by which information, meanings, and feelings are shared by persons through the exchange of verbal and non-verbal messages' (2).

'Not something that people do to one another, but rather it is a process in which they create a relationship by interacting with each other' (3).

---

## Defining communication

There are a variety of definitions of communication (Box 24.1).

Within these multiple definitions are regularly reported facilitative attitudes and traits of: empathy, genuineness, respect, unconditional positive regard, and reflexivity (4,5) (Table 24.1).

The need for and value of early conversations about future care, how their condition might affect them in the future, treatment preferences, and opportunities to record wishes and decisions for people with incurable illness is well documented (6). Conversations not only give information and treatment or care decisions, they also accompany individuals as they live with, prepare, and plan for dying. Communication is a fundamental part of ACP (7) and core business for anyone involved in palliative care.

## Benefits

Studies report benefits such as meaningful and trusting relationships, accurate identification of problems (8), increased patient satisfaction, understanding, adherence, recall and health outcomes (9). Overlapping topics are reported (Table 24.2) illustrates the breadth of conversations.

The value of honesty, clarity, and sensitivity is well documented. Conversations do not necessarily increase patient distress or remove hope (11) including patient-centred communication through engaging with prognosis discussions, responding to emotion, informing about opinions and perspectives as well as framing uncertainty (12). Studies show awareness of prognosis increases satisfaction with care as well as lowering levels of depression (13).

## Empathetic listening

ACP is a series of discussions e.g. exploratory conversations as well as decision-making ones (14). Of value is paying attention to the considering, contemplating, and discussing side of conversations rather than just a focus on the decision, documentation, and implementation (15). The context of people's lives becomes a core catalyst, motivation, and therapeutic intent of conversations. For clinicians, this means paying equal weight to a person within their social world as well

**Table 24.1** Key communication attitudes, behaviours, and traits (4,5)

| | |
|---|---|
| Empathy | The ability to understand a person's experiences and feelings accurately including demonstrating that understanding |
| Genuineness | The ability to be yourself despite your professional role. |
| Respect | The ability to accept the patient as he or she is. |
| Unconditional positive regard | The ability to take a non-judgemental approach. |
| Reflexivity | Immediate, dynamic, and continuing self awareness and reflection. |

**Table 24.2** Examples of end of life and advance care planning conversation topics (10,11)

| | |
|---|---|
| Shared decision making, transition from curative to palliative treatment, commencing or changing treatment, recurrence, survivorship, withholding and withdrawing treatment, preferred place of care or death, prognostication and life expectancy, future symptoms and management, communicating risk | Assessing and managing depression and anxiety, maintaining hope, understanding fears and goals, breaking bad news, responding to emotions, denial and collusion, talking with family members, family conflicts, spirituality, assisted dying, awareness of dying, and the process of dying |

Source: data from Russell S (2016) *Advance care planning and living with dying: the views of hospice patients* [Internet], University of Hertfordshire, http://hdl.handle.net/2299/17474

as being a patient; enabling a wider spectrum of people to be part of conversations. For example, the health support worker who provides a non-judgemental space for a patient to express their concerns or the physiotherapist who explores a person's fears about being a future burden. The domiciliary care home worker who listens to a worry about what happens if another chest infection occurs or the care home staff who wonders if the resident wants to talk again about what happens when they die.

## Barriers and blocks

Barriers and blocks to communication can lead to a failure to recognise or agree patients' concerns, underate patient distress, increase psychological morbidity, as well as hinder a doctor-centred approach to information gathering and giving (16). This leads to underestimating information needs (17) with patients anxious, uncertain, and dissatisfied with care (18). Problematic communication also contributes to clinicians' increased stress, high malpractice claims, emotional burn out, low personal accomplishment, lack of job satisfaction, and high psychological morbidity (19).

Barriers; or reasons why good communication does not happen can range from individual lack of skills, competence, knowledge, and confidence to organisational systems and bureaucracy (Box 24.2).

Blocking behaviour—verbal or nonverbal behaviours that inhibit conversations (Table 24.3) lead to the avoidance of honest, detailed discussion, poorer patient satisfaction, and increased psychological distress (23). Also reported is a desire to maintain hope, belief that patients are not ready or willing to have conversations as well as prognostic uncertainty, lack of confidence

## Box 24.2 Examples of barriers to communication (19–21)

Fear of being blamed, being untaught, eliciting a reaction, not knowing what to say, expressing own emotion, own death awareness, and medical hierarchy
Fear of taking away hope and the work environment

Professional-led conversations
'Bystander effect' where patients and clinicians await the other to start conversations

Underestimating patients' need for information whilst overestimating his or her understanding of prognosis and awareness, lack of time to have conversations, difficulty knowing when it is the right time for conversations. Concerns over managing emotional responses, uncertainty about prognostication and impact of family dynamics

Source: data from Russell S (2016) *Advance care planning and living with dying: the views of hospice patients* [Internet], University of Hertfordshire, http://hdl.handle.net/2299/17474

**Table 24.3** Blocking behaviour examples (10,19)

| | |
|---|---|
| Clinician rather than patient led agenda, poor eye contact, body language, avoidance, missing cues, premature or false reassurance, jumping to conclusions, explaining away distress as normal (normalisation), lack of empathetic response, collusion, lecturing, poor information giving, withholding information, non-disclosure, jargon | Multiple questions, leading or closed questions, focussing on the physical, switching topic, person or timeframe, removing the emotion, ignoring psychological aspects, blaming, being defensive, judgemental, 'jollying' along, language difficulties, cultural mismatches |

Source: data from Russell S (2016) *Advance care planning and living with dying: the views of hospice patients* [Internet], University of Hertfordshire, http://hdl.handle.net/2299/17474

with different diagnosis, dying trajectories, and a reluctance to give bad news (24). Clinicians are concerned about their own communication skills (7) and timing of conversations such as; when, where, and from whom.

What these behaviours illustrate is the potentially negative impact of clinicians' behaviours on conversations, see (Table 24.4).

**Table 24.4** Further examples of blocking behaviour

*Closed questions*
Whilst closed questions (those answered with 'yes' or 'no') certainly have their place in clinical encounters, using only closed questions gives little opportunity for patients to explain their ideas, concerns, and expectations in their own words.

*Leading questions*
Leading questions tend to include the expected answer in some way, for example, 'You've got on very well at the day hospice, haven't you?' This can discourage patients from giving an honest response.

*Focus only on physical aspects*
Like closed questions, questions with a physical focus are an essential part of many consultations and assessments. However, staying with the physical side can be an effective way of avoiding discussing more sensitive issues.

*Premature advice or reassurance*
When a patient introduces a problem, it can be tempting to go into advice or reassurance mode before that it has been fully explored. This effectively inhibits any further discussion of the problem and significant information may be suppressed. Premature reassurance may give false hope.

*Explaining away distress as normal*
It may seem helpful to respond to a patient's fears, for example, about going into a nursing home by saying something like, 'Everyone feels like that when they give up their home'. However, this can lead to the patient feeling that their concerns have been dismissed and prevent them from explaining further.

*'Jollying' patients along*
Encouraging patients to 'look on the bright side' or to 'keep positive' may be counter productive if it stops them from discussing their concerns.

*Switching the topic*
When we feel uncomfortable discussing emotional issues, we might change the subject as an avoiding strategy e.g.

| *Switching Person* | *Switching Time Frame* | *Removing the Emotion* |
|---|---|---|
| My husband is worried about me being at home. What did your doctor say about that? | I felt really down yesterday. Lets talk about this morning. | The pain makes me feel so helpless. Have you been taking the painkillers? |

# Facilitative communication skills

Facilitative communication skills are conversation catalysts (Table 24.5).

Valued skills include truth telling (25), balancing hope, honesty, and knowledge of future death (26). Also reported is encouraging questions, hence clarifying and negotiating the individual's information needs and level of understanding (22). A relationship with a confident expert may be preferred (19). Dias (27) reports how good communication is both personally satisfying and professionally rewarding for clinicians with studies reporting the impact on competency, self-awareness of and confidence in conversations.

**Table 24.5** Facilitating behaviours

| Behaviour | Rationale |
|---|---|
| Body Language | Non-verbal communication conveys emotions and meaning. Communication practices other than words encourage discussion. e.g. Paying attention to body language and positioning as well as the flow of a conversation. |
| Open directive questions | Open in that they allow the patient to give information in their own way, but directive in that they focus on one aspect of the patient's experience. *'Can you tell me how things have been for you over the past few weeks?'* |
| Questions with a psychological focus | A focus on emotional and psychological aspects helps to find out how people feel about the events that are occurring in their life at this time. *'What are your feelings about going into the hospice?'* |
| Questions which explore answers to psychological questions | The initial response to a psychological question may be brief, even consisting of one word, and this requires some clarification if we are to understand what is meant. *'You say you are frightened about going into the hospice . . . can you tell me more?'* |
| Empathic statements | We can never really know what another person is going through, but we can signal that we care and that we are eager to understand. We can acknowledge that their situation is difficult; reflect what we see or stay silent for a while to allow someone to talk. *'From what you have said, this has been a worrying time for you.'* |
| Screening questions | Finding out whether there are any other concerns is important because clinicians sometimes offer advice before patients have managed to say everything that matters to them (23). Screening questions ('what else' questions) can help here. *'You have mentioned some concerns already—what else is on your mind?'* |
| Summarising | In a conversation we might receive a good deal of information from the patient. It is useful to summarise at intervals and at the end of a conversation to check that what we understand is what the patient actually meant and that we have picked up the important points. *'So, we have talked about x and y . . . is that right?'* |
| Cues | Cues include words and body language that hint at emotions not yet expressed which may be helpful to explore with the person. |

## Communication models

Over the years there have been a variety of conversation models (Table 24.6). SPIKES (20) was originally intended as a protocol for breaking bad news, but is usefully adapted for ACP discussions. Calgary-Cambridge (28) is a generic model for structuring a medical consultation, containing elements that can be applied to an end of life setting. PREPARED (19) and SAGE and THYME (29) were developed to help clinicians deal with the challenges of discussing with patients how they would like to be cared for. Whilst 'one size does not fit all' there is a common emphasis on a person-centered approach which explores the patient's perspective, conveys visible empathy in

**Table 24.6** Models that can lend structure to advance care planning discussions

| SPIKES | PREPARED | SAGE & THYME | CALGARY-CAMBRIDGE |
|---|---|---|---|
| **Setting**: includes privacy, involving significant others, listening mode and body language | **Prepare for the discussion**: check patient's diagnosis and results; privacy; significant others | **Setting**: create privacy and choose right time to discuss emotions and concerns | **Initiating the session**: establish initial rapport; identify reason for consultation with open questions; listen without interrupting; confirm and screen for further problems; negotiate agenda |
| | **Relate to the person**: develop rapport and show empathy | | |
| **Perception**: the 'before you tell, ask' principle; you should glean a fairly accurate picture of the patient's perception of their medical condition | **Elicit patient and caregiver preferences**: clarify aim of meeting. Elicit patient's understanding and expectations | **Ask**: specific questions about feelings <br> **Gather**: make a list of things the patient tells you <br> **Empathy**: see below <br> **Talk**: ask if patient has anyone they can talk to <br> **Help**: 'Have they been helped in the past?' <br> **You**: 'What do you think would help?' <br> **Me**: 'Would you like me to do anything?' | **Gathering information**: explore patient's problems; open to closed questions; listen attentively; facilitate patient responses; pick up cues; clarify unclear statements; summarise periodically; use clear questions; establish sequence of events; explore patient's ideas, concerns, expectations, and feelings |
| **Invitation**: check how much patient wants to know about diagnosis and treatment; obtaining overt permission respects the patient's right to know (or not to know) | **Provide information**: offer to discuss issues, giving patient option not to discuss it | | |

**Table 24.6** Continued

| SPIKES | PREPARED | SAGE & THYME | CALGARY-CAMBRIDGE |
|---|---|---|---|
| | | | **Providing structure**: summarise appropriately; signpost; use logical sequence; keep to time |
| | | | **Building relationship**: appropriate non-verbal behaviour; develop rapport, use empathy, provide support; involve patient |
| **Knowledge**: give information at patient's pace using the same language as them; 'chunk and check'. | **Provide information**: give information at patient's pace, using clear language; explain uncertainty; consider caregiver's and family's information needs | | **Explanation and planning**: correct amount and type of information; aid recall and understanding; shared understanding; shared decision-making |
| **Empathy**: listen for, identify, acknowledge and validate emotions | **Acknowledge emotions and concerns**: explore, acknowledge and respond to fears, concerns and emotions | **Empathy**: use silence, give space, reflect patient's feelings | |
| | **(Foster) Realistic hope**: be honest, offering appropriate reassurance, but not false hope | | |
| | **Encourage questions and further discussions**: check understanding; emphasise discussion can be ongoing | | |
| **Strategy and summary**: summarise discussion, give chance for questions or concerns; clarify next steps | **Document**: write summary of discussion; contact other relevant healthcare providers | **End**: reflect, acknowledge and conclude meeting, emphasising main points | **Closing and planning**: forward planning; summary; final check |

both information giving and the hearing of their story, as well as summarises and plans at the end of the conversation.

Another example is the Serious Illness Conversation Guide (30), with advice about clinicians steps (Set up—Guide—Act) and conversations (understanding, information preferences, prognosis, goals, fears/worries, function, trade-offs, and family). Further sugg]estions include Gawande's (31) five questions:

1. What is your understanding of your current health or condition?

2. If your current condition worsens, what are your goals?

3. What are your fears?

4. Are there any trade-offs you are willing to make or not?

5. What would a good day be like?

In addition some on-line video clips for the public can be of help in understanding, normalising and introducing such discussions, such as the GSF 5 steps to Advance Care Planning (32).

## End of life conversation cards

Internationally, there are a number of end of life conversation cards with an overall aim of helping to start, continue, or share conversations (Table 24.7). Their value is that they can be used by patients with their families and friends as well as by healthcare professionals.

**Table 24.7** End of life Conversation Cards Examples

| | |
|---|---|
| **The Conversation Game** | Originally developed by the CODA Alliance (USA). Includes a deck of 36 cards and instruction leaflet. Objective is to be an easy and entertaining way to think and talk about how you want to be treated if you became seriously ill. www.conversationsforlife.co.uk |
| **Heart2Hearts: Advance Care Planning Cards** | Heart2Hearts® (USA) deck of cards invented to provide 52 conversation starters about end of life healthcare issues. Also, includes a work book. http://www.discussdirectives.com/heart2hearts-acp.html |
| **Go Wish Cards** | A deck of 36 cards (USA) to help start end of life discussions. http://codaalliance.org/go-wish/ |
| **My Gift of Grace** | A conversation game (USA) with 47 Question Cards, and 32 Thank You Chips. Players have a chance to share their answers to the same question, trading chips as part of the game play. http://www.mygiftofgrace.com/ |
| **Just Ask Conversation Card** | Advance care planning conversation guide from Speak Up (Canada) http://www.advancecareplanning.ca/resource/just-ask/ |
| **Fink Advance Care Planning Cards** | Developed by Helen Sanderson Associates and Sarah Russell (UK). Includes a deck of cards divided into four categories (how I like to talk about things, who and what matters to me, advance care planning/still to do and as I die/celebrating my life). Cards are used to start, share or continue advance care planning conversations. www.finkcards.com |
| **Grave Talk Cards** | A resource from the Church of England (UK) of 50 unique cards for use in small groups, each with a thought-provoking question to get the conversation started. Topics covered include: Life, Death, Society, Funerals, Grief. Also used in death café scenarios. https://www.chpublishing.co.uk/books/9780715147030/grave-talk-cards |

These communication models and tools offer accessible guides to navigate the uncertainty of end of life conversations whilst being flexible enough to respond to the individual context of each persons' life. For example, conversations do not only include the discussion and documentation of future care or medical intervention decisions (e.g. advance decisions or statements). Discussions are also a contemplative space to manage the uncertainty as the person lives with, prepares, and plans for their dying. Patients may wish to discuss and reflect with you the impact of dying on their lives. For example, concerns may include practical issues such as ensuring a will has been completed or financial arrangements are in place. There may be questions about what dying is like and what help and support is available for family members. Future care decisions can be motivated by concern for others (e.g. being a burden) as well as personal preparation for dying (15).

## Communication skills in practice

There are a variety of communication education programmes available. Self-awareness and understanding of one's own skills enhance the confidence of clinicians in conversations. Knowing about models is not enough—being able to use the most appropriate model in response to individual patient needs enables patients to gather the information and support they need as well as clinicians being able to coordinate care, honour wishes, and decisions.

### Case study

June is a 79-year-old grandmother with advanced breast cancer. She has increasing symptoms. You would not be surprised if she died in the next six months. She is the main carer of her 83-year-old husband with Alzheimer's. You have met June before, see (Table 24.8).

**Table 24.8** Example Scenario

**'See the person; not just the process and paperwork'**
Communication skills are not just about what is said,
but also how and when they are said within a conversation.

**Starting conversations**
It is not always easy to start conversations. The Calgary-Cambridge Guide recommends identifying the reason for the consultation/conversation. This also helps to negotiate the agenda and ensure that what matters to the patient is discussed.

| Good Enough | Not Good Enough |
|---|---|
| 'June, now that we have discussed your pain I wondered if there was anything else you wanted to talk about?' | 'June, we must talk about your advance care planning.' |
| This encourages and invites June to say what she understands or wants to talk about. | This is blunt, uses jargon and the agenda is the healthcare professionals. |

**Other suggestions**
'I wonder if we could discuss what might happen in the future
I have been wondering if we could talk about if your illness got worse?'

**Discussing advance care planning**
The Prepared Model reminds us to foster realistic hope, to be honest, offering appropriate reassurance. The model advises giving information at the patient's pace, clear language; explain uncertainty and consider caregiver's and family's information needs.

*(continued)*

**Table 24.8** Continued

| | |
|---|---|
| 'I **wish** we could slow down the growth of your cancer. But I **worry** that you and your family won't be prepared. I **wonder** if we can discuss a "what if" plan today.' | 'We need to talk about your advance care planning.' |
| The Serious Illness Conversation Guide includes the 'I wish, I worry, I wonder' framework which enables practitioners to align with patient's hopes (wish) whilst allowing for being truthful (worry) and to be able to make a recommendation (wonder). | This is jargon and blunt. |

**Other suggestions**
'June, I wonder if we could talk about something called "advance care planning".
Some people find it helpful to think and talk about the end of their life—would you like to?'

**Continuing the Conversation**
Picking up cues and listening to the concerns from the person is crucial to understanding the context of what matters to them. The SPIKES model advocates a *'before you tell, ask'* approach which enables you to gather information about the persons' life.

| | |
|---|---|
| 'You mentioned before about your husband . . .can you tell me a little more?' | 'Let's talk about your worries for your husband.' |
| This picks up on a previous cue about June's husband but encourages her to explain what she is worried about. | This tells June what she is worried about rather than explore what they might be. |
| 'Is there anything that you are worried or fearful about?' | 'Tell me your fears.' |
| This encourages a conversation about fears or worries. | This assumes that June has fears. |

**Other suggestions**
'This may be difficult to talk about—are you ok to go on?'

**Tailoring Information**
The Serious Illness Conversation Guide suggests that information preferences should always be tailored to the individual e.g. some people like to know about time, others like to know what to expect, others want to plan in detail, others less so.

| | |
|---|---|
| 'What detail/information would you like to know?' | 'Long description of the details of a document.' |
| Enables tailored information—should include giving chunks of information and then checking if understood or if want to continue. | Too much information, too quickly. |

**Other suggestions**
'What would be most helpful for you to talk about?'

**Discussing documentation**
Documentation of wishes and decisions is only one part of advance care planning. The PREPARED model advises offering to discuss issues as well as giving the option not to discuss.

| | |
|---|---|
| 'June, you just mentioned a few things that were important to you– can you say a bit more?' | 'These forms will stop you going into hospital.' |
| 'June—you mentioned about not wanting anything "unnecessary" in the future—can we discuss what could help?' | |
| This encourages discussion of June's wishes and decisions which can then be documented. | This focuses on the process of documentation. |

**Table 24.8** Continued

---

### Other suggestions
'Some people find it helpful to write down their wishes and decisions so that their family, friends, doctors and nurses know about them  . . . .'

---

### Discussing specific documentation or decisions
The PREPARED model reminds us to give information at patient's pace, using clear language.

| | |
|---|---|
| 'You have mentioned several things that you don't want to happen. | 'Here is the Advance Statement and ADRT form.' |
| Would you like to do something more to record and share your wishes/decisions?' | |
| The focus is on June's wishes and the pace of the conversation rather than the documents. | The focus is on the form not the person. |

### Other suggestions
'I have some suggestions about paperwork which could help.'

---

### Difficult Topics e.g.
' "just put me down", "don't tell anyone", "I just want to die", "there is no point to this" '
The Calgary-Cambridge Guide recommends exploring patient's ideas, concerns, expectations and feelings. Sometimes conversations may be a contemplative space for a person to reflect and share their feelings and thinking.

| | |
|---|---|
| 'Can you help me understand your thinking?' | 'You mustn't feel like that.' |
| 'Can you help me understand what kind of thinking and planning you would find helpful . . .' | 'I can't do that.' |
| This is a non-judgemental way to encourage further expression of feelings. | This does not allow expression of the persons' feelings or thinking. |

### Other suggestions
'I'd like to know more . . . please tell me.'

---

### When conversations go wrong
All conversations will go through patches where they seem to go wrong. The discussion may dry up or the person may seem offended or fearful about what you have said. Apologies about the impact of the conversation is always helpful.

| | |
|---|---|
| 'I wish that things were better so we didn't need to talk about this.' | 'That's not what I meant/said.' |
| Apologising and conveying empathy about the impact of the conversation is appropriate! | This introduces argument into the conversation. |

### Other suggestions
'I'm sorry, can we start again?'

---

### Finishing the conversation
The Sage and Thyme model reminds us to reflect, acknowledge and conclude meeting, emphasising main points

| | |
|---|---|
| 'I know this was probably not an easy conversation. | 'We have finished now. Thank you for your time.' |
| I would like to talk again with you about your illness and medical care as treatment continues. Is that okay?' | |
| This conveys empathy and clarifies what the action plan is. | Whilst this is polite—it does not convey empathy or summarise the conversation or next steps. |

### Other suggestions
'Do you have any thoughts or questions about what we have discussed?'

## Summary

Good communication is a core part of all clinicians' role. Communication skills are not just about what is said, but also how and when things are said within a conversation. Person-centred communication in ACP sees the person not just the paperwork, prognosis, or process. This enables people to explore and express their feelings about their future death as well as discuss and share their wishes and decisions.

## References

1. **Russell S** (2016). *Advance care planning and living with dying: the views of hospice patients* [Internet]. University of Hertfordshire. Available from: http://hdl.handle.net/2299/17474

2. **Brooks W** and **Heath R** (1985). *Speech Communication*. 7th edn. Madison: Oxford.

3. **Groogan S** (1999). 'Setting the scene'. In: Long A, ed. *Interaction for Practice in Community Nursing*. Macmillan: London.

4. **Coulehan J** and **Block M** (2006). *The Medical Interview: Mastering Skills for Clinical Practice*. 5th ed. Philadelphia: F.A. Davies Co.

5. **Finlay L** and **Gough B** (2003). *Reflexivity: A Practical Guide for Researcers in Health and Social Sciences*. Finlay L, Gough B, eds Oxford: Blackwell Publishing.

6. **Parry R**, **Land V**, and **Seymour J** (Dec 2014). 'How to communicate with patients about future illness progression and end of life: a systematic review'. *BMJ Support Palliat Care* **4**(4): 331–41.

7. **Institute of Medicine of the National Academies** (2014). *Dying in America: Improving Quality and Honouring Individual preferences Near End of Life*. doi: org/10.17226/18748.

8. **Libert Y**, **Merckaert I**, **Reynaert C**, **Delvaux N**, **Marchal S**, **Etienne A-M**, et al. (Jun 2007). 'Physicians are different when they learn communication skills: influence of the locus of control'. *Psychooncology* **16**(6): 553–62.

9. **King A** and **Hoppe RB** (2013). ' "Best practice" for patient-centered communication: a narrative review'. *J Gr Med Educ* [Internet]. **5**(3): 385–93. Available from: http://www.pubmedcentral.nih.gov/articlerender.fcgi?artid=3771166&tool=pmcentrez&rendertype=abstract

10. **Walczak A**, **Butow PN**, **Clayton JM**, **Tattersall MHN**, **Davidson PM**, **Young J**, et al. (2014). 'Discussing prognosis and end-of-life care in the final year of life: a randomised controlled trial of a nurse-led communication support programme for patients and caregivers'. *BMJ Open* [Internet] **4**(6): e005745–e005745. Available from: http://bmjopen.bmj.com/cgi/doi/10.1136/bmjopen-2014-005745

11. **Bernacki RE** and **Block SD** (Dec 2014). 'Communication about serious illness care goals: a review and synthesis of best practices'. *JAMA Intern Med* **174**(12): 1994–2003.

12. **Gramling R**, **Stanek S**, **Ladwig S**, **Gajary-Coots E**, **Cimino J**, **Anderson W**, et al. (Nov 2015). 'Feeling heard and understood: A patient-reported quality measure for the inpatient palliative care setting'. *J Pain Symptom Manage*. doi: org/10.1016/j.jpainsymman.

13. **Chochinov HM**, **Tataryn DJ**, **Wilson KG**, **Ennis M**, and **Lander S**. 'Prognostic awareness and the terminally ill'. *Psychosomatics* 2000; **41**(6): 500–4.

14. **Seymour J**, **Gott M**, **Bellamy G**, **Ahmedzai SH**, and **Clark D** (Jul 2004). 'Planning for the end of life: the views of older people about advance care statements'. *Soc Sci Med* **59**(1): 57–68.

15. **Russell S**. 'Preparing and Planning for Dying: What's the Difference?' In: *11th Palliative Care Congress* [Internet]. Glasgow: Palliative Care Congress; 2016. Available from: http://www.pccongress.org.uk/

16. **Maguire P** and **Pitceathly C** (2002). 'Key communication skills and how to acquire them'. *Br Med J* **325**(7366): 697–700.

17. **Fallowfield LJ**, **Jenkins VA**, and **Beveridge HA** (Jul 2002). 'Truth may hurt but deceit hurts more: communication in palliative care'. *Palliat Med* **16**(4): 297–303.

18. **Commission Audit** (1993). *What seems to matter? Commmunication between Hospitals and Patients*. London.

19. **Clayton JM, Hancock KM, Butow PN, Tattersall MHN, Currow DC, Adler J**, et al. (Jun 2007). 'Clinical practice guidelines for communicating prognosis and end-of-life issues with adults in the advanced stages of a life-limiting illness, and their caregivers'. *Med J Aust* **186**(12 Suppl): S77, S79, S83–108.

20. **Kurtz SM, Silverman DJ, Draper J, van Dalen J**, and **Platt F** (2005). *Teaching and learning communication skills in medicine*. Radcliffe Publications: Oxford.

21. **Baile WF, Buckman R, Lenzi R, Glober G, Beale E**, and **Kudelka P** (2000). 'SPIKES-A six-step protocol for delivering bad news: application to the patient with cancer'. *Oncologist* **5**: 302–11.

22. **Parker SM, Clayton JM, Hancock K, Walder S, Butow PN, Carrick S**, et al. (2007). 'A systematic review of prognostic/end-of-life communication with adults in the advanced stages of a life-limiting illness: patient/caregiver preferences for the content, style, and timing of information'. *J Pain Symptom Manage* [Internet]. **34**(1): 81–93. Available from: http://linkinghub.elsevier.com/retrieve/pii/S0885392407002606

23. **Clayton JM, Butow PN, Arnold RM**, and **Tattersall MHN** (May 2005). Fostering coping and nurturing hope when discussing the future with terminally ill cancer patients and their caregivers. *Cancer* **103**(9): 1965–75.

24. **De Vleminck A, Pardon K, Beernaert K, Deschepper R, Houttekier D, Van Audenhove C**, et al. (2014). 'Barriers to Advance Care Planning in Cancer, Heart Failure and Dementia Patients: A Focus Group Study on General Practitioners' Views and Experiences'. *PLoS One* [Internet]. **9**(1): e84905. Available from: http://dx.plos.org/10.1371/journal.pone.0084905

25. **Hancock K, Clayton JM, Parker SM, Wal der S, Butow PN, Carrick S**, et al. 'Truth-telling in discussing prognosis in advanced life-limiting illnesses: a systematic review'. *Palliat Med* [Internet]. 2007; **21**(6): 507–17. Available from: http://pmj.sagepub.com/cgi/doi/10.1177/0269216307080823

26. **Clayton JM, Hancock K, Parker S, Butow PN, Walder S, Carrick S**, et al. (Jul 2008). 'Sustaining hope when communicating with terminally ill patients and their families: a systematic review'. *Psychooncology* **17**(7): 641–59.

27. **Dias L** (2003). 'Breaking bad news: a patient's perspective'. *Oncologist* **8**: 587–96.

28. **Kurtz SM, Silverman DJ, Draper J, van Dalen J**, and **Platt F** (2005). *Teaching and learning communication skills in medicine*. Oxford: Radcliffe Publishing.

29. **Griffiths J, Wilson C, Ewing G, Connolly M**, and **Grande G** (2015). 'Improving communication with palliative care cancer patients at home—a pilot study of SAGE & THYME communication skills model'. *Eur J Oncol Nurs* **19**(5): 465–72.

30. **Bernacki RE** and **Block SD** (2014). 'Communication about serious illness care goals' [Internet]. *JAMA Internal Medicine* **174**: 1994. Available from: http://archinte.jamanetwork.com/article.aspx?doi=10.1001/jamainternmed.2014.5271

31. **Gawande A** (2014). *Being Mortal: Medicine and What Matters in the End*. 1st ed. New York: Metropolitian Books, Henery Holt and Company.

32. GSF 5 Steps to Advance Care Planning video http://www.goldstandardsframework.org.uk/new-5-steps-advance-care-planning-film or https://www.youtube.com/watch?v=i2k6U6inIjQ

# Chapter 25

# Advance care planning in chronic disease: finding the known in the midst of the unknown

Karen Detering, Elizabeth Sutton, and Scott Fraser

'The good physician treats the disease, the great physician treats the patient who has the disease'
*William Osler*

---

**This chapter includes**

- An outline of the disease trajectories in chronic kidney disease, chronic obstructive pulmonary disease, and chronic heart failure
- The evidence pertaining to the current situation regarding advance care planning (ACP) in these conditions
- Considerations as to how and why ACP is important in these conditions
- Practical guidance as to how to have ACP discussions under these conditions

---

**Key Points**

- Advances such as new technologies and medications for chronic diseases mean that people are living longer lives with greater burden of disease
- ACP helps to clarify patient values beliefs and treatment goals and has positive effects on patients and carers
- ACP is achievable for many people with chronic disease, despite prognostic uncertainty
- ACP should occur early in the care of a person with chronic disease, and be revisited regularly
- Documentation is not the only outcome of successful ACP conversations. Conversations are useful in their own right, however, documentation is helpful

---

**Key Message**

ACP must become an important part of routine care for patients with chronic disease. The current under-provision of ACP may reflect concerns regarding prognosis given the uncertain illness trajectory, failure to recognise and discuss symptom control, lack of clinician skills in how to have ACP conversations, and a greater emphasis on providing ACP and palliative care for patients with malignant rather than non-malignant disease. An awareness of the importance to patients of holding these discussions in a timely fashion may assist in ensuring that healthcare professionals prioritise these discussions relative to their scope of practice, earlier in routine care, thereby improving patient care.

## Introduction

With aging populations, and technological advances, people live longer lives, with a greater burden of disease. Three diseases that contribute to this burden are chronic kidney disease, chronic obstructive pulmonary disease and heart failure—both right and left sided. While technology has provided treatments that can prolong life, patients with these disease types have known life-limiting illnesses.

Patients are mostly keen to understand more about their disease. Healthcare professionals should ensure that patient information needs are met, including fully informed consent, and that all likely scenarios are discussed. This cannot occur until healthcare professionals become adept at talking to patients about their disease and its impact on life span and quality. Healthcare professionals need to know what kind of care a person wants in order to plan future care. Advance care planning (ACP) is a process that facilitates this and should be introduced early and regularly reviewed during a patient's care journey.

## Chronic diseases with life-limiting implications

### Chronic kidney disease, chronic obstructive pulmonary disease and heart failure

Chronic kidney disease (CKD) is a progressive, life–limiting condition caused by damage to both kidneys. In 2013, CKD caused 956,000 deaths globally (1). Treating CKD is not aimed at cure except when transplantation is possible. Rather, treatment aims to slow disease progression and manage symptoms. In developed countries haemodialysis has become the default treatment for people with end-stage kidney disease. Dialysis is not curative but can sustain life. Many people who are now commencing dialysis are elderly. For example, Australian data shows over half of new dialysis patients are aged over 65 years and 26% of people currently on dialysis are aged over 75 years (2). Importantly elderly people who receive dialysis—as compared to those with malignancy or heart failure—experience very high rates of hospitalisation, and numerous invasive procedures during the final month of life (3).

Chronic obstructive pulmonary disease (COPD) is a chronic progressive lung disease. The typical disease trajectory in COPD is a gradual decline in health status and physical capacities over many years, punctuated by episodic acute exacerbations that may require hospitalisation. These exacerbations are associated with increased risk of dying (4,5). In-hospital mortality following an exacerbation of COPD is as high as 25%, while of those who survive, 25–55% will be readmitted, and 25–50% will die within one year (6). Patients usually survive many acute episodes before death. This episodic course of COPD makes predicting death difficult and it often seems unexpected when it occurs. It is therefore essential that ACP is introduced early in the disease course.

The degree of lung function impairment is often not correlated to the patients' symptom burden or disease course, and objective measures of lung function alone are not good predictors. Factors which may be more prognostically useful include advanced age, prior admissions for exacerbations, severity of lung disease, significant comorbidities, severity of dyspnoea, low body-mass-index, and degree of functional impairment (7).

Heart failure, the inability of the heart to maintain the workload required of it to oxygenate tissues and organs in the body, may be left or right sided or both. Heart failure patients experience a similar disease trajectory and symptom burden to COPD patients (8). Patients also face treatment decisions and dilemmas similar to CKD patients with implantable devices available to assist the heart function. In some patients, this therapy is used to sustain life while awaiting transplant; in many, the insertion of a device is the likely final treatment. In these instances it is referred to as destination therapy and careful consideration and discussion is required between doctor, patient, and family/carers before commencement, regarding the appropriateness of such treatment, now and in the future.

Healthcare professionals need to be ready to have conversations with patients regarding the commencement of therapy, and whether it is appropriate, and at what point (if any) it ought to be ceased. This should be revisited. It is inappropriate to wait to initiate these conversations until a very advanced stage of the illnesses. Prognostication in these diseases can be difficult, and this inability to determine when death is nearing has been identified as a barrier to ACP (9). Whilst tools have been developed to assist with prognostication, the usefulness of these tools is limited in individual people (7). Rather, as mortality is an inevitable consequence of living and becomes less distant in chronic disease, preferences for care now and in the future, should be a critical and ongoing conversation commenced early in the treatment journey. These conversations must take into account patient's information wants and needs (10,11).

Advance care planning and its benefits is a coordinated communication process between a person, their family, and healthcare providers. It aims to clarify the person's values, treatment preferences, and goals of medical treatment, should the person lose capacity to make or communicate such decisions in the future (10). Although completion of documents (advance directives) setting out the person's preferences is desirable, the ACP discussions, are valuable in their own right (12). These discussions help to identify patient's goals for treatment and care.

ACP is not a single event, and should be revisited often during the course of a person's life, particularly as health status changes. The main focus of ACP should be on preparing patients and surrogate decision-makers to participate with clinicians in making the best possible 'in-the-moment' decisions (13). This means that complex health decisions are based on a complete set of considerations, such as the current clinical context, shifting and evolving goals, the patient's preferences, and finally, the decision-makers' needs (13). This is especially relevant for patients with CKD, COPD, and HF where prognostication is difficult. Importantly, ACP also provides an opportunity to introduce palliative care early in the disease process for people with these diseases, which is particularly important for symptom management.

## Why should we do advance care planning?

ACP has been shown to significantly improve outcomes for patients and their families. ACP improves the quality of care, including end of life care (14,15). It is associated with an increase in utilisation of hospice services, and reduction in hospitalisation and the use of unwanted intensive treatments at the end of life (12,14,15). Importantly, ACP has been shown to improve psychological outcomes in both surviving relatives (14,15) and treating healthcare providers. Data show that ACP reduces the cost of end of life care, (15,16) without increasing mortality. A 2014 review on the efficacy of ACP (12) concluded that 'considering the positive effects of ACP on multiple outcomes, implementation into regular clinical care is recommended'.

# ACP in long term conditions—every patient's right to know

## Hope

Contrary to the view of destroying hope, studies have found that patients want to be informed about prognosis and life expectancy (17) and discussing their prognosis and life expectancy can be empowering as it enables patients to determine future goals for their care.

## Prognosis and planning

In a survey of 500 Canadian CKD patients many were unaware of the likelihood of clinical deterioration or their expected prognosis. However, these patients felt it was important to receive this information and plan for future death (18). Similarly, patients with advanced COPD experience severe morbidity, disability, and increased healthcare resource utilisation, and want information (7).

## Symptom burden

These patient groups may have shortness of breath, fatigue, difficulty sleeping, and dyspnoea during their last months of life. These symptoms affect the person's ability to attend to their daily activities of living and serve to isolate them socially. This debility can cause severe anxiety and depression.

## Technology and future care

For patients undergoing life-sustaining treatments such as ventricular assist devices and dialysis, clinical decisions need to be made about the commencement and continued use, and when and under what circumstances these treatments are to be withdrawn.

# Current state of advance care planning in patients with lifelimiting illnesses

CKD, COPD, and HF patients have likely life-limiting illnesses, and thus should have access to ACP.

A 2016 study compared existing European Union COPD and HF guidelines and pathways. Of 19 documents (17 guidelines and two pathways) 18 discussed reduction of suffering, 15 talked about prognostication of illness and its limitations and discussing this with the patient, but ACP was only mentioned in 11 (19). This begs the question that for those documents that did not mention ACP and prognostication, how did they suggest patient care goals be identified and delivered upon?

Even when ACP is known about and available it may not be offered, or the outcomes of it may not be of sufficient quality to be useful. A survey of renal health professionals in Australia found that two thirds of respondents reported that ACP was done 'poorly' or 'very poorly'. Furthermore, whilst 80% thought that ACP discussions should occur prior to starting dialysis, only a third reported that ACP was offered *prior to commencement* of dialysis (20). Even less encouragingly, although COPD is a common condition that entails complex care needs and a significant symptom burden, one study found that only 23% of patients with COPD had discussed their wishes regarding cardiopulmonary resuscitation before being hospitalised (21). Further, patients with COPD were found to be more likely to receive aggressive care including intensive care admission at the end of life than cancer patients, even though patients often stated that they wanted to avoid these treatments (22).

**Table 25.1** Barriers, enablers and benefits of advance care planning

| Barrier | Enablers |
| --- | --- |
| Lack of studies on how to implement ACP into certain disease groups—timing and issues to discuss | ◆ ACP knowledge and skill<br>◆ Incorporating ACP into routine care<br>◆ Similarities that chronic illnesses have on patients and families even if the diseases are different |
| Staff lack confidence and knowledge relating to ACP (24) | ◆ Understanding that a patient with a chronic disease will need information to make informed decisions (25)<br>◆ Education improves outcomes (26) |
| Clinicians feeling poorly prepared and not proficient in discussing death and dying (9) | ◆ Being aware that patients wish to receive information about their disease and providing it does not destroy hope or increase anxiety (7)<br>◆ Start discussions early and as part of routine care (7,24) |
| ACP conversation will lead to conflict (27,28) | ◆ Being aware that carers of people with a chronic disease wish to receive information about their loved one's likely pathway (29)<br>◆ Conflict also occurs commonly due to lack of ACP |
| Initiating the initial ACP conversation in a time of crisis when a patient is critically ill and a family stressed (9) | ◆ Being aware that both patients and family/carers want information about death and dying (30,31) |

# Barriers/enablers and benefits of advance care planning

Key issues relating to the provision of ACP relate to the difficulty in identifying the right timing for ACP, reluctance to raise ACP for fear of upsetting patients, lack of support from senior staff (23), lack of skills, and a need for ACP training and education (20). However patients report wanting information regarding prognosis and life expectancy and this can be empowering, and enables them some control over their lives. ACP should therefore be a key component of care for people with chronic disease, see (Table 25.1).

# The advance care planning process—demystified for patients with chronic disease

An ACP conversation is a semi-structured discussion. The order the ACP discussion follows will vary depending on the patient and physician, the current clinical situation, and how the discussion progresses (32). Patients and family need time to reflect, so it is expected that the ACP process will extend over time. The key components of an ACP discussion, and other important elements to consider are outlined here (7).

## Key outcomes of advance care planning discussion

1. Establishing how decisions are to be made, if the person themselves does not wish to, or is unable, to make their own decisions.
   - ◆ Often involves appointment of surrogate decision maker/s
   - ◆ Establishing how surrogates will make decisions—discuss how much scope or 'leeway' the patient would like the decision maker to have. Patients and surrogates may not be aware of importance of preparing for future decision-making

2. Exploring the person's values and beliefs and what it means to live well.
   - These components are important as they form the basis of the person's decisions. Focus on living well is vital, makes ACP a positive, empowering experience. Discussion of current/future goals and what would be a 'reasonable treatment outcome' is included

3. Understanding illness, treatment and prognosis (where desired)
   - Assess current understanding of the illness, likely trajectory, and prognosis. Provide disease-specific information. Acknowledge uncertainty and the difficulty this causes. There may be specific treatments not wanted under any circumstance, and trials of treatment may be appropriate. Discuss these

4. Documenting and Sharing
   - Documentation is not essential in ACP, however it may be beneficial as it increases the likelihood of a person's preferences being known and respected. Even if a surrogate has been appointed, documentation can support them in their role and importantly is available if the surrogate is not contactable in an emergency

Conversion of a person's wishes as outlined in advance directives into clear and actionable medical orders may be especially important for patients with advanced disease.

## Advance care planning conversations with patients who have chronic, life-limiting illnesses

With these components in mind, a guide to the key actions clinicians need to follow in order to have successful ACP conversations is given.

- First—obtain permission

Patients may not wish to have an ACP discussion, (now or at any time) and differ in the extent to which they want to receive information regarding their prognosis (25).

- Second—ensure relevant people are present during discussions

Having others, including surrogates involved in discussions provides support for the patient, and provides opportunity to receive disease-related information first hand, treatments, and likely disease course. When surrogates are present, completion of advance directives is more likely (33). Surrogates are therefore better able to follow a person's wishes (34).

- Third—giving information whilst being mindful of the delivery and receptiveness of the patient and others present

Studies have shown accurate information is preferred providing it is not delivered bluntly, or with too much hard factual, or detailed information (35). Therefore it is best to balance sensitivity and honesty when discussing prognosis or delivering bad news (30,36). Patients also vary in how they like to receive prognostic information.

When discussing their disease it is important to acknowledge there is a degree of uncertainty. Clinicians should also be mindful of the important interaction between preferences for hope, and the desire for prognostic information (37). One way to address this is to consider the dual agendas of 'hoping for the best and planning for the worst' (38).

- Fourth—reassure that the patient is not being abandoned

Patients and caregivers want health professionals to provide empathy, consistency, and a sense that they will not be abandoned as the illness progresses (35,36).

◆ Fifth—fostering realistic hope

This may be facilitated by emphasising what can be done (particularly when disease specific treatments are no longer working). Patients may hope for many things, not just cure. Exploring this with patients may help to facilitate setting realistic goals. Be honest without being blunt (36).

◆ Finally—review and update as required

Advance care plans should be reviewed and revisited as the patient's needs and preferences change and as their condition changes. For those patients who initially refuse ACP, reintroduction of the concept is part of good care to ensure that they are given opportunity to undertake ACP if they are now ready to do so. Further, review of an ACP means that patients can change their preferences and surrogate decision-maker appointments should they choose to do so.

## Conclusion

In order to deliver person-centred care, improve the quality of life, and reduce the suffering of people with CKD, COPD and HF and their families, ACP and palliative care need to be incorporated earlier into the trajectory of illness. Currently, clinicians and patients/families are waiting until identification of the terminal phase of illness. This creates major difficulties given that the terminal phase is often indistinguishable from the slow chronic decline punctuated by repeated acute exacerbations that are typically seen in these diseases.

Frontline healthcare providers should focus on symptom management, ACP and support for patients as part of usual, comprehensive care for patients with these diseases. Patients presenting with these conditions have serious likely life-limiting illness(es) that are not curable and that often cause a significant burden of symptoms and a dramatic reduction in quality of life. Patients with these diseases and their families seldom have a complete understanding of the conditions and prognosis. Whilst prognosticating can be difficult, mortality is ultimately high and patient education regarding the implications of diagnosis is often lacking.

ACP must become an important part of routine care for patients with chronic disease. The current under-provision of ACP may reflect a combination of difficulty in predicting when a patient with these diseases is near or at the end of life, particularly given the uncertain illness trajectory, failure to recognise and discuss symptom control and reduced quality of life, lack of clinician skills in how to have ACP conversations, and a greater emphasis on providing ACP and palliative care for patients with malignant rather than non-malignant disease. An awareness of the importance to patients of holding these discussions in a timely fashion may assist in ensuring that healthcare professionals prioritise these discussions relative to their scope of practice, earlier in routine care.

## References

1. GBD (2013). 'Mortality, Causes of Death Collaborators', regional, and national age-sex specific all-cause and cause-specific mortality for 240 causes of death, 1990–2013: a systematic analysis for the Global Burden of Disease Study 2013'. *Lancet* **385**(9963): 117–71.
2. Jose M (2016). ANZDATA Overview—Australian Society of Nephrology Annual Scientific Meeting. (http://www.anzdata.org.au/v1/presentations_ANZSN.html. (Accessed 20 January 2017.)
3. Wong SP, Kreuter W, and O'Hare AM (2012). 'Treatment intensity at the end of life in older adults receiving long-term dialysis'. *Arch Intern Med* **172**(8): 661–3; discussion 3–4.
4. Murray SA, Kendall M, Boyd K, and Sheikh A (2005). 'Illness trajectories and palliative care'. *BMJ* **330**(7498): 1007–11.
5. Lyn J and Adamson, D (2003). 'Living Well at the End of Life'. *RAND Health*, white paper, Santa Monica CA.

6. **Steer J, Gibson GJ**, and **Bourke SC** (2010). 'Predicting outcomes following hospitalization for acute exacerbations of COPD'. *QJM: monthly journal of the Association of Physicians* **103**(11): 817–29.

7. **Detering K, Sutton E**, and **MacDonald C** (2016). 'Recognising advanced disease, advance care planning and recognition of dying for people with COPD'. In: Bausewein C, Currow D, Johnson M, eds ERS Monograph—*Palliative Care in Respiratory Disease*. European Respiratory Society UK, pp. 204–20.

8. **Gavazzi A, De Maria R, Manzoli L, Bocconcelli P, Di Leonardo A, Frigerio M**, et al. (2015). 'Palliative needs for heart failure or chronic obstructive pulmonary disease: Results of a multicenter observational registry'. *Int J Cardiol* **184**: 552–8.

9. **Gott M, Gardiner C, Small N, Payne S, Seamark D, Barnes S**, et al. (2009). 'Barriers to advance care planning in chronic obstructive pulmonary disease'. *Palliat Med* **23**(7): 642–8.

10. **The Australian Commission of Quality and Safety in Health Care** (2015). *The National Consensus Statement: Essential elements for safe and high-quality end-of-life care* www.safetyandqualitygovau/ publications/national-consensus-statement-essential-elements-for-safe-high-quality-end-of-life-care/ (Accessed 20 January 2017.)

11. **Fried TR, Bradley EH, Towle VR**, and **Allore H** (2002). 'Understanding the treatment preferences of seriously ill patients'. *N Engl J Med* **346**(14): 1061–6.

12. **Houben CH, Spruit MA, Groenen MT, Wouters EF**, and **Janssen DJ** (2014). 'Efficacy of advance care planning: a systematic review and meta-analysis. Journal of the American Medical Directors Association'. **15**(7): 477–89.

13. **Sudore RL** and **Fried TR** (2010). 'Redefining the "planning" in advance care planning: preparing for end-of-life decision making'. *Ann Intern Med* **153**(4): 256–61.

14. **Brinkman-Stoppelenburg A, Rietjens JA**, and **van der Heide A** (2014). The effects of advance care planning on end-of-life care: A systematic review. *Palliat Med* **28**(8): 1000–25.

15. **Teno JM, Gruneir A, Schwartz Z, Nanda A**, and **Wetle T** (2007). 'Association between advance directives and quality of end-of-life care: a national study'. *J Am Geriatr Soc* **55**(2): 189–94.

16. **Zhang B, Wright AA, Huskamp HA, Nilsson ME, Maciejewski ML, Earle CC**, et al. (2009). 'Health care costs in the last week of life: associations with end-of-life conversations'. *Archives of internal medicine* **169**(5): 480–8.

17. **Davison SN** and **Simpson C** (2006). 'Hope and advance care planning in patients with end stage renal disease: qualitative interview study'. *BMJ* **333**(7574): 886.

18. **Davison SN** (2010). End-of-life care preferences and needs: perceptions of patients with chronic kidney disease. *Clin J Am Soc Nephrol* **5**(2): 195–204.

19. **Siouta N, van Beek K, Preston N, Hasselaar J, Hughes S, Payne S**, et al. 'Towards integration of palliative care in patients with chronic heart failure and chronic obstructive pulmonary disease: a systematic literature review of European guidelines and pathways'. *BMC Palliat Care* **15**: 18.

20. **Luckett T, Spencer L, Morton RL, Pollock CA, Lam L, Silvester W**, et al. (2017). 'Advance care planning in chronic kidney disease: A survey of current practice in Australia'. *Nephrology* (Carlton) **22**: 139–49.

21. **Hofmann JC, Wenger NS, Davis RB, Teno J, Connors AF, Jr., Desbiens N**, et al. (1997). 'Patient preferences for communication with physicians about end-of-life decisions. SUPPORT Investigators. Study to Understand Prognoses and Preference for Outcomes and Risks of Treatment'. *Ann Intern Med* **127**(1): 1–12.

22. **Claessens MT, Lynn J, Zhong Z, Desbiens NA, Phillips RS, Wu AW**, et al. (2000). 'Dying with lung cancer or chronic obstructive pulmonary disease: insights from SUPPORT. Study to Understand Prognoses and Preferences for Outcomes and Risks of Treatments'. *J Am Geriatr Soc* **48**(5 Suppl): S146–53.

23. **Perry E, Swartz R, Smith-Wheelock L, Westbrook J**, and **Buck C** (1996). 'Why is it difficult for staff to discuss advance directives with chronic dialysis patients?' *J Am Soc Nephrol* **7**(10): 2160–8.

24. **Luckett T, Bhattarai P, Phillips J, Agar M, Currow D, Krastev Y**, et al. (2015). Advance care planning in 21st century Australia: a systematic review and appraisal of online advance care directive templates against national framework criteria. *Aust Health Rev* **39**(5): 552–60.

25. Gardiner C, Gott M, Small N, Payne S, Seamark D, Barnes S, et al. (2009). 'Living with advanced chronic obstructive pulmonary disease: patients concerns regarding death and dying'. *Palliat Med* **23**(8): 691–7.

26. Detering K, Silvester W, Corke C, Milnes S, Fullam R, Lewis V, et al. (2014). 'Teaching general practitioners and doctors-in-training to discuss advance care planning: evaluation of a brief multimodality education programme'. *BMJ Supportive & Palliative Care* bmjspcare-2013-000450.

27. Morrison RS, Morrison EW, and Glickman DF (1994). 'Physician reluctance to discuss advance directives. An empiric investigation of potential barriers'. *Arch Intern Med* **154**(20): 2311–8.

28. Patel K, Janssen DJ, and Curtis JR (2012). 'Advance care planning in COPD'. *Respirology* **17**(1): 72–8.

29. Elkington H, White P, Addington-Hall J, Higgs R, and Edmonds P (2005). 'The healthcare needs of chronic obstructive pulmonary disease patients in the last year of life'. *Palliat Med* **19**(6): 485–91.

30. Parker SM, Clayton JM, Hancock K, Walder S, Butow PN, Carrick S, et al. (2007). 'A systematic review of prognostic/end-of-life communication with adults in the advanced stages of a life-limiting illness: patient/caregiver preferences for the content, style, and timing of information. Journal of pain and symptom management'. **34**(1): 81–93.

31. Currow DC, Ward A, Clark K, Burns CM, and Abernethy AP (2008). 'Caregivers for people with end-stage lung disease: characteristics and unmet needs in the whole population'. *International journal of chronic obstructive pulmonary disease* **3**(4): 753–62.

32. Advance Care Planning Australia (2017). Available from: http://advancecareplanning.org.au/advance-care-planning. (Accessed 20 December 2016.)

33. Detering KM, Hancock AD, Reade MC, and Silvester W (2010). 'The impact of advance care planning on end of life care in elderly patients: randomised controlled trial'. *BMJ* **340**: c1345.

34. Silveira MJ, Kim SY, and Langa KM (2010). 'Advance directives and outcomes of surrogate decision making before death'. *The New England journal of medicine* **362**(13): 1211–8.

35. Jones I, Kirby A, Ormiston P, Loomba Y, Chan KK, Rout J, et al. (2004). 'The needs of patients dying of chronic obstructive pulmonary disease in the community'. *Family practice* **21**(3): 310–3.

36. Wenrich MD, Curtis JR, Shannon SE, Carline JD, Ambrozy DM, and Ramsey PG (2001). 'Communicating with dying patients within the spectrum of medical care from terminal diagnosis to death'. *Arch Intern Med* **161**(6): 868–74.

37. Curtis JR, Engelberg R, Young JP, Vig LK, Reinke LF, Wenrich MD, et al. (2008). 'An approach to understanding the interaction of hope and desire for explicit prognostic information among individuals with severe chronic obstructive pulmonary disease or advanced cancer'. *J Palliat Med* **11**(4): 610–20.

38. Back AL, Arnold RM, and Quill TE (2003). 'Hope for the best, and prepare for the worst'. *Ann Intern Med* **138**(5): 439–43.

# Chapter 26

# Planning ahead in all areas

Nigel Mathers and Craig Sinclair

'I can make the last stage of my life as good as possible because everyone works together confidently, honestly and consistently to help me and the people who are important to me, including my carer(s)'

---

**This chapter includes**

- A brief overview of the policy context that has informed the development of advance care planning (ACP) as part of end of life care in the United Kingdom and Australia
- A discussion regarding how an medicalised approach to ACP can potentially conflict with person-centred care principles
- Consideration of the benefits of a broader, holistic approach to ACP
- Discussion as to how some of the challenges associated with the practical implementation of this approach can be addressed, with a particular focus on practitioners working in primary care settings

---

**Key Points**

- With an ageing society and changing patterns of illness more people will live for longer and with increasing co-morbidities. This means the role of the general practitioner (GP) and other healthcare professionals in planning and palliative and end of life care becomes ever more challenging
- ACP should commence early in the course of a life-limiting illness, be an ongoing process, and encompass goals and values from a broad range of domains (e.g. cultural, spiritual, life-style, and/or financial)
- This broad approach has a number of benefits including a reduced focus on end of life care, alignment with person-centred care principles, and a greater capacity for incorporating 'future planning' discussions into routine care
- Additionally, this broad type approach may be accessible to a wider range of patients enabling meaningful discussions to commence prior to, or soon after, the diagnosis of a life-limiting illness

> **Key Message**
>
> A 'medicalised' approach to ACP has resulted in the tendency to delay ACP discussion until late in the course of a person's illness and led to concerns about the implementation of advance directives in real-world clinical situations. By adopting a more holistic approach to planning, the needs of many more people will be met with the likelihood of improved outcomes for the population.

## Introduction

Advance care planning (ACP) has been defined as an ongoing process of discussion, aimed at clarifying a person's goals, values, and preferences for future care, particularly in the context of a time in which they may be unable to communicate their wishes (1,2). ACP evolved out of a desire to promote autonomy and person-centred care for patients at the end of life. However, the implicit alignment of ACP with end of life care, and the often vexing issues of substitute decision-making in relation to medical treatments, have led to a tendency for ACP to focus on facilitating anticipatory decisions about healthcare and medical treatments, rather than broader, holistic approaches to planning, which might also include lifestyle, financial, cultural, or spiritual aspects. This 'medicalised' approach to ACP has led to a number of difficulties, including the tendency to delay ACP discussion until late in the course of a person's illness and concerns about the implementation of advance directives in real-world clinical situations. It also appears to be poorly matched to the needs of the growing demographic of patients living with chronic conditions, who experience an accumulating symptom burden, and for which prognosis can be uncertain. These difficulties lead to a mismatch between the needs of consumers and those implementing ACP, and may explain the sub-optimal levels of ACP uptake. This chapter outlines the policy context that has informed the development of ACP as part of end of life care in the United Kingdom and Australia, and argues that a medicalised approach to ACP can potentially conflict with person-centred care principles. We outline the benefits of a broader, holistic approach to ACP, and address some of the challenges associated with practically implementing this approach, with a particular focus on practitioners working in primary care settings.

## Background

The United Kingdom and Australia share a number of similarities in the organisation of the healthcare systems which must meet these changing population needs. Both are organised around the general practitioner (GP), who provides primary care in community settings, and functions as both a coordinator of other primary care services, and a 'gatekeeper' to specialist services. Acute care services are provided by networks of secondary and tertiary hospitals, and are accessed either through GP referral, or by attending hospital emergency departments. Access to GPs and other approved health services are provided by nationally funded schemes (National Health Service in the United Kingdom, and Medicare in Australia).

These changing population demographics and patterns of illness have created challenges for the acute care system, which was designed around the common scenario of short episodes of acute, hospital-based care. The contemporary acute care system has struggled to meet the needs of a growing cohort of patients with incurable chronic conditions, an ongoing symptom burden, and unpredictable prognoses. Residential aged care facilities meet some of these needs, however it can be difficult to access places when required.

In Australia, the introduction of the 'Living Longer Living Better' policy provides access to home and community care packages for older people assessed as being eligible. A key aim of this policy is to enable older people living with chronic or life-limiting illnesses to remain in their home for as long as possible, by providing access to relevant community care and supports. Future policy directions include the introduction and embedding of 'consumer-directed care' across the aged-care sector. This policy direction aims to give 'choice and control' to recipients of aged care funding packages, enabling these consumers to choose their preferred providers and allocate funding to their preferred services. Such a policy direction comes with the implicit assumption of informed and empowered 'consumers' of healthcare services, who are able to choose their preferred level and type of care.

Parallel with this move towards community-based care, and efforts to promote greater choice and control for consumers, has been a growing discussion about the importance of better meeting the end of life care needs of patients and their family members. The hospice movement, established in the 1960s in an attempt to better meet the needs of dying cancer patients, has been refocused to meet the needs of a growing demographic of patients with non-malignant disease. For patients with chronic conditions, the extended illness trajectory, variable symptom burden, and uncertain prognosis have been seen to require a 'palliative approach' to care. This is a tailored approach that may incorporate palliative and supportive care principles, alongside ongoing curative care aimed at prolonging life.

In addition to a shift towards the palliative approach to care, there have been shifts in broader ethical principles underpinning healthcare decision making. Historically 'paternalistic' attitudes of healthcare professionals have been challenged by changing community expectations, which support an increased respect for patient autonomy in decision making about healthcare and medical treatments.

These changes in population demographics, patterns of illness, and policy direction, along with a growing attention to palliative care and personal autonomy, have provided a basis for increasing attention to the topic of ACP. Current approaches to ACP in the UK and Australia, along with some of the established research relating to its implementation in different settings are covered in this chapter.

## Personalised care and support planning

The Royal College of General Practitioners is committed to promoting *personalised care and support planning* across the UK. With a rapidly ageing society and changing patterns of illness many more people will live for longer and with increasing co-morbidities. Each year more of us will die and many more of us will face the challenges of dying, death, and bereavement (3,4). As patterns of illness change due to advances in medical treatment and technology, the role of the GP and other healthcare professionals in palliative and end of life care becomes ever more challenging—not only is the prevalence of multi-morbidity and complexity rising but more people of all ages with a wide range of conditions may be considered to have *palliative care needs*—these may be physical, psychological, social, and spiritual (4). The particular challenge for health professionals is to develop *practical solutions* to the clinical, ethical, and moral challenges that caring for patients with complex needs and frequent fluctuations in their clinical condition can present. It is also important to recognise that local communities are essential partners in providing sustainable palliative and end of life care in the future.

There is good evidence that people with personalised care plans for their end of life care experience a better quality of life near death, fewer hospital admissions, and more hospice admissions (5). Compassionate and effective *communication* is fundamental to supporting people and those important to them to help make decisions of their journey of care—in addition to their under-standing of the relevant legal issues and documentation.

*So what is personalised care and support planning and how does it fit with ideas around advance directives?*

## Personalised care and support planning

ACP is used to describe the process of discussing and planning ahead in end of life care. For example, when there is anticipation of some deterioration in a patient's condition, a template to facilitate discussion of this with patients and carers can be found on the Gold Standards Framework website (6).

**An advance statement** is a general statement of views and wishes and allows the person com-pleting the statement to indicate their preferences for receiving or refusing forms of treatment in the future. They may express these preferences in the form of a 'values history' which is com-monly completed as a series of scenarios in which varying degrees of disability or death are given negative or positive scores in comparison with death itself. These documents are not considered legally binding (7).

**An advance directive** may be known in lay terms as a 'living will' and are generally used to indicate a person's specific wish to refuse all or certain forms of medical treatment and the circumstances under which these wishes would apply. It is important to note that advanced directives cannot specify a par-ticular treatment which a person requests. They can only indicate a refusal of a specific treatment. They are not wills in the traditional sense in that they do not allow for the disposal of assets, nor are they valid after a person's death. An advance directive is considered legally binding on the treating medical team assuming that it is valid and applicable to circumstances that then arise (7).

*Everyone approaching the end of life should be offered the chance to create a personalised care plan (8).*

This UK national partnership (8) outlines six ambitions for end of life care which are as follows:

◆ Each person is seen as an individual

◆ Each person gets fair access to care

◆ Maximisation of comfort and wellbeing

◆ Care is coordinated

◆ All staff are prepared to care

◆ Each community is prepared to help

Underpinning all of these six ambitions are eight foundations, one of which is **personalised care planning**. Many people with long-term conditions or complex needs will already have a care plan and this should be updated to reflect their changing needs. Although participation should be voluntary (unless a person is no longer competent), the opportunity for informed discussion and planning should be universal and these discussions should be between the per-son nearing the end of their life, those important to them (as they wish), as well as their pro-fessional carers.

Such ACP should commence early in the course of a life-limiting illness, be an ongoing process, and encompass goals and values from a broad range of domains (e.g. cultural, spiritual, life-style, and/or financial). This broad approach has a number of benefits including a reduced focus on end of life care, alignment with person-centred care principles and a greater capacity for incorporating 'future planning' discussions into routine care. In addition, such an approach may be accessible to a broader range of patients enabling meaningful discussions to commence prior to, or soon after, the diagnosis of a life-limiting illness.

# Advance care planning

The benefits of ACP are supported by a growing body of research evidence. In the Australian context, a randomised controlled trial of the Respecting Patient Choices* intervention recruited older, hospitalised inpatients, who were offered a facilitated ACP intervention, led by trained, non-medical facilitators (9). This study found that those who received the intervention and died during the follow up period were more likely to have their wishes known and respected. Follow-up data collected from family caregivers of the enrolled patients also indicated lower likelihood of depression, anxiety, or post-traumatic stress disorder among those who received the intervention. Internationally, two recent systematic reviews support the results from this trial concluding that ACP interventions are associated with increased likelihood that patients will receive their preferred type of end of life care (10,11).

ACP is also associated with a lower likelihood of in-hospital death, and increased likelihood of planned hospice admission at the end of life (12).

Despite these benefits associated with ACP, research has typically shown low levels of community uptake, which may be explained by a number of 'barrier' factors (13,14).

Patients often express discomfort in talking about end of life care and dying expressing a preference to maintain a present focus or take 'one day at a time' (15).

It is also common for patients to report difficulties in planning ahead for hypothetical future scenarios, and particularly with documenting these plans on legally binding advance directives (16). This is often associated with concerns about changing preferences, or fear of 'binding' their family members or healthcare team to anticipatory treatment decisions, which turn out to be inappropriate or poorly matched to the complexities of the actual clinical situation when it arises. This concern is often associated with a desire to make decisions 'when the time comes', even if this means delegating decision-making to family members or healthcare professionals (17).

Additional concerns relate to difficulties identifying the right time to start discussing ACP, lack of access to trusted and supportive health professionals (18), family or relationship concerns that make ACP discussions difficult (16) and the complexity of paperwork associated with ACP. For patients experiencing chronic conditions, in which prognosis is uncertain and symptom burden and treatment options may develop and change over an extended period of time, these concerns may be further exacerbated.

**Personalised care and support planning discussions** need, therefore, to include not only treatment escalation plans including elements such as cardiopulmonary resuscitation, but they should also allow people to express their preferences for care and to set personal goals highlighting what matters most to them. A comprehensive six-stage process provides a model for such a care plan (19). This process may be summarised as:

1. **Context.** This includes understanding the local care pathways and service options, establishing methods for identifying relevant people and embedding care planning processes within systems which can ensure that planning meets agreed quality standards.

2. **Preparation**. This includes organising the processes of care, performing assessments, providing feedback to the person, and ensuring that the individual and their families/carers have sufficient information, support, and time to prepare for the discussion.

3. **Conversation/discussion**. The care planning meeting should allow for a longer conversation (usually between 20 and 40 minutes) where the individual's goals and psychosocial needs are given equal prominence to their biomedical needs. Such conversations should be with the most appropriate person who may or may not be a health professional. Many models exist with people producing their own plan with support from family and peers, health coaches, and 'health navigators' allied to a clinical team.

If a health professional is the most appropriate person this could be the GP but it could equally be the practice nurse, a social care professional, or one of the other allied health professionals. The conversation needs to cover what people can do themselves to live well and maintain their independence as well as what support they might need to help them achieve their goals. The *most important thing is that the conversation is tailored to be appropriate to that person.*

The discussion needs to provide an opportunity to consider the individual's future needs. These will include contingency planning in the case of deterioration in their health and wellbeing.

4. **Recording/documentation**. The care plan is written up, owned by the person, and included in their health records. Relevant documents are shared with team members to enable coordination of care around patients' preferences and goals.

5. **Making it happen.** This stage is about coordinating and supporting the actions agreed in the conversation. It may include ongoing support such as booking appointments, managing medicines, and, if appropriate, the finances and processes around obtaining a personal health budget (where appropriate and available).

6. **Review.** The frequency of reviews reflects the person's needs and wishes. The care plan will need to be reviewed both in terms of success and recording actions against goals as well as recording the individuals changing needs.

Some of these issues with the medicalised approach have led to a revision of the aims and conceptual foundations of ACP, to better match the needs of patients and their families. Sudore and Fried have argued that the 'planning' aspect of ACP should focus more on preparing patients and family members for better quality 'in the moment' decision making (2). A number of other authors propose that a broader, values-based approach to ACP yields a number of benefits, and is preferable to the medicalised approach (15,20).

The next section explores a number of considerations that are relevant to adopting a broader approach to 'planning ahead in all areas'.

## Advance care planning—an 'holistic' approach

Contemporary approaches to ACP have emphasised the need to approach ACP as an ongoing process of conversation, which explores a broad range of domains, and attempts to understand patient goals and values in relation to decision making. This approach acknowledges that patient perspectives on their condition, and their preferred approach for decision-making about medical treatments, are informed by a range of factors, including social, interpersonal, financial, logistical, cultural, and spiritual considerations. Instead of seeing these perspectives as an 'add on' to the medical aspects of a person's care, practitioners can instead understand these various domains as intertwining, and informing a patient's overall approach to decision making and future planning. For example, a patient's preference for a certain type of care may have significant financial implications, which might impact on the person's estate, and conflict with the expectations of other family members. Such complexity could lead to family conflict or an impasse in decision-making, perhaps hindering engagement in ACP. By incorporating a broader perspective, practitioners may be able to facilitate more timely and productive ACP discussions, which better meet patient and family member needs. The principles underpinning this broader approach to ACP include:

◆ Seeing the person, not just the illness

◆ Validating patient and family member concerns

◆ Exploring current concerns, and their relationship to goals, values and future planning

◆ Taking a multi-disciplinary approach

## Seeing the person, not just the illness

While this principle is something that a practitioner would always aspire to, it is particularly important when trying to facilitate a broad and holistic approach to ACP. This approach asks the practitioner to understand and acknowledge the whole person, not just the illness that might be causing that person to present and/or seek treatment. While an illness may result in a set of physical or emotional symptoms and functional impacts, the aim is to understand these in reference to the person's broader experiences, identities, roles, values, and goals. It may also be helpful to actively explore a person's life 'beyond' the impact of a particular illness, even if the illness is serious and/or life-threatening. To do so may validate a person's efforts to maintain a focus on 'normal' or 'everyday' experiences of life, something that has been shown to be important among people with life-limiting illness (15). To develop a broader understanding of the person, a practitioner may consider asking a number of questions:

- How has this illness affected you?
- Aside from this illness, what is important for you?
- What are your goals right now?

Adopting this mindset and perspective towards the person and the therapeutic relationship can be seen as a first step in facilitating a broader perspective on planning for the future.

## Validating patient and family member concerns

The next step in this process is to validate the importance and relevance of concerns raised by the patient and/or family members, even when these reach beyond the direct impacts of the person's illness. This might include financial, social, or interpersonal, logistical, cultural, or spiritual concerns. These concerns are important when considering future planning, as they:

- Demonstrate the person's broader priorities
- Enable better understanding of how a person's wishes exist within a broader social context
- May identify the goals, values, relationships, social contexts, and/or constraints that inform or impact on decision making or future planning
- Enable consideration of the broader impact of a person's illness, and any treatment decisions they might make

Validating the person's broader concerns thus plays an important and practical role in facilitating future planning, as it 'opens up' the conversation to include the broader factors that might facilitate or hinder engagement in such planning. It is important to acknowledge that exploring these broader concerns can raise complex issues, which may extend beyond a practitioner's scope of practice or capacity to respond. To validate such concerns, even where organisational policy or professional scope of practice might limit the responses that can be made to these concerns, demonstrates their importance, and can encourage the patient and/or family member to mobilise existing resources, and seek additional help where required, to address these concerns (see 'Taking a multidisciplinary approach').

## Exploring current concerns and their relationship to goals, values, and future planning

This step asks that the practitioner explore the person's current concerns to generate engagement in the process of planning for the future. It may seem counter intuitive to focus on the present as a means of encouraging future planning. The aim of this step is to first 'meet the patient where they are at'. This acknowledges the patient's current experience of their illness, and the principles of person-centred care. A person's current concerns might seem, at first glance, to have little direct relationship to future planning. We advise that practitioners work with patients and family members to explore these concerns, from both a practical (problem solving) and reflective (philosophical) perspective. In some cases, it may be that a person's concerns cannot be alleviated. However in exploring the nature of the concern, the potential solutions or coping mechanisms, and understanding the person's preferred approach to managing the concern, the practitioner has access to rich information about the person's goals, values, and preferred approaches to making decisions that are relevant to their life. This material can be harnessed in ongoing discussion about future planning, as it enables the practitioner to frame future planning considerations with reference to what is known to be relevant and important to the person. Some possible approaches to understanding a person's goals and values from their approaches to managing current concerns are given below:

◆ From what you have told me, it seems really important to you that . . .

◆ Based on what you have told me, am I right in thinking that if [situation] arose, some of these issues would be important for you?

◆ Of the things we have discussed today, what would be important to you in terms of planning for the future?

## Taking a multidisciplinary approach

Armed with a suitably broad understanding of a person's key concerns, and a knowledge of how these link to their goals, values, and preferred approaches to decision making and/or future planning, the practitioner may now be better placed to address these concerns and/or identify necessary resources for gathering further relevant information. It is important to acknowledge the potential complexity of these issues, including their medical, legal, financial, interpersonal, logistical, cultural, or spiritual considerations. Any of these factors might take a patient's concerns outside the remit of organisational policy, or beyond a practitioner's scope of practice. In these cases, it is useful to access multi-disciplinary perspectives, and in some cases to be able to refer patients to further resources and/or other professionals or organisations. These might include medical sub-specialists, social workers, psychologists, or counsellors, representatives of relevant service provider organisations (e.g. home nursing care, residential care facilities, or hospice), legal practitioners, advocacy or mediation services, accountants, financial or estate planners, social services, cultural community leaders or cultural liaison officers, spiritual advisers, or funeral providers, among others. The practitioner has the opportunity to remain involved in the process of accessing these further resources, addressing any concerns raised by the involvement of specific professionals, advocating for the patient's needs, and coordinating follow up and further referrals, as well as the documentation of any ACP discussions arising.

## Challenges and practical strategies

The broader approach to ACP already outlined is purposefully general in focus, in the hope of being applicable to practitioners in a wide range of contexts. Of course, this broad approach may not be feasible in all situations due to practical constraints. The challenges in adopting a broad approach might include:

◆ Patient or family member beliefs or stereotypes about the role of a particular practitioner or organisation

- Interactions between different decision-making domains (e.g. accessing a certain type of care may have financial implications which requires financial decision making)
- Legal complexities associated with decision making (e.g. a patient may have decision-making capacity for general decisions about their healthcare, but lack the capacity to make decisions about sale of property or management of their estate)
- Limitations in time or funding
- Organisational remit, service eligibility criteria, and/or professional scope of practice
- Lack of access to particular desired professionals or service providers (e.g. due to distance, cost or patient functional limitations)

The responses to these challenges will likely depend on the local service provision context and models of care. In developing practical strategies to overcome these challenges, we recommend the following key principles:

- Understand the local context of service provision, including resource limitations, and potential sources of support
- Inform patients about access to public services, as well as making relevant referrals to private practitioners
- Work proactively to address patient and family member concerns relating to the involvement of additional professionals and/or organisations (e.g. specialist palliative care providers)
- Where possible, integrate a broad approach to ACP into routine care
- Use everyday clinical history taking and discussion relating to treatment options as an opportunity to explore patient goals and values for care

Everyday clinical history taking and discussion relating to treatment options can provide a number of opportunities to explore patient values and goals for care. This can enable a broadening of focus to a discussion of more holistic aspects of care, and can also aim to understand the aspects of a decision that might reflect a patient's enduring goals, the principles that might guide decision making if the patient is unable to communicate their wishes at the time. It also provides an opportunity to explore the factors that constrain a person's decision making, and whether these might be addressed through more holistic approaches to care. Acknowledging these resource limitations, and mobilising additional resources from relevant professionals or service providers, can be an important way of addressing the practical constraints that can otherwise hinder patient engagement in ACP. In different jurisdictions there may be funding schemes in place to enable practitioners to provide broad and/or multidisciplinary approaches to care. Practitioners can also work to better understand the local service provision context, and develop referral pathways or information packs for patients and/or family members who express particular concerns (see Figure 26.1).

## House of care

The model of care places 'holistic' person-centred care at its heart with the conversation as key and the other elements of the house being present to support it (21). All the elements are needed to make collaborative care and support planning a reality. Without engaged patients there would be no demand. Without organisation processes such as call and recall, the plan cannot be delivered. If professionals do not commit to partnership working there cannot be the necessary continuity of care. Fundamental system change is often required to implement such models.

For the model to be implemented successfully it needs to be constructed around the person not the disease(s).

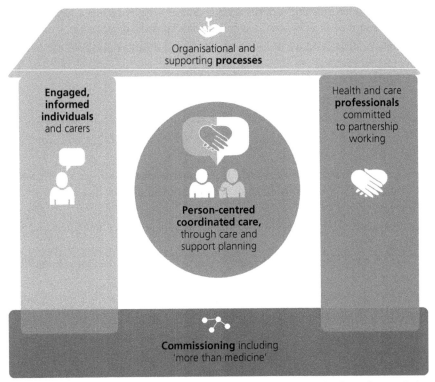

**Figure 26.1** A model for collaborative care and support planning (CC and SP) requires a whole system approach as illustrated by the House of Care (21)

Reproduced with the permission of the Coalition for Collaborative Care, www.coalitionforcollaborativecare.org.uk

The 2012 National Voices 'I statements' express how successful person-centred integration of services should look to a person living with a life-limiting condition (22).

The statements show that people wish to be empowered and have all the information they need to make decisions about their care. They want to experience continuity of care and communication across the system as well as to be supported to develop the confidence to share decision making and self manage where appropriate. An integrated approach is required—one planning process across a person's whole needs rather than separate ones for health and social care. The process needs to be designed in partnership with people in organisations who work towards the goals and outcomes that they want to achieve rather than assumptions about their needs by healthcare professionals.

## Evidence-based guidelines

A flexible approach to evidence-based guidelines also needs to be encouraged. Current models tend to follow disease-specific guidelines formed from a biomedical evidence-base. Such guidelines have real value and should not be lost but need to be incorporated into a new way of working around the individual and their priorities and needs. The importance of *patient values and preferences* in shaping decisions about decisions cannot be underestimated. With the increasing complexity of conditions and comorbidities (particularly towards the end of life); mental health issues and functional problems may outweigh biomedical issues for people. This is a consideration that needs to be built into shared decision making frameworks and it is essential to create mechanisms for discussion across professional groups—for example, with multidisciplinary teams—especially when decisions about reducing or stopping treatment are being made.

To reiterate, for collaborative care and support planning to be successful in the care of people approaching the end of their lives, a whole system-integrated model for the delivery of care is essential. Providers of care need to work together to ensure seamless, joined up delivery of services that are organised around the patient and their carers. The delivery of such care depends on breaking down the current disease and organisation-based working silos and opening up the system to better communication. In essence, patients and their carers should only have to tell their story once (23).

## Conclusion

ACP is one component of personalised care and support planning and should be considered when deemed appropriate by the clinician and patient. This is not a 'tick box' exercise. As a person progresses along their journey of care, personalised care planning conversations can be incremental with the valuable information recorded at the person's pace over several conversations. Holistic and person-centred approaches to ACP and 'future planning' may enable greater engagement and participation by patients and their family members. This requires excellent communication; a broad, multi-disciplinary approach; exploration and validation of patient and family values and goals, and the use of these values in applying evidence-based guidelines. The result may be a broader approach to planning ahead in all areas, which better meets patient and family needs, and contributes to a more consistent delivery of person-centred care. A recent UK government document provides a framework and a set of principles for developing policy in this area (24).

## Acknowledgements

The epigraph at the beginning of this chapter was reproduced from National Voices, 'Every moment counts: a narrative of person-centred coordinated care for people near the end of life', March 2015, www.nationalvoices.org.uk, Copyright © 2015 National Council for Palliative Care. It has been reprinted here with permission from Hospice UK, which has now merged with the NCPC.

## References

1. 'Every moment counts: a narrative of person-centred coordinated care for people near the end of life'. (March 2015) *National Voices*. Available at: http://www.nationalvoices.org.uk/

2. **Sudore RL** and **Fried TR** (2010). 'Redefining the "Planning" in advance care planning: preparing for end-of-life decision making'. *Annals of Internal Medicine* **153**(4): 256–61.

3. **Gomes B** and **Higginson IJ** (2008). 'When people die (1974–2030): past trends, future projections and implications for care'. *Pall Med* **22**(1): 33–41.

4. **Calanzani N**, **Higginson IJ** and **Gomes B.** (2013). 'Current and future needs of hospice care: an evidence-based report'. *London Hospice UK*. Available at: https://www.hospiceuk.org/what-we-offer/commission-into-the-future-of-hospice-care/commission-resources].

5. **Mullick A**, **Martin K**, and **Sallnow l.** (2013). 'An introduction to advanced care planning in practice'. *BMJ* 347: 60–64.

6. Gold Standards Framework. Available at: http://www.goldstandardsframework.org.uk/cd-content/uploads/files/ACP/Thinking%20Ahead%20(3).pdf. (Accessed 18 January 2017.)

7. **Lunan C** (October 2008). 'Advance Directive: A basic guide for GPs'. *Royal College of General Practitioners report.*

8. 'Ambitions for Palliative and End of Life Care. A national framework for local action 2015–2020'. *National Palliative and End of Life Care Partnership.* Available at: www.endoflifecareambitions.org.uk. (Accessed December 2016.)

9. **Detering KM, Hancock AD, Reade MC, and Silvester W** (2010). 'The impact of advance care planning on end of life care in elderly patients: Randomised controlled trial'. *British Medical Journal* **340**: 1136–345.

10. **Houben CHM, Spruit MA, Groenen MTJ, Wouters EFM, and Janssen DJA** (2014). 'Efficacy of advance care planning: A systematic review and meta-analysis'. *Journal of the American Medical Directors Association* **15**: 477–89.

11. **Brinkman-Stoppelenburg A, Rietjens JA, and van der Heide A** (2014). 'The effects of advance care planning on end-of-life care: A systematic review'. *Palliative Med* **28**(8): 1000–25. doi: 10.1177/0269216314526272.

12. **Bischoff KE, Sudore R, Miao YH, Boscardin WJ, and Smith AK** (2013). 'Advance care planning and the quality of end-of-life care in older adults'. *Journal of the American Geriatrics Society* **61**(2): 209–14. 10.1111/jgs.12105.

13. **Bradley SL, Woodman RJ, Tieman JJ, and Phillips PA** (2014).' Use of advance directives by South Australians: results from the Health Omnibus Survey Spring 2012'. *The Medical journal of Australia* **201**(8): 467–9.

14. **White B, Tilse C, Wilson J, Rosenman L, Strub T, Feeney R, et al.** (2014). 'Prevalence and predictors of advance directives in Australia'. *Internal Medicine Journal* **44**(10): 975–80. doi: 10.1111/imj.12549.

15. **Horne G, Seymour J, Payne S** (2012). 'Maintaining integrity in the face of death: A grounded theory to explain the perspectives of people affected by lung cancer about the expression of wishes for end of life care'. *Int J Nurs Stud* **49**(6): 718–26. doi: 10.1016/j.ijnurstu.2011.12.003.

16. **Schickedanz AD, Schillinger D, Landefeld CS, Knight SJ, Williams BA, and Sudore RL** (2009). 'A clinical framework for improving the advance care planning process: start with patients' self-identified barriers'. *Journal of the American Geriatrics Society* **57**(1): 31–9. doi: 10.1111/j.1532-5415.2008.02093.x.

17. **Chiu C, Feuz MA, McMahan RD, Miao Y, and Sudore RL** (2016). ' "Doctor, make my decisions": decision control preferences, advance care planning, and satisfaction with communication among diverse older adults'. *J Pain Symptom Manag* **51**(1): 33–40. Available at: http://dx.doi.org/10.1016/j.jpainsymman.2015.07.018.

18. **Sinclair C, Auret KA, and Burgess A** (2013). 'The balancing point: understanding uptake of advance directive forms in a rural Australian community'. *BMJ Supportive & Palliative Care* **3**: 358–65. doi: 10.1136/bmjspcare-2012-000256.

19. **Think Local, Act Personal. Personalised care and support planning tool**. Available at: http://www.thinklocalactpersonal.org.uk/personalised-care-and-support-planning-tool/. (Accessed 18 January 2017.)

20. **Prommer EE** (2010). 'Using the values-based history to fine-tune advance care planning for oncology patients'. *Journal of Cancer Education* **25**(1): 66–9. doi: 10.1007/s13187-009-0014-0.

21. **House of Care**. 'Coalition for Collaborative Care'. House of Care. Available at: www.coalitionforcollaborativecare.org.uk/aboutus/houseofcare

22. **National Voices** (2013). 'A narrative for person-centred co-ordinated care'. Available at: www.england.nhs.uk/wp-content/uploads/2013/05/nv-narrative-cc.pdf. (Accessed 18 January 2017.)

23. **Royal College of General Practitioners** (2015). 'Stepping Forward'. *Commissioning principles for collaborative care and support planning.* Available at: http://www.rcgp.org.uk/clinical-and-research/our-programmes/collaborative-care-and-support-planning.aspx. (Accessed 18 January 2017.)

24. **UK Government report** (June 2014). 'One chance to get it right: improving people's experience of care in the last few days and hours of life'. Available at: https://www.gov.uk/government/uploads/system/uploads/attachment_data/file/323188/One_chance_to_get_it_right.pdf. (Accessed 18 January 2017.)

# Chapter 27

# A population-based approach to end of life care and advance care planning

Rammya Mathew, Muir Gray, and Keri Thomas

It is vain to talk of the interest of the community, without understanding what is the interest of the individual
*Jeremy Bentham*

---

**This chapter includes**

- Introduction to population based approach to healthcare
- Population health and end of life care
- Values, value based healthcare and end of life care
- The importance of early advance care planning (ACP) as a high-value intervention
- Person-centred care and population healthcare: two sides of the same coin
- Conclusion and next steps

---

**Key Points**

- Within a resource-confined system we need to consider how to maximise value for both the individual and the population
- Population-based healthcare aims to reduce variation by reducing the use of low-value interventions and increasing the use of high-value interventions
- ACP should be viewed as a high-value intervention, given its potential to deliver person-centred care and reduce the use of resources that are not in line with the person's wishes
- ACP needs appropriate investment if it is to deliver these potential benefits and achieve maximum value

---

**Key Message**

A population based approach takes account of the needs of the people within a given population. This type of approach is becoming of increasing importance as we grapple with the rising cost of healthcare and the increasing health needs of an ageing population. ACP is a means by which we can maintain a person-centred approach to care at the end of life and achieve maximum 'value' for the population. It does so by enabling people to receive the care that they want and not undergo treatments and interventions that are not in line with their wishes. In doing so, ACP facilitates the appropriate allocation of resources for those in their last years of life, and it is therefore a low-cost means of addressing the current ethical and economic challenges in healthcare.

## Introduction to a population-based approach to healthcare

Population healthcare focuses primarily on populations defined by a common need, which may be a symptom such as breathlessness, a condition such as arthritis, or a common characteristic such as being at the end of life. It does not focus on institutions, specialities or technologies. Its aim is to maximise value for those populations and the individuals within them, and clinicians practicing population medicine can and must play a leading part in achieving this.

Clinicians in the twenty-first century are expected to act as stewards of the allocated resources, and to become conscious not only of the people who could benefit, but also of the 'benefit foregone' by the whole population—not just to the patients who happen to have made contact with their services but also for all the people whose needs could have been met, directly or indirectly, by their service (1).

The ageing population is the greatest single challenge to our health and social care system. At the time of writing, the average age in Britain has hit 40 for the first time (compared to the worldwide average of 30) and life expectancy continues to soar (2). In addition, in the UK, more baby-boomers than ever are 70, reflecting post-war demographic surges. The increasing life expectancy reflects the significant advances made in the spheres of public health and medicine over the last 50 years, see (Box 27.1).

In recent years amazing progress has also been made in end of life care, with a clear focus on communication with the people affected and their relatives, supported by the development of

## Box 27.1 The skills of population-based medicine (2)

The skills for population medicine
- Maximising value
- Reducing waste and increasing sustainability
- Mitigating inequity
- Promoting health and preventing disease
- Creating systems
- Building networks
- Clarifying pathways
- Developing budgets
- Managing knowledge
- Engaging the population and patients
- Changing the culture

Reproduced courtesy of Muir Gray

training programmes designed to improve the quality of care. However, at the end of these years of progress, end of life care, like every other type of care, still has three huge problems. The first is huge and unwarranted variation in access, quality, cost, and outcome, which is directly related to the second and third problems, which are the underuse of high-value interventions and the overuse of low-value interventions.

1. **Unwarranted variation** was defined by Jack Wennberg in his ground-breaking Dartmouth Atlas of Healthcare as 'variation that cannot be explained by variation in need or explicit preferences of patients and the public.' The variation in the proportion of people dying at home is relatively small; only 1.7-fold compared with much larger variations for interventions like hip replacement or prescribed medication. However, a 1.7-fold variation is still a variation from 45 to 75% and when the map of England is looked at, as it is from the NHS Atlas of Variation (3); there is no obvious reason for the rate in one population being different from another population.

It is important to point out that the people responsible for providing services have been rarely aware of the variation. They are so focused on providing high quality care for the patients who reach their service that the appropriateness of those who do reach their service, and the potential benefit to those who do not, is not high on their agenda.

2. **Underuse** is when unwarranted variation arises in part from the underuse of high-value interventions, and perhaps the single most important intervention which is needed in great amounts is nursing at home, both by trained nurses and by people who are less-highly trained but who are compassionate and empathic, sometimes called care assistants or nursing assistants. There is also of course underuse of effective pain control and the control of other symptoms, in spite of the excellent work being done to spread these skills much more widely. It is worth noting that these resources are high value, not only because they are low cost, but because they have shown to be effective in improving quality of life and relieving symptoms at the end of life.

3. **Overuse** is the second problem revealed by unwarranted variation, namely the overuse of lower-value interventions. This is now receiving much more attention, although not yet in care in the last year of life. The key issue in thinking about people in the last year or two of life is not really the overuse of hospice beds or specialised palliative care nursing; it is the overuse of technologies and interventions provided by other services, for example intensive care or surgical services.

Although the technological revolution has lent itself to many medical marvels, it has also made it infinitely more challenging to decide when to forgo active treatment and change the focus to best supportive care. 'Just because we can doesn't mean we should', particularly if it is not in line with the person's wishes. It often feels unnatural to make the conscious decision to stop active treatment, particularly when surrounded by medicines and technologies that offer the potential to prolong life. This applies, for example, to cancer patients with non-curative disease who are being offered aggressive chemotherapy, but also in people with frailty, dementia, and multimorbidity, where decisions need to be made as to whether the repeated use of interventions and antibiotics are actually in the best interests of the person.

## Population health and end of life care

If we consider the Donabedian curve in the context of end of life care (see Figure 27.1), the investment of resources has a positive impact on the health of the population up to a certain point (this is referred to as the point of optimality), but beyond that, there is no further improvement in

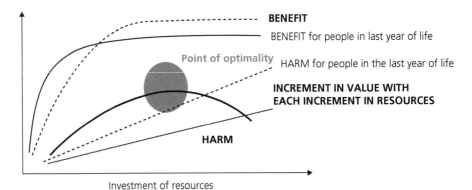

**Figure 27.1** The Donabedian curve for people in their last year of life versus the general population

Adapted with permission from NHS Confederation: a culture of stewardship—the responsibility of NHS leaders to deliver better value healthcare. September 2015

population outcomes, whereas the harms associated with intervention continue to increase. This is the case for interventions of all types, whether they are high or low value.

If for example, we take the general population of people with cancer, the benefits of chemotherapy plateau after a certain number of people within the population receive this treatment. The harms also increase in a linear fashion; the more people who have chemotherapy, the greater the cumulative risk of harm. However, if we consider this paradigm for people in their last year of life with a diagnosis of cancer, the benefits of chemotherapy may plateau earlier (i.e fewer people in their last year of life will benefit from this treatment) and the cumulative harm is greater with each incremental increase in the use of chemotherapy.

Even if we consider high-value interventions such as home nursing, there still comes a point at which the benefits tail off with further investment, as it is likely that people with the greatest need will be offered the service first and then subsequently people who have lesser needs. As with any intervention, there is also a risk of 'harm', which is cumulative. For example, it might be that home nursing takes away a person's independence or interrupts valuable time with friends and family at the end of life. Therefore, even high-value interventions need to be allocated appropriately.

What is needed is a population-based approach remembering always that the other side of the coin from population healthcare is personalised care.

## Values, value-based healthcare and end of life care

One of the great achievements of the paradigm shift brought about by the movement led by hospices and palliative care has been the recognition that the values of the patient are of central importance in the design and delivery of care. This chapter focuses on the use of the term in the singular, the definition more closely related to economics, but of course, values—ethical and philosophical, are also central to decisions about the allocation and use of resources. This approach is now called value-based healthcare in many countries (4,5) but different countries use different language, RightCare is the term used in England with Scotland using the term Realistic Medicine and Wales the term Prudent Healthcare. They all emphasise the importance of shared decision making and eliciting what matters most to the patient. However, at the end of life, people are commonly unable to express their choices and the only way that their choices can be incorporated into clinical decision making is through the use of advance care planning (ACP).

## Value-based healthcare

Using the population as the denominator, as opposed to the patients who are treated by a service forces us to think about value and there are three types of value, two of them related to the population and one to the individual.

In some way, the simplest form of value is that which relates to the individual and it is here that the specialty of palliative care and the hospice movement have made such a major impact. We now know that we need to deliver services that are deemed to be of value to the individual and their family.

There are however two aspects of value that relate to the population served. The first of these is what is called **allocative value.** In economics there has been a long-standing interest in resource allocation. The aim is to optimize allocative value, sometimes called allocative efficiency. Aiming for optimal allocation is aiming for the point at which not a single pound can be reallocated from one budget to another to get more value for the population as a whole. Needless to say no service has yet achieved this. The NHS in England uses programme budgeting with the programmes focused on sub-groups of the population defined by their principal diagnosis. This approach, called programme budgeting, has therefore led to budgets for people with cancer or people with mental health problems and this is certainly an advance on simply deciding how much to spend on 'acute' or 'community' which is the way most health services have operated in the past. Having to think about the right balance of resources between, for example, care for people with musculoskeletal disease, care for people with mental illness, care for people with respiratory disease, and care for people with failing vision, to give but four of the twenty programmes brings up very difficult issues.

The second aspect of population-based value is sometimes called **technical value or utilisation value** which is much more than simply assessing the efficiency with which patients are treated. It is certainly important to measure outcomes against the costs but this is usually classified as efficiency. To measure value, it is also necessary to consider:

◆ Whether there are people who would benefit from the service who are not being treated, or even referred to the service because of social or language difficulties

◆ If there are people being treated who are being over-treated, thus offering the opportunity to switch resources to provide treatment for those people who are at present not being met

These are the factors that distinguish efficiency from value.

## The importance of early advance care planning as a high-value intervention

Analysis of US medical care expenditure indicates that there has been steady progress in addressing the value agenda in advanced illness and at end of life. Historically, approximately a quarter of Medicare expenses were attributed to the last year of life, but with increasing age, there is a trend towards decreasing expenditure (6). This is thought to be due to decisions reached by patients, their families, and by doctors to avoid aggressive treatments that often lack any significant benefit to this cohort of the population.

ACP is key in ensuring that we achieve high-value person-centred care. Statistics show that to date, the uptake of ACP in the UK has been poor; in a survey of more than 2000 British adults commissioned by Dying Matters, only 4% said they had set out how they would want to be cared for at the end of life in the event that they were unable to make decisions themselves (7).

ACP should be considered a high-value intervention in itself, if it allows people to receive the care they want. If we are serious about ACP and making it work, then we must invest in the process by raising awareness, and developing platforms which allow the information from advance care plans to be shared and implemented. Much like home deaths, ACP can be dismissed as idealistic, but with appropriate investment, it may prove to be one of the most effective ways of ensuring limited resources are allocated in a way which allows us to achieve the maximum benefit for both the individual and the population.

The main priority of ACP discussions are to discuss personal needs, values, wishes, and preferences for both living and dying. Sometimes, however, the more person-focused ACP discussion sets the scene for a clinically focussed shared decision-making conversation related to deciding on best treatment options.

### Advance care planning for individuals and for the wider community—developing a programme budget for the last two years of life determined by people's preferences

To deliver the system of care for older people in need, it is necessary for resources to be switched from lower-value to higher-value care, and one way to do this would be to develop a programme budget for people with these characteristics.

Supposing for example that all the resources used in the last two years of end of life were put in the one budget, would it not be appropriate to switch some of the resources from lower-value interventions such as chemotherapy, to high-value nursing and social care that is often under provided and therefore too often results in people being inappropriately admitted to hospital? Of course once having been inappropriately admitted to hospital it may be that they will be inappropriately admitted to intensive care because it is not clear what their preferences actually are. These issues require a radical new approach to end of life care, the first stage of which is the widespread adoption of ACP at an individual level, and the second of which is the development of a population-based healthcare system, based on the cumulate expressed wishes and needs of the wider population.

Camden Clinical Commissioning group is an example of an organisation who have attempted to deliver high-value population-based care by asking elderly frail patients and their caregivers, 'what matters most to you?' (8). Their response was 'time spent at home and out of hospital' and therefore in Camden they commissioned local services based on this particular outcome measure. Their experience of innovating around a core outcome is that it enabled all involved to change how they work together to prevent hospitalisation, and when hospitalisation was necessary, to get patients home faster. It seems that focusing on a particular segment of the population and using patient-defined measures creates powerful clarity of purpose.

The practice of population-based medicine also has implications for people with specialist knowledge about end of life care, see (Figure 27.2).

### Implications for specialists and palliative care in the hospice movement

Healthcare is complex and one aspect of complexity is the way in which individuals reach the services most likely to be of benefit to them. Need arising from trauma is relatively straight forward at least in its presentation because all the people in need get to the right service but for people approaching the end of life and who would benefit from the skills and knowledge of specialists the problems are illustrated in Figure 27.2.

This means that the people working in a specialist unit (because that is where most specialists are based) need to see themselves as **people who are not only managing a specialist unit but as people who are relating to a population and as people who provide knowledge**. At present the

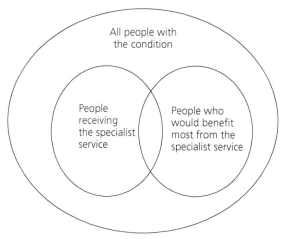

**Figure 27.2** The population paradigm
Reproduced courtesy of Muir Gray

knowledge confers benefit on the patients referred to the specialist service or hospice but if we are to regard the National Health Service as a knowledge service rather than real estate service then we need to think of ways in which the knowledge reaches all those people who would benefit from it. One way of course is to greatly expand the number of people working in specialist end of life care. However another way is to increase the work that is already taking place to ensure that everybody who encounters someone in the last years, weeks, or month is aware not only of what they can do but also very clear about appropriate referrals to specialists. This is the basis of the expanding area of generalist palliative/ end of life care training, recommended in all national UK EOLC policy and by NICE (9), and exemplified by the GSF training (10) and several others, to enable and upskill teams in primary care, hospitals, care homes, and other settings (cf. as in Chapters 11, 12, and 13). This ensures that staff are able to recognise patients in the last years of life, assess clinical needs, and refer when appropriate, but also allow space for discussion of personal needs through ACP discussions.

# The issues of personal care alongside population care, systems, and accountability

Personal care focusses on the needs and wishes of the individual and those close to them—this is obviously important as we all only die once. But alongside this, is consideration of the needs of the population as a whole, which includes the chance that more of the population will receive high standards of care and, in this case, will live well and die well. Is it right that we have a top class service for some and are lacking basic provisions for others—a Rolls Royce service for some or a bicycle for all?

## Population-based systems

We need to think of ways in which this system of care can be accountable to the population served for the value delivered as well as for the quality of care provided.

There has been increasing debate about end of life care for the last twenty years, and rightly so. This debate is focused on the quality of care received by people in the last year, months, weeks, and days of life. One proxy measure of this has been the proportion of people dying at home, but place of death is only one aspect of the quality of care provided. More important has been the development of quality standards initially pioneered by the hospice movement and the medical specialty of palliative care. The importance of quality standards cannot be questioned, but simply to focus on quality alone does not cover the issue of value. What is needed is not only to ask what is the quality of service provided to this person or this group of people, for example people who die in a hospice or who die in a hospital ward but also to ask how good is the care provided to those who are dying in Bedfordshire, or Manchester, or Wales?

For each objective one or more outcome criteria should be chosen so that progress, or the lack of it can be measured. For each activity it is also helpful to set standards so that the service, and the people served in the population can ask questions such as the questions set out below

Is the service for the people in our population at the end of life?

a) Below the minimal acceptable standard
b) Of high quality, i.e. in the top quartile
c) In the middle of the range

This might include developing measures related to wider populations such as the numbers of people identified to be the last year of life, the proportion offerd ACP discissions, the numbers dying where they choose, in addition to measures of wellbeing and quality of life. Such measures are being tested in various parts of the country, and several areas are beginning to be able to monitor progress and watch for variation, largely due to the use of the digital records or Electronic Palliative Care Co-ordination Systems (EPaCCS) (11).

## Population accountability

Bureaucracies are accountable to the superior level in the administration, ultimately to NHS Improvement or the Department of Health depending upon which country the bureaucracy is based on. However population-based systems should be accountable to the population they serve allowing people in that population to contribute not only by holding the service to account but also by playing a part in decision making.

The population can campaign for more resources for their service but the population in need also needs to have a view on the balance of the resources that are available. For example they need to ask if there is overuse of interventions of low value, for example by the inappropriate admission of people with multiple morbidity to hospital or intensive care, who had expressed a wish to die in their own homes.

The population can raise these important managerial and ethical issues in a way that is difficult for the service itself to raise. End of life care needs a population-based systems approach and in England this is starting to evolve. The populations often relate to traditional patterns of referral from general practice to hospital service rather than to jurisdictions namely the organisations responsible for managing the NHS and finance. These population-based systems of care will work together as a single community of practice learning from one another and supporting one another in getting more value for people in the last year of life from the resources available.

This should be done by raising awareness, spreading training and use, monitoring increasing routine uptake and developing platforms, and creating systems which allow the information from advance care plans to be gathered as part of normal practice, shared and then implemented.

# Conclusion

As we face the challenges of the spiralling needs of our ageing populations across the developing world we also face the parallel issue of increasingly limited resources in all countries. Whilst medical advances support longer life, they don't always confer better quality life. We need to balance the personal perspective along with the population-based approach, based on conferring better value in our use of resources for the wider population whilst ensuring individual needs are met.

The process of ACP can be seen as a high-value means of securing better quality of life with better use of limited resources. It enhances a value-based approach that balances the needs of both the person and the population as a whole to ensure that more can attain care in line with their preferences and live well and die well in the place and manner of their choosing.

If we are serious about ACP and making it work, then we must invest in the process. The effects of systematically mainstreaming ACP as part of normal life for every person and normal practice for every care provider could be huge. If it receives appropriate investment, and national support for implementation, it may prove to be one of the most effective ways of ensuring that limited resources are allocated in a way which allows us to achieve the maximum benefit for both the individual and the population.

# References

1. *Daily Mail*. Available at: http://www.dailymail.co.uk/news/article-3138853/Britain-s-mid-life-crisis-UK-average-age-hits-40-time-population-jumps-500-000-64-6-million.html
2. **Muir, JA** (2013). *How to Practice Population Medicine*. Oxford: Gray Offox Press.
3. **Public Health England** (September 2016). *The NHS Atlas of Variation in Healthcare*.
4. **Department of Health** (July 2008). *End of Life Care Strategy: promoting high quality care for all adults at the end of life*. DH, London.
5. **NHS England**. *NHS Ambitions for Palliative and End of life care 2015*. Available at: http://endoflifecareambitions.org.uk/
6. **Calfo, S. Smith J**, and **Zezza, M** (2008). *Last year of Life Study*. Centers for Medicare and Medicaid Services.
7. **Dying Matters**. *Survey reveals our reluctance to discuss own death*. Available at: http://www.dyingmatters.org/page/survey-reveals-our-reluctance-discuss-own-death
8. **Sayer C** (April 2016). 'Time spent at home: A patient defined outcome measure'. *NEJM Catalyst* **375**: 1610–12.
9. **NICE National Institute for Health and care Excellence** (NICE). *End of Life care for Adults*. Available at: https://www.nice.org.uk/guidance/qs13
10. **Gold Standards Framework**. *Evidence of impact of GSF training programmes enabling generalists*. Available at: http://www.goldstandardsframework.org.uk/evidence
11. **EPaCCs in England**. Available at: http://www.endoflifecare-intelligence.org.uk/resources/publications/epaccs_in_england

# Useful websites and resources

There are continually new advance care planning resources being produced internationally—these are a selection of useful websites and resources. When using them, consideration should always be given to the cultural and legal frameworks within which the resources operate.

## UK based resources

**All Wales Paediatric Palliative Care Network**
http://advancecareplan.org.uk/wp-content/uploads/2017/04/PAC-Plan-leaflet.pdf

**Advance Care Planning Resources for England and Wales**
http://advancecareplan.org.uk/

**Advance Care Planning—The Gold Standards Framework Centre**
http://www.goldstandardsframework.org.uk/advance-care-planning

**Age UK**
http://www.ageuk.org.uk/health-wellbeing/relationships-and-family/end-of-life/difficult-conversations/
https://www.bhf.org.uk/publications/living-with-a-heart-condition/difficult-conversations—talking-to-people-with-heart-failure-about-the-end-of-life

**Ambitions for Palliative and End of life care 2015 NHS England**
http://endoflifecareambitions.org.uk/wp-content/uploads/2015/09/Ambitions-for-Palliative-and-End-of-Life-Care.pdf

**Ambitions for Palliative and End of Life Care 2015 NHS England Resources**
http://endoflifecareambitions.org.uk/category/general/

**Ambitions for Palliative and End of Life Care 2015 NHS England Useful Links**
http://endoflifecareambitions.org.uk/useful-links/

**Atul Gawande—Being Mortal—Medicine and what matters in the end**
http://atulgawande.com/book/being-mortal/

**British Lung Foundation**
https://www.blf.org.uk/support-for-you/end-of-life

**BMJ—Supportive and palliative care—Courageous conversations**
ACP with teens with serious medical conditions and their families

◆ http://spcare.bmj.com/content/2/2/187.3.abstract

**Compassion in Dying—campaign 'Make it Your Decision'**
https://www.makeityourdecision.org.uk/?utm_source=stakeholder&utm_campaign=makeityourdecision&utm_medium=email

**Compassion in Dying—understanding your legal rights in EOLC**
http://compassionindying.org.uk/

**Decisions relating to cardiopulmonary resuscitation:**
A joint statement from the British Medical Association, the Resuscitation Council (UK), and the Royal College of Nursing www.resus.org.uk/pages/dnar.pdf

**Dead Social**
http://www.deadsocial.org/features/about-us

**Digital Legacy Association**
https://digitallegacyassociation.org/for-the-public/

**Dying Matters UK**
http://www.dyingmatters.org/overview/resources

**Electronic Palliative Care Co-ordination Systems in England**
http://www.endoflifecare-intelligence.org.uk/resources/publications/epaccs_in_england

**GMC (General Medical Council) guidance on ACP, consent and other issues in end of life care**
http://www.gmc-uk.org/guidance/ethical_guidance/end_of_life_advance_care_planning.asp

**GMC Treatment and Care towards the end of life**
http://www.gmc-uk.org/static/documents/content/Treatment_and_care_towards_the_end_of_life_-_English_1015.pdf

**GMC/Age UK September 2015**
http://www.gmc-uk.org/Age_UK_GMC___Advance_Care_Planning___Final_report.pdf_64693525.pdf

**Gold Standards Framework**
http:// www.goldstandardsframework.org.uk
General guidance and information on the use of advance care planning as part of the Gold Standards Framework programmes in end of life care, primary care, care homes, acute hospitals, and other settings.

**GSF Proactive Identification Guidance—guidance on early recognition of decline, prompting ACP discussions**
http://www.goldstandardsframework.org.uk/pig

**GSF 5 Steps to Advance Care Planning—a public facing animated video encouraging earlier ACP discussions**
available at http://www.goldstandardsframework.org.uk/new-5-steps-advancecare-planning or on You Tube on https://www.youtube.com/watch?v=i2k6U6inIjQ (Google GSF 5 Steps ACP)

**GSF Evidence-Improving Advance Care Planning Discussions in different settings**
http://tinyurl.com/hlvh4bz

**Health Talk UK**
http://www.healthtalk.org/peoples-experiences/dying-bereavement

**Ireland—Irish Hospice Foundation**
http://hospicefoundation.ie/programmes/public-awareness/think-ahead/

**Ireland—Northern Ireland**
https://www.macmillan.org.uk/information-and-support/organising/planning-for-the-future-with-advanced-cancer/advance-care-planning-ni

**Northern Ireland Advance Decisions**
http://www.niassembly.gov.uk/globalassets/documents/raise/publications/2015/hssps/11815.pdf

**Macmillan Cancer Support**
http://be.macmillan.org.uk/Downloads/CancerInformation/LivingWithAndAfterCancer/MAC136160115Your-life-and-choices-ADRT-formFP20160823.pdf

**Macmillan ACP**
https://www.macmillan.org.uk/information-and-support/organising/planning-for-the-future-with-advanced-cancer/advance-care-planning-england-wales

**Marie Curie**
https://www.mariecurie.org.uk/help/support/terminal-illness/planning-ahead/advance-care-planning

**Mental Capacity Act 2005**: Information booklets
Current information is available from: http://www.justice.gov.uk/guidance/mental-capacity.htm

**Motor Neurone Association**
https://www.mndassociation.org/wp-content/uploads/2015/07/eol03-difficult-conversations-with-professionals.pdf

**my Decisions**
https://mydecisions.org.uk/

**NHS—Planning for your future care—a guide**
https://www.nhs.uk/Livewell/Endoflifecare/Documents/Planning_your_future_care%5B1%5D.pdf or http://www.dyingmatters.org/page/planning-your-future-care

**Office of the Public Guardian—GOV.UK**
https://www.gov.uk/government/organisations/office-of-the-public-guardian

**Recommended Summary Plan for Emergency Care and Treatment**
http://www.respectprocess.org.uk/

**Resuscitation Council UK**
https://www.resus.org.uk/information-for-the-public/

**Royal College of Physicians: National Guidelines Advance Care Planning**
Concise guidance to good practice, number 12. An excellent guidance document produced by the Royal College of Physicians on the benefits and uses of ACP in England
http://www.rcplondon.ac.uk

**Scotland—Making an Anticipatory Care Plan Good Life Good Death Good Grief (Scotland)**
https://www.goodlifedeathgrief.org.uk/content/anticipatory_care_plan/

**Sue Ryder Care**
https://support.sueryder.org/practical-emotional-advice?field_info_page_topic_tid%255b%255d=14

**The National Council for Palliative Care**
www.ncpc.org.uk/publications

- The Mental Capacity Act in Practice
- Good Decision Making: The Mental Capacity Act and End of Life Care

http://www.ncpc.org.uk/sites/default/files/AdvanceCarePlanning.pdf

- ACP A guide for health and social care staff

**Transforming your Care Northern Ireland Health and Social care** http://www.transformingyourcare.hscni.net/?s=advance+care+planning

**Together for Short Lives**
http://www.togetherforshortlives.org.uk/professionals/resources

**Palliative Care Hub**
http://www.adultpalliativehub.com/about-us

**Wales—A Framework for Advance Care Planning in Wales IPADS Palliative Care Wales**
http://wales.pallcare.info/index.php?p=sections&sid=68

**Wales—Talk CPR Wales**
http://talkcpr.wales/

**Winston's Wish**
https://www.winstonswish.org.uk/

## International resources

**Some examples from other countries** (others are included in the relevant chapters)

**Australian**

ACP Talk: http://www.acptalk.com.au/

Advance Care Planning Australia: An Australian national hub of education and resources for health and care workers, and consumers. Austin Health, Melbourne. This website links to many other Australian initiatives:

◆ www.advancecareplanning.org.au

Decision Assist: A national specialist palliative care and advance care planning advisory services website

◆ www.decisionassist.org.au

Australian Centre for Health Law Research. It is designed to be used by patients, families, health and legal practitioners, the media, policymakers and the broader community to access information about Australian laws relating to death, dying and decision-making at the end of life.

◆ https://end-of-life.qut.edu.au/

**Canada**

National ACP website: Speak up www.advancecareplanning.ca/

**New Zealand**

Advance Care Planning NZ: www.advancecareplanning.org.nz/
http://www.advancecareplanning.org.nz/
https://www.healthnavigator.org.nz/health-topics/advance-care-planning/

**Five Wishes**

https://www.agingwithdignity.org/
https://www.cdc.gov/aging/advancecareplanning/index.htm

**USA**

Literature Review on advance directives. Wilkinson AM, Wenger N, Shugarman LR. (2007).

◆ Available at: http://aspe.hhs.gov/daltcp/reports/2007/advdirlr.pdf

https://www.ariadnelabs.org/areas-of-work/serious-illness-care/

Communication about Serious Illness Care Goals PDF

◆ http://www.conversationsofalifetime.org/downloads/Article-Communication
  AboutSeriousIllnessCareGoals.pdf

**Singapore**

http://www.livingmatters.sg/

# Index

Tables, figures and boxes are indicated by an italic *t*, *f*, and *b* following the page number